Surveillance and Evaluation of Global Health Emergencies - Lessons from the Social Sciences Perspective

Covid-19, HIV/AIDS, Ebola: Two Decades in the early 2000s at Global and Local Levels with Communities

Surveillance and Evaluation of Global Health Emergencies - Lessons from the Social Sciences Perspective

Covid-19, HIV/AIDS, Ebola: Two Decades in the early 2000s at Global and Local Levels with Communities

Cyril Pervilhac

ELIVA PRESS

ISBN: 978-99949-8-849-5

Cover Design: Eliva Press
Cover Image: Ingimage
Email: info@elivapress.com
Website: www.elivapress.com

This Eliva Press imprint is published by the registered company Eliva Press Global Ltd. part of Eliva Press S.R.L. Publishing Group

The registered company address is: Pope Hennessy Street Level 2, Hennessy Tower Port Louis, Mauritius
Eliva Press S.R.L. Publishing Group address is: Bulevardul Moscova 21, Chisinau, Moldova, Europe

Table of contents

1

Planning high COVID-19 vaccination among aged population in Switzerland: how can social sciences make a difference?

Cyril Pervilhac, Tina Draser

Cyril Pervilhac, Retiree, WHO HQ Geneva, pervilhacc@gmail.com

Tina Draser, Retiree, The Global Fund to fight AIDS, TB and Malaria, Geneva

https://smw.ch/op-eds/post/planning-high-covid-19-vaccination-uptake

Introduction

The national strategy for Switzerland to confront the epidemic is based on three pillars: the increase of vaccination coverage, screening and non-pharmaceutical interventions (NPIs). For vaccination, however, the Swiss National COVID-19 Science Task Force (NCS-TF) had signaled insufficient coverage (67.24%, December 2021). As of mid-February 2022, 70% of the Swiss population had been vaccinated at least once against SARS-CoV-2,[1] and 41% with an additional dose[2]. Last October 2021, while planning the new massive vaccination promotion campaign, the plan stated that *"based on current knowledge, it is likely that the vaccination rate for the over-65s would have to be between 90 and 95% before measures could be lifted. At present, only 88.5% of this age group have received at least one vaccine."* [3] The elderly population[4] has been vaccinated as a first priority and remains the prime target for second and booster doses to maintain full immunization. This is in synchrony with broader recent international recommendations[5] as an on-going post-Omicron strategy for the global COVID-19 response to reach among aged population, typically older than

---

[1] https://sciencetaskforce.ch/fr/rapport-scientifique-15-fevrier-2022/
Swiss National COVID-19 Science Task Force, "Aspects de la gestion du SARS-CoV-2 au cours des 12 prochains mois. Scénarios, option d'action et préparation d'un point de vue scientifique, » 15 février 2022
[2] https://www.covid19.admin.ch/fr/vaccination/persons (p. 1)
[3] https://www.uvek.admin.ch/uvek/en/home/detec/media/press-releases.msg-id-85336.html
BAG, « Coronavirus_ Federal Council plans new vaccination drive", Bern, 01.10.2021
[4] https://www.bag.admin.ch/dam/bag/de/dokumente/mt/k-und-i/aktuelle-ausbrueche-pandemien/2019-nCoV/sur-bericht-juli-2022.pdf.download.pdf/2022_07_report_DE_2022_07_27.pdf
Schweizerische Eidgenossenschaft, FOPH, "Demographic characteristics by immune status", in Bericht zum spitalbasierten COVID-19-Sentinel - überwachungssystem» , 25 Juli 2022, p. 14
[5] https://apps.who.int/iris/rest/bitstreams/1406385/retrieve
WHO SAGE Roadmap for Prioritizing Use of COVID-19 Vaccines, "Highest priority-use group, Older adults", latest update: 21 January 2022, p. 16

60 years of age (60+), high and full vaccination coverage beyond the first dose, including boosters (90-95% coverage including the most at risk population) next autumn/ winter months 2022/23.[6]

The NCS-TF expects seasonal waves during the upcoming winter months based on the past 24 months data from Central Europe. At the European level, the European Centre for Disease Prevention and Control (ECDC) [7] recommended the planning of future campaigns based on taking stock of earlier phases of the vaccination program and behavioral insights. The NCS-TF clarified with *"options for action"* the strategies for the management of SARS-COV-2 in the next 12 months in order to reach a high vaccination rate.

In this opinion paper, in addition to a few primary sources of key informants and journal news, we reviewed essentially secondary sources of data: Covid-19 Social Monitor, Corona Immunitas Research Program, Swiss Corona Stress Study, scientific reports/ publications based on those, socio-demographic/ economic studies (Geneva).

Our findings and discussion are limited by the rapidly changing epidemiological evolution of the variants and the still on-going data analysis with pending results, and we could not here report on social media evaluations or the Federal Office of Public Health (FOPH) communication package. Upcoming findings (second semester 2022) of external reviews and experiences at federal and cantonal levels may clarify further this first insight into existing gaps and solutions. For example, the evaluation from the Canton of Geneva could not yet be exploited due to the "political agenda" delaying substantially its dissemination (Aglaé Tardin, communication personnelle, 24 juin 2022).

For the end of the pandemic, the World Health Organization (WHO) [8] highlighted the importance of using robust social science data for the preparedness plans. Early findings on the importance of public health but the oversight of social sciences were already reported for the pandemic in France,[9]

---

[6] https://www.rockefellerfoundation.org/wp-content/uploads/2022/03/The-Path-Forward-A-Post-Omicron-Strategy-for-the-Global-Covid-19-Response.pdf
COVIDGAP, "The Path Forward: A Post-Omicron Strategy for the Global COVID-19 Response", Updates: 30 March 2022, p. 2
[7] https://www.ecdc.europa.eu/sites/default/files/documents/Public-health-considerations-to-support-decisions-on-implementing-a-second-mRNA-COVID-19-vaccine-booster-dose.pdf
ECDC, "Public health considerations and evidence to support decisions on the implementation of a second mRNA COVID-19 vaccine booster dose", 28 April 2022
[8] https://apps.who.int/iris/rest/bitstreams/1416547/retrieve
WHO, "Strategic preparedness, readiness and response plan to end the global COVID-19 emergency in 2022." Geneva: World Health Organization; 2022 (WHO/WHE/ SPP/2022.01), p. 11
[9] https://thescipub.com/pdf/jssp.2022.6.18.pdf

with a historical perspective in Switzerland[10], and various communications[11] about Switzerland.[12] Bio-medical experts are preparing actively their response for the next autumn/winter seasons with the development of new vaccines and logistics. In turn, social scientists need to contribute[13] with the refinement of their already available tool kits and activities for an improved targeted community response at primary health care level. Given this context, how can we nevertheless take stock of the lessons learned over the past year and activities related to full coverage among the most impacted vulnerable and aged population with the lens of social sciences in order to better prepare the vaccination strategy in the autumn/winter 2022/23?

Findings and discussion

Given the neglect of social sciences, we utilise therefore this lens to analyze more in-depth the findings, limitations and potential solutions of two existing robust tools. This will allow an increase in vaccination coverage among the 60+ population for the preparatory weeks ahead in order to reach at least 90-95% coverage next autumn/winter. We then consider additional strategic views on the upcoming FOPH plan and its goal.

"The Covid-19 Social Monitor"[14] is a longitudinal online panel[15] of a random sample of the Swiss population (aged 18-79 years). It allows the monitoring of

Maria Verykiou, Laurent Denis, Cyril Pervilhac, "Social sciences and social justice in the design, implementation, and evaluation of measures against COVID-19 - the case study of France in 2020", J. of Social Sciences, 17 Jan. 2022

[10] https://www.horizons-mag.ch/2022/06/02/heres-to-their-health/
Nicolas Gattlen, "In sickness and in health", Horizons, 02/06/2022
[11] C. Pervilhac, "Social sciences and social justice in the complex equation of measures against COVID-19 - the case study of France in 2020", the Congress of Swiss Sociological Association, 29 June 2021
[12] https://www.tdg.ch/role-central-de-la-sante-publique-257345481213
Cyril Pervilhac, Tina Draser, « Contrecarrer la pandémie et cinquième vague de COVID-19 en Suisse : un changement de paradigme avec la santé publique », Tribune de Genève, Lettre du jour, 10 décembre 2021
[13] https://smw.ch/op-eds/post/a-paradigm-shift-with-public-health-to-counteract-the-pandemic-and-fifth-wave-of-covid-19-in-switzerland
C. Pervilhac, T. Draser, "Beyond the November 28, 2021 vote: a paradigm shift with public health to counteract the pandemic and fifth wave of COVID-19 in Switzerland?", Swiss Medical Weekly, 28th Dec. 2021
[14] https://www.sgs-sss.ch/wp-content/uploads/2021/01/SGS-Bulletin-157.pdf
Höglinger, M. & Heiniger, S., "The Covid-19 Social Monitor: A panel study providing evidence about the social and public health impact of the pandemic," in The Covid-19 pandemic, health and medicine: Sociological investigations and perspectives, Bulletin of the Swiss Sociological Association, Bulletin 157, Dec. 2020, pp. 14-19
[15] https://www.zhaw.ch/en/sml/institutes-centres/wig/projekte/covid-19-social-monitor/
Marc Höglinger, et. al., « Covid-19 Social Monitor -Monitoring the Social and Public Health Impact of the Pandemic, Results of Survey Wave 22, March 14 to 24, 2022, Reporting for FOPH, March 2022» (Zürich University of Applied Sciences, ZWAH and Epidemiology, Biostatistics and Prevention Institute, University of Zürich, Clinical Trial Unit, University of Bern)

15 topics of key societal level indicators[16] (e. g. mental health, general health, adherence to Covid-19 measures, health services use and non-use). Using the Social Monitor data (March 2020 – Dec. 2021), a detailed analysis of the COVID-19 vaccination uptake[17] among the study population living largely in urban area (80%) has shown that the elderly aged 60-79 years shared a *"much earlier and faster uptake"*. This study showed higher uptakes than the data from the official vaccination rates from the FOPH: a vaccination uptake of 93% among the 60-69 year old (vs. 86%, FOPH figure), and 95% among the 70-79 year old (vs. 91%, FOPH figure). These discrepancies are largely due to a more representative sample of the national population for the FOPH data. Following the first twelve months of the vaccination strategy, a separate analysis had already highlighted two main causes of vaccine hesitancy, with the need for special attention for future vaccination campaigns: the fears of unwanted vaccine effects and doubts regarding vaccine effectiveness (Heiniger S., op. cit., p. 1). This was also reported earlier in the results from the data in spring 2021 the "COVID-19 MOSAiCH survey".[18] An additional analysis of the data specific to elderly people[19] from the "COVID-19 Social Monitor" revealed the need to improve prevention and communication efforts between linguistic regions in Switzerland. The rural German speaking cantons have the lowest COVID-19 vaccination coverage.[20]

Yet, as acknowledged in the methodology, the study has several limitations which need to be addressed for a full picture of the aged population group: the *"selectivity of the sample with on-line affinity and education to be addressed by statistical adjustment"*, and the *"possible under- or even non-representation of specific subpopulations (individuals with chronic diseases, lower education level, vulnerable groups, persons with serious health conditions)"* (M.

---

[16] https://journals.plos.org/plosone/article?id=10.1371/journal.pone.0242129
Moser, A., Carlander, M., Wieser, S., Hämmig, O., Puhan, M. A., & Höglinger, M. (2020). "The COVID-19 Social Monitor longitudinal online panel: Real-time monitoring of social and public health consequences of the COVID-19 emergency in Switzerland." PLoS ONE, 15(11), e0242129
[17] https://smw.ch/article/doi/smw.2022.w30162
Heiniger S. et. al., "Differences in COVID-19 vaccination uptake in the first 12 months of vaccine availability in Switzerland – a prospective cohort study", Swiss Medical Weekly, 8th Apr. 2022; 152:w30162, p. 4, 6
[18] https://forscenter.ch/wp-content/uploads/2021/07/willigness-to-receive-the-covid_19-vaccine.pdf
Gian-Andrea Monsch, et. al., "Willingness to receive the COVID-19 vaccine in Switzerland: Who wants it, who does not, and why
[19] https://www.researchgate.net/publication/347369658_Social_mixing_and_risk_exposures_for_SARS-CoV-2_infections_in_elderly_persons
H. Christina, et. al., "Social mixing and risk exposures for SARS-CoV-2 infections in elderly persons", Swiss Medical Weekly, 05 Dec. 2020, p. 7
[20] https://www.watson.ch/schweiz/international/195039641-corona-wieso-die-impfquote-in-deutschsprachigen-laendern-so-tief-ist
Watson (blog), «Impfen? Nein, danke – deutschsprachige Regionen haben ein Problem mit der Spritze», 13.11.2021 (accessed on 5 July 2022)

Höglinger, "Limitations", op. cit., March 2022). The latter are two key factors of importance among the small proportions of the still hard-to-reach 60+ population who may have a lower full coverage (beyond the first dose). The study analyzed self-reported vaccination uptake (first dose or a proxy for access to vaccination services). The data may largely underestimate the second dose or full vaccination status (second and booster dose).

Exploiting further the "COVID-19 Social Monitor", the sampling should be adjusted by including the rural population (approximately one fourth of the total population in Switzerland); additional sampling can be provided by the Social & Market Research Institute at reasonable costs (Von Wyl, personal communication, June 2022). Other limitations mentioned above can be addressed by monitoring as well the additional doses beyond the first one, and by analyzing additional retrospective data collected over the past 12 months which the study offers at present.

The "**Corona Immunitas – Digital Follow-up Cohort**"[21] is a study focusing on vaccination uptake with large samples of people 65-74 and 75+ who have been followed over time in 2021. At first sight, the *Vaccination Status stratified by Age and Gender*" (op. cit., Fig. 3, p. 8) is encouraging, with more than 80% of those aged 65-74 and 75+ vaccinated. "Corona-Immunitas" has produced general seroprevalence data at the end of 2021. (NCS-TF, 15 Feb. 2022, p. 9) The "Corona Immunitas" network is pursuing some analysis relevant to the upcoming vaccination strategies, for example disaggregated data on vaccination coverage for the second and booster doses, in particular among aged population (Von Wyl, personal communication, 1 June and 4 July 2022). In the next phase in June/July 2022, [22] the network will assess to what extent the immunity in the Swiss population reached high rates (90% or more) among those aged 65+ in several Cantons (e.g., Vaud, Valais, Zurich, Ticino).

There are several limitations of the "Corona-Immunitas" study. The potential biases in the study sample signal that the population selected may be more adherent to recommendations and obligations during the COVID-19 pandemic than the general Swiss population (op. cit., p. 4). The disaggregation is not matching the more useful age breakdowns of the "Covid-19 Social Monitor",

---

[21] https://www.corona-immunitas.ch/media/qrnlmrqp/report_on_status_of_vaccination_commented_122021_2021-12-10.pdf
Corona Immunitas Resarch Group, "Report on status of vaccination in Switzerland," 2021-12-10
[22] https://www.corona-immunitas.ch/en/news/seroprevalence-in-the-swiss-population-after-the-5th-test-phase/
Corona Immunitas (11.05.2022), "Seroprevalence in the Swiss population after the 5th test phase" (accessed on 28 Jun. 2022)

and the "*vaccinated*" are limited to those who received at least one vaccine injection for SARS-CoV-2. The NCS-TF noted that in the general population, the additional information about the second dose reports a limited 41% coverage at national level (mid-February 2022); this shows that the population is neither fully protected against the evolution to a serious outcome (hospitalization or death), nor taking stock of the importance of the second dose (NCS-TF, Rapport scientifique, 26 Oct. 2022 p. 2).

For the "Corona-Immunitas", the general findings leave many interpretations still open to programmatic questions. It merits further exploitation, particularly in terms of the existing interpretations of graphs and summary of findings, for example, in relation to vaccine hesitancy and vaccination campaign messages. Studies pushing their findings to recommendations are rare. A good example is the recent prospective cohort study that formulated the following sound "implications": early planning of vaccination campaigns encompassing lower education levels and lower health literacy with the support of local/ cantonal authorities with actors other than government agencies and scientists to overcome the low trust in government and science (Heineger S. et. al., op. cit., p. 8). Building up and translating practical recommendations into operations is a challenge that the various levels of health authorities need to tackle.

Antoine Flahault suggested[23] the need to engage the anthropologists' perspective as a potential solution to improve the understanding behind the non-vaccinated and to boost the vaccination rates when these were stagnating at the end of 2021. "Corona Immunitas" was able to establish quickly a national cooperation with more than 40 studies related to immunity in the country; the Swiss School of Public Health (SSPH+)[24] offers access to close to 400 doctoral students with 50 fellowships through its multidisciplinary academic structures. The "Corona Immunitas" network can further advance the understanding of Covid-19 (also combined with Influenza) vaccination completeness and vaccine hesitancy with an improved commitment of the SSPH+ network (involving half a dozen Universities across the country) with an anthropological research focus.

---

[23] https://www.tdg.ch/cinq-pistes-pour-booster-la-lutte-anti-covid-en-suisse-252662340746
Antoine Flahault, « Cinq pistes pour booster la lutte anti-Covid en Suisse », Tribune de Genève, 18.11.2021
[24] https://medicalforum.ch/fr/detail/doi/fms.2021.08959
Nino Künzli, "Plus forts ensemble – Swiss School of Public Health", Swiss Medical Forum – Forum Médical Suisse, 2021; 21(51-52): 869-871

A socioeconomic position paper[25] recommended that *"Governments and health-care systems should address this pandemic of inequality by taking measures to reduce health inequities in response to the SARS-CoV-2 pandemic."* Triangulation with additional data sources is necessary. Along these lines, based on existing studies (e. g. Swiss neighborhood index of socio-economic position, Geneva neighborhood socio-economic vulnerability index), the strategic use of socio-economic mapping would allow a rapid identification of areas with lower coverage among disadvantaged social classes or neighborhoods in order to increase vaccination coverage among these hard-to-reach populations. This research will include urban and rural populations using a mix of quantitative/ qualitative study via well-known anthropological methods. The latter combines focus groups and semi-structured interviews (closed questionnaires with representative samples encompassing more vulnerable socioeconomic status pockets).

Several of these anthropological methods have been used in this pandemic by young researchers from Swiss Universities.[26] The engagement of social scientists (i.e. social epidemiologists, anthropologists, sociologists, psychologists, and economists) is an opportunity to exploit the diverse research areas and bring in the expertise needed.

Complementary to these studies and findings, additional strategic considerations may further feed into the upcoming plan. The experiences gathered over more than one year suggest continuous and sustained communication campaigns for vaccination (i. e. several weeks vs. one week) adapted to the vulnerable groups (including the 80+ years). The changing epidemiology of the pandemic will necessitate adjusting vaccination strategies from large campaigns through vaccination centers to on-going health services. This builds on the lessons learnt from the review about "Mapping the Swiss Supply Chain"[27] which suggests targeting elderly patients with their family physicians and tailoring individual communication. In addition, it recommends collaborating with the cantonal public health authorities who are in charge of the vaccination campaign implementation. In this context, the bridge between chronic and infectious diseases at the primary health care level and their medical services (medical

---

[25] https://www.thelancet.com/journals/lanpub/article/PIIS2468-2667(21)00160-2/fulltext
J. Riou et. al., « Socioeconomic position and the COVID-19 care cascade from testing to mortality in Switzerland: a population-based analysis", The Lancet, July 9, 2021
[26] "Covid-19 through the lens of social sciences in Switzerland", AMADES Conference, Lausanne, June 3rd 2022
[27] https://www.frontiersin.org/articles/10.3389/fpubh.2022.935400/full
Thakur-Weigold B, Buerki P, Frei P and Wagner SM (2022) Mapping the Swiss Vaccine Supply Chain. Front. Public Health 10:935400. doi: 10.3389/fpubh.2022.935400

doctors' offices) is more than ever necessary, particularly for the aged population. It is necessary to identify factors influencing individuals' clinical vulnerability such as obesity or diabetes which increase the risk of COVID and the need for booster shots. Weight excess inequities linked to socioeconomic vulnerabilities is more common among individuals with low educational status, [28] low revenue and belonging to some professional categories. Primary healthcare attention on the connection between infectious and chronic diseases is an opportunity to extend the links and the impact of public health services both at community and at tertiary hospital service level to end the pandemic. Injecting both the influenza vaccine and the COVID-19 vaccine during the same visit for a double protection is a sustainable strategy, which may allow future routine services to be better accepted among the aged-population. Such granular research and considerations are an investment into the potential improvement of other vaccination strategies and antigens (e. g. measles) for present and future pandemics.

Finally, the NCS-TF noted that the National Research Program (NPR) will support advanced research and improve the understanding of inequities with the "Covid-19 and society" call for research[29] (Jan. 2022). Yet the final recipients (approximately forty) for this call were still to be selected at mid-year (June 2022). Consequently, the research will only be implemented in 2023 with at best expected findings in 2024. The social science-based innovative approach proposed could leverage in the next few weeks fast-track funds of the NPR for a rapid and robust design. Preliminary findings could then be available during the autumn 2022 allowing refinement of the strategies, interventions and targeted vaccination campaigns among the 60+ at federal and canton levels.

Conclusion

Promoting the importance of studies that are social science driven with the determinants of health (vs. biomedical and mortality focused) is critical to advance the understanding of preventive measures, including vaccination. Furthermore, equity and well-being have been recognized by the international community[30] at the heart of the COVID-19 sustainable response with better

---

[28] https://www.bmj.com/content/373/bmj.n1158
A. Chiolero, "Body mass index as socioeconomic indicator", BMJ, 2021;373:n1158
[29] https://www.nfp80.ch/fr/
[30] https://apps.who.int/iris/bitstream/handle/10665/351798/PMC8795854.pdf?sequence=1
Oscar J. Mujica et. al., "Health inequity focus in pandemic preparedness and response plans", Editorials, Bull World Health Organ 2022, 100:91-91A

governance encompassing the interdependencies between health, social, environmental and economic systems. Benefitting from the well-rounded tools offered by social science is essential to achieve this goal.

Stimulating further partnerships between researchers in large networks (e. g. SSPH+) and local levels (cantons and "communes"/ local authorities) as well as advocating for financial support are essential to making a difference for the upcoming unfinished vaccination agenda. This approach is a worthwhile and relatively low-cost investment in ending the pandemic, taking into account the personnel and material costs,[31] which reached CHF 352 million for five university hospitals in 2020 and 2021.

We hope our additional specific options for action for Switzerland may better inform the upcoming strategy towards the end of the pandemic for the aged population with the COVID-19 vaccines and for applications to all non-pharmaceutical interventions. Although the focus here is on Switzerland, the findings are largely applicable to other countries in Europe, for the long term (e. g. new Omicron variants BA.4 and BA.5, new waves, upcoming ARN Moderna and Pfizer-BioNTech ARN vaccines), and for future pandemics. A broader perspective of the importance of social sciences focusing on various measures to improve the responses and to counteract inequities with examples from Switzerland, Italy and Germany has been presented at the European Society for Health and Medical Sociology (ESHMS) conference.[32]

Special thanks to the in charges of the Covid-19 Social Monitor, and Corona Immunitas, the Taskforce BAG Covid-19, Social Media Communication (FOPH), as well as for and to Stephane Cullati for reviews.
(This paper is based on preliminary findings presented by Cyril Pervilhac, Tina Draser, "COVID-19 Vaccination Coverage in Switzerland: How can Social Sciences Make a Difference in an Agenda Yet to be Fully Accomplished?", Conférence suisse de l'AMADES, Lausanne, « Covid-19 sous l'angle des sciences sociales en Suisse », 3 juin 2022)

---

[31] https://www.tdg.ch/le-covid-revele-le-defi-du-financement-des-hopitaux-universitaires-315259052461
Tribune de Genève, « Bilan provisoire: Le Covid révèle le défi du financement des hôpitaux universitaires », 12 mai 2022
[32] M. Verykiou, M. Marx, C. Pervilhac, "What role can social sciences play in evaluating COVID-19 responses and addressing inequities? A European perspective", 19th Biennial European Society for Health and Medical Sociology (ESHMS) Conference, Bologna, 25-27th August 2022

Beyond the November 28, 2021 vote: a paradigm shift with public health to counteract the pandemic and fifth wave of COVID-19 in Switzerland?

28 December 2021

Cyril Pervilhac, Retiree, WHO HQ Geneva, pervilhacc[at]gmail.com

Tina Draser, Retiree, The Global Fund to fight AIDS, TB and Malaria, Geneva

The vote of November 28, 2021 on the modification of the law and the COVID certificate in Switzerland, far from ending the debate, reopens it as to the measures to be pursued.[1] The rate of infection has risen dramatically in recent weeks (doubling of cases every two weeks), whereas the vaccination rate (66%) is only slowly increasing.[2] The measures taken at present are accompanied by a certain scepticism of experts with the containment pointing at the horizon as a possible consequence.[3] But what are the solutions and avenues offered by public health and prevention to overcome the fifth wave but also this pandemic in 2022 and beyond? Are they fully exploited?

The background to these figures in Switzerland has already been well documented in recent weeks:

- Austria has shown similar trends to Switzerland,[4] but a few days ahead, as reported by members of the Covid-19 task force: insufficient and similar vaccination rates between the two countries, infection curves with identical trends, recent high incidence of the virus in three cantons bordering Austria.
- The German-speaking cantons suffer from a tighter situation and lower vaccination coverage than the French-speaking cantons; [5] to recall that in addition to vaccination, the Federal Council will not be able to avoid seriously considering a new set of measures in the coming weeks.
- With only a little over two-thirds of the population fully vaccinated as of a few days ago and the failure of the recent National Immunization Week in

---

[1] Lise Bailat, "Ce que change le oui à la loi Covid", TdG, 29.11.2021

[2] OFSP, 1 December 2021

[3] Julien Vicky, et. al, "Combien de temps avant le prochain tour de vis?", TdG, 3.12.2021

[4] Yannick Weber, " Avec vingt jours de retard, la Suisse prend exactement la voie de l'Autriche ", 20mn.ch, 16 November 2021

[5] F. Giroud, "Cinquième vague de Covid-19 - Pourquoi les cantons romands font mieux que les alémaniques", 16 November 2021

November accompanied by underestimation of popular anger, the situation is serious. [6]

- The causes and degree of rejection of vaccination are complex.[7] A recent analysis grouped them into six social categories: "natural medicine followers, primitive Swiss, conspiracists, politicians, moderates, and populists".

- Vaccine refusal or hesitancy is a well-known and long-standing phenomenon throughout the world, with an average of 13% expressing some degree of scepticism.[8]

Faced with this situation, there is no reason to despair, however: public health measures offer us clear paths to overcome this pandemic in the weeks and months to come.

Lessons learned from other countries with high vaccination rates (e.g. Portugal, Italy, Spain) with a Latin culture of collective responsibility logic (vs. individual responsibility for German-speaking countries) indicate how culturally adapted communication played a key role. These campaigns took place weeks before and during the launch of the vaccination programmes so that the population would adhere to them. The "*seven good reasons to get vaccinated*" [9] for Switzerland are a good example:

1. *You protecting yourself from COVID-19 and getting very sick.*
2. *You get immunized the safe way.*
3. *You help to reduce the number of cases.*
4. *You help combat the effects of the pandemic.*
5. *You prevent potential long-term debilitating effects of COVID-19 (long-term effects of COVID-19)*
6. *You help relieve pressure on the healthcare system.*
7. *You help us get our everyday freedom back.*

But these remain very general and insufficiently convincing in terms of their formulation and simplified messages which need to be regularly updated and targeted to different populations and ages using the wide range of multimedia available.

---

[6] Serge Enderlin, "Covid-19 : en Suisse, la cinquième vague déferle sur la population la moins vaccinée d'Europe de l'Ouest", Le Monde, 17 November 2021

[7] Dominique Botti, Lise Bailat, " Contre la loi COVID, l'alliance de tribus que tout oppose " Le Matin Dimanche, 7 November 2021, pp. 17-19

[8] Larson et. al, in Hans Rosling et al, Factfulness, 2018

[9] Source :https://www.bag.admin.ch/bag/fr/home/krankheiten/ausbrueche-epidemien-pandemien/aktuelle-ausbrueche-epidemien/novel-cov/impfen.html

In Spain, the cultural context, the importance of intergenerational family ties and solidarity, played a fundamental role. They are accompanied by close social contacts with consequent mutual responsibility to be vaccinated. [10] At the same time, in Switzerland, the Christmas and New Year's holidays encourage the population to protect close family members. This could be an opportunity to launch a sustained and massive media campaign on family solidarity and thus convince a few hesitant people.

In addition, there is now an urgent need to use tailored communication campaigns targeting some of the six groups identified above as hesitant with education and training interventions.[11] This will help to gain a few more critical percentages. Exploitation of all communication channels to disseminate the vaccination and barrier messages with posters and pamphlets, audio-visuals and social media is needed. The vaccinated can in turn use them in their own communities where counter-campaigns take place. Prior to the referendum, anti-vaccination materials flourished and were already being massively distributed in many public places such as hotel entrances, small shops, weekly markets, or entertainment sites, or in mailboxes with sophisticated anti-vaccination newspapers and messages. Future targeted communication campaigns should be based on detailed mapping of current immunisation coverage and incidences of new infections and their diverse populations.

At the local level, the involvement of the community and their local medical doctors' offices is crucial. Confidence in local doctors and the public health system are key factors in the willingness to be vaccinated. They should therefore be equipped accordingly. We can also take advantage of the situation to offer messages for the whole family, for example on the measles vaccine for children, which is also meeting resistance.

Communication is essential in prevention, but accessibility to services is another challenge. It is ironic that for both, and from our international professional experience, we have much to learn from public health programs in Africa that, over the years, have achieved sustained rates of immunization coverage of 80-90% or higher, achieving herd immunity. Social decision-making is an open and complex process, but immediate investment can pay off in the short term and will be beneficial from a long-term public health perspective. Facilitating access for different populations is essential, especially in sites that are not easily accessible by mobile strategies or services offered in public places (e.g. schools,

---

[10] Agencia SINC, « Por qué somos uno de los líderes mundiales en vacunación COVID », El Pais, 01/09/2021
[11] ECDC, "Rapid literature review on motivating hesitant population groups in Europe to vaccinate", October 2015, p. 8

supermarkets). Access to the third dose for the elderly should be aided with nearby sites, mobile facilities or walk-in centres. Other age cohorts will follow and will also require easier access.

It is encouraging to know that cantons are currently launching initiatives to evaluate their own strategies since the beginning of the pandemic. However, will this opportunity be fully exploited with sufficient financial support and multidisciplinary expertise to fully assess the impact of the various measures and factors of resistance to vaccination, or will it be a simple exercise of a few days by one or two epidemiological experts[12] to study statistical data already known? For example, an international panel of experts on pandemic preparedness points out that systemic, behavioural, environmental and social interventions also need to be better understood. These interventions, beyond the strict biomedical ones that are currently the focus of debate and strategy, are too few in number and insufficiently financed.

Based on the lessons learned from failures and successes, an innovative platform for exchange between the cantons could stimulate more appropriate strategies for rapid and dynamic adaptations according to local situations.

Consequently, in order to get out of the paradigm that favours only the biomedical interventions, it is necessary to counteract this pandemic that will leave COVID-19 endemic in the years to come: it is therefore necessary to give a central role to public health and prevention strategies. These must be adapted to each canton, with support at the federal level, and focused on reducing the circulation of the virus through the rapid achievement of high vaccination rates combined with the continuation of proven effective barrier measures[13] such as hand hygiene, wearing masks, and physical distancing and ventilation.

---

[12] www.bessi-collab.net
[13] Stella Talic, et. al, "Effectiveness of public health measures in reducing the incidence of covid-19, SARS-CoV-2 transmission, and covid-19 mortality: systematic review and meta-analysis," BMJ, 17 November 2021

Social sciences and social justice in the design, implementation, and evaluation of measures against COVID-19 - the case study of France in 2020

Maria Verykiou, MSc[1], Laurent Denis, MSc[2], Cyril Pervilhac, DrPH, MPH*[,3]

*Corresponding author

Author Affiliations

1. CERGAS, Center for Research on Health and Social Care Management, SDA Bocconi School of Management, Bocconi University, Via Sarfatti 25, 20136 Milano (MI), Italy

2. Director of Monitoring, Evaluation and Learning for an international NGO, USA

3. Independent international Public Health consultant, WHO retiree, 300 Chemin Rousseau, 01280 Prévessin-Moëns, France

Maria Verykiou: maria.verykiou@sdabocconi.it
Laurent Denis: laurentdenislaus@gmail.com
Cyril Pervilhac: pervilhacc@gmail.com

Keywords: COVID-19, social sciences, evaluation, policy, inequities, France

ABSTRACT

Background: The social impact of the COVID-19 pandemic has been profound. This paper uses France as a case-study to analyze the role of social sciences in the COVID-19 response from March 2020 to February 2021.

Methods: France's national evaluation reports as well as other secondary sources were used to examine five social science aspects: i) basic public health measures in response to COVID-19, ii) mental health, and cross sectoral issues in social justice, such as iii) communication, iv) civil society and community involvement in decision-making, and v) inequities.

Results: Findings indicate poor consideration of inequities in the conception of basic measures such as wearing facemasks, hand hygiene, and social distancing, especially for vulnerable populations, while social components such as mental health, communication, and community engagement lacked in the evaluation of France's COVID-19 response.

Conclusion: Pandemic responses and evaluations of interventions must integrate social science aspects. To this effect, practical recommendations with policy implications are provided to pave the way towards social justice.

1. BACKGROUND

As observed across the world over the past year, the COVID-19 pandemic highlighted the inadequacy of health system preparedness. It has been termed a "total social event" (Pittet et al., 2021) and the social sciences' support in the response to the pandemic outbreak during the first year in France is documented (Gaille et al., 2020). However, despite COVID-19's major historical and social component, and representatives of sociology and anthropology signaling early-on the health, economic, but also psychosocial risks of the pandemic (Deroche et al., 2020) (Brooks et al., 2020), the social sciences remained in a "secondary position in the public arena" (Ferreira et al., 2020) both in terms of the response to and evaluation of the health crisis.

In terms of the response, experiences with pandemic control (i.e., HIV / AIDS, SARS, Ebola), particularly in Africa but also in the Global North, including France for the case of HIV/AIDS, have demonstrated the instrumental role of social sciences in the adaptation, implementation, and acceptance of containment measures. Epidemics are "social as well as biological phenomena" (Shah, 2020) (Silk & Fefferman, 2021) as illustrated by anthropologists in Africa's Ebola epidemic who recommended the replacement of traditional burial practices that favored the spread of the disease, with safer ones (Nielsen et al., 2015). In the case of COVID-19, the implementation of Non-Pharmaceutical Intervention (NPI) strategies, which targeted a person or community to prevent the transmission of the pathogen, did not account for different forms of inequalities (Berkhout et al., 2021) or cultural variations. Despite the signaled importance of collecting and reporting data on socioeconomic determinants as well as race and ethnicity to identify high-risk populations for the development of equitable public health measures (Khalatbari-Soltani et. al., 2020), in France, as in other countries, NPIs were driven by limited indicators such as hospitalization and mortality rates, putting forward a biomedical model in the pandemic response (Pittet et al., 2020) (Pittet et al., 2021) (Deroche et al., 2020), and initially included lockdowns, curfews, and social distancing restrictions. While the rapid mobilization and response of the French health system actors, from administration to citizens, and the resilience of the social protection system are acknowledged (Pittet et al., 2021), such measures impacted social aspects such as mental health (Phiri et al., 2021), household relationships, adverse alcohol use (Niedzwiedz et al., 2020), caregiving for dependents, as well as organizational and educational aspects. As a result, COVID-19 altered the living conditions of populations, introduced strain and instability (Van Bavel et al.,

2020), and exacerbated social inequalities by shrinking the social safety net, monopolizing public resources, and leaving many unemployed (Ferreira et al., 2020). The risks following this initial response of confinement and restrictive measures included economic and social upheaval as well as "lost generations". In an Oxfam survey of 295 economists from 79 countries, most respondents felt that gender and racial inequalities are likely to increase as a result of the pandemic, and that their governments do not have plans in place to combat them (Berkhout et al., 2021).

Our goal in this case study is to demonstrate how the pandemic presents an opportunity to rethink social sciences' role and contribution in decision-making and health system preparedness. The objectives are to (i) analyze the results of the essential COVID-19 assessments conducted between March 2020 to February 2021 in France with an emphasis on social sciences, ii) discuss the reasons why the latter are of importance and, iii) suggest ways to better exploit existing evidence with practical policy recommendations in the context of the existing and future pandemics. Emphasis is placed on the pandemic's effect on vulnerable populations and addressing inequities.

2. METHODS

2.1. Sources

This case-study is based on five key-secondary sources of information on the evaluation of France's COVID-19 response which took place during the period between March 2020 and February 2021. These sources, outlined below, were selected based on their relevance and in-depth analysis of the topic:

i) The national evaluation of the COVID-19 crisis management and anticipated pandemic risks was commissioned by the President of the French Republic, E. Macron, on the 25th of June 2020 to D. Pittet, Chief Medical Doctor in charge of the prevention and infection control service (HUG Geneva). A mid-term report of this evaluation, released on 13th October 2020, was used for this study, hereafter referred to as the **Mid-term report** (Pittet et al., 2020) as well as the 179-pages final report with 40 recommendations, completed in March 2021 and released in May 2021, hereafter referred to as the **Final report** (Pittet et al., 2021). The evaluation focuses on the first and second semesters of 2020 until February 2021, with an impact analysis of mortality and an in-depth macro socio-economic analysis for France, including comparative analyses in Europe.

ii) The 1072-page report to the Senate from the national evaluation of public policies related to big pandemics in light of the COVID-19 health crisis and its management, published in December 2020, hereafter referred to as the **Senate report** (Deroche et al., 2020). This is based on interviews with more than thirty high-level key informants and six roundtables with minutes of key meetings.

iii) A review on the current status and perspectives on social inequalities in France in relation to COVID-19 by the Direction de Recherche des Etudes de l'Evaluation et des Statistiques (**DREES**) (Dubost et al., 2020), published in July 2020, presenting a review of the international and French literature, complementing it with statistical analysis of the data for France.

iv) The preliminary results, published in October 2020, from the national survey "Epidemiology and Living Conditions" (**EpiCoV**) (Warszawski et al., 2020) by DREES were also considered.

v) An in-depth analysis of inequities during the pandemic by the Institut De Recherche en Santé Publique (**IReSP**) (Bajos et al., 2021), released in October 2020. The team comprised of epidemiologists, sociologists, demographers, and economists, whose objective was to estimate the dynamics of the epidemic at the national and departmental levels in order to measure the effect of living conditions on exposure to the virus, and vice-versa. The survey aimed to follow the evolution of the epidemic by interviewing the same populations over several waves.

Additional secondary sources were explored based on a scoping review, to complement the above sources which addressed the same principal themes on the French COVID-19 response in terms of public health measures, mental health, communication, civil society engagement and inequities from a social sciences perspective. These included newspaper articles, case-studies, scientific publications (meta-analysis that provided review of the scientific literature on the subject). Recently released Non-Governmental Organizations (NGOs) reports for 2020, such as from Fondation l'Abbé Pierre (FAP) and Secours Populaire, were also reviewed, referring to inequalities. Finally, personal experience on the management of epidemics and pandemics in Africa was drawn upon to put into perspective this case-study of France and to provide relevant practical conclusions for future reference.

2.2. Analysis

A Qualitative Secondary Analysis (QSA) methodology was followed (Tate & Happ, 2018), in which the role of social sciences (sociology, anthropology, psychology) in the pandemic response was documented in terms of policy design and their evaluation. An evaluation of the economic aspects was out of scope of our study and was thus excluded from the analysis since it was extensively accounted in the key sources, in particular the Final report (Pittet et al., 2021).

The analysis focused on five aspects in total, comprising of two preventive NPIs addressing: i) basic public health measures against COVID-19 (excluding testing) and ii) mental health, as well as three cross-sectoral issues: iii) communication, iv) civil society and community involvement, and v) inequities. This selection is based on the 2020 WHO guidelines that informed the pillars of public health measures against COVID-19 (WHO, 2021). For each, operational recommendations are provided in the Discussion section to address the gaps observed in the evaluation process and to inform present and future political agendas.

3. RESULTS

3.1. Basic measures

A trend analysis of the basic hygiene measures observed in France between March 2020-July 2021 is provided by the research agency Santé Publique France (2021) (Figure 1).

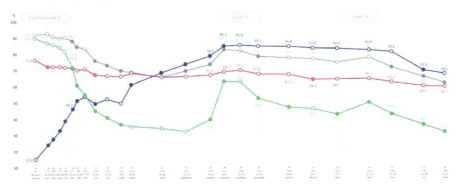

Figure 1: Trend of the declared systematic adoption of prevention measures (weighted %) between 30th March 2020 – 21st July 2021 (Santé Publique France, 2021). Legend: social greetings without using handshaking or kissing (grey), mask-wearing in public (blue), regular hand-washing (pink), avoid group gatherings and face-to-face meetings (green).

For the key measures analyzed in this paper, during the period of March-November 2020 corresponding to that examined in the Final Report: (i) Social distancing by avoiding group and in-person gatherings (green) was adopted strictly as France entered the peak of the first wave on 30th Mar.-1st Apr. 2020 at 84.7%; however, during the proceeding summer and early fall periods, this percentage ranged between 50-60%, while even at the second confinement in November 2020, physical distancing is still maintained at a lower rate of 63%. Further, the practice of (ii) hand hygiene (pink) decreased between 76% at the first confinement and 70% at the second confinement, indicating approximately a quarter of the French population not observing this measure. Finally, the controversy on (iii) wearing a mask (blue) is depicted by an antithetic trend starting from a rate of 15.1% at the onset of the pandemic and reaching 80% by the time of the second confinement, with the majority of the population adopting the measure during the summer (70% on 24-26th Aug. 2020). Although excluded from the time-period analyzed, it is worth mentioning that in view of the ramp-up of the vaccination campaign after the third lockdown, the new variants and the relaxation of restriction measures, the trends for basic hygiene practices such as the ones described above show a systematic decrease.

While the data point to accomplishments and gaps in the adoption of these measures, it may be subject to high variation between the general and vulnerable populations. In terms of their evaluation, critics from the political bench argue for the relative effect of these measures on impact and transmission rates, as these must evolve in relation to the evolution of the virus and its variants' behavior (Deroche et al., 2020). Further, the Mid-term report, even if the trends were not yet complete, did not analyze how much the populations used these basic measures (i.e., wearing masks, social distancing, hand hygiene), and the Final report did not provide any recommendations on how to improve access and compliance to these basic measures at present in view of new waves or future pandemics, and used a narrow trend period.

3.1.1. Social distancing

The spectrum of the relative enforcement of social distancing in France, from the absolute closure of all restaurant services to the closure of bars at 10 pm, and the permission to remove masks in cafés and restaurants during the day, has dichotomized the political scene. Some claimed that these measures have put at a disadvantage certain business more than others and questioned the lack of intermediate and equitable solutions (Deroche et al., 2020). Social distancing was identified as a challenging measure to implement, especially during the spring and summer seasons, which might have contributed to the measure's severity and extent, affecting mostly caregivers and employees in tourism, construction, and commerce (Pittet et al., 2020). Furthermore, the terminology that was used may have affected the extent to which the measure was adopted, as "social distancing" implies the "cut-off of meaningful interactions". Anthropologists argue that the term "physical distancing" may be better suited to reflect the necessity of avoiding physical rather than social contact to prevent the spread of the virus (Deroche et al., 2020).

3.1.2. Hand hygiene

The national evaluation concluded that hand hygiene and social distancing in addition to mask wearing were essential. These represent moderate measures that must form the core of public communication strategies in the prevention of future surges. However, the trend for hand-washing remains constant over time (Figure 1), which can be explained by the population coming into and getting out of supermarkets, who are encouraged to disinfect, but not having spontaneously acquired the hand hygiene practice (Pittet et al., 2021). Further, an overall 6% decrease in the practice was reported between the first and the second lockdown over a nine-month period, despite extensive public health messaging delivered in that period. This suggests a gap in the effective application or design of the measure. The Minister of Health highlighted that the debate on the effectiveness of mask wearing may have affected public attention towards observing the practice correctly (Deroche et al., 2020). However, questions around why the practice is not performed or done so poorly and by whom, remain.

3.1.3. Use of masks

The Mid-term and Final reports highlight that extensive debates and contradictory opinions on mask-wearing have been important challenges, while they identify as accomplishments the scientific, industrial, and public solidarity in the provision of masks and their effective adoption through internet tutorials. At the time of the national evaluation, their effectiveness in public spaces had not yet been demonstrated and there were fears that these provided a false sense of security that may jeopardize the application of other measures (Pittet et al., 2021). Furthermore, the focus on masks was concentrated on logistics (i.e., orders and manufacturing, management of stocks and shortages, types of masks and users, distribution, messages), rather than on quantifying access, identifying target mask users, measuring demand, determining utilization rates, and addressing potential cultural barriers for wide uptake. Despite the early activation of all the mechanisms to combat influenza during COVID-19, several other approaches could have been used to achieve wider adoption of mask-wearing, such as better use of networks and associations (Deroche et al., 2020) or promotion activities for wearing masks as conducted in 26 neighborhoods in Guyana. Further, research into the reasons for the use or non-use of a mask could be pursued, as was done with condoms for HIV/AIDS, leveraging on behavioral surveillance to monitor and link the behaviors with prevalence and incidence among young people as well as other populations (Rehle et al., 2004).

3.2. Mental health

Early in the pandemic, China called for the inclusion of mental health services in the package of prevention measures (Zhou et al., 2020) and the international community called for collaborations in order *to provide high-quality, timely crisis psychological services to community-dwelling older adults"* (Yang et al., 2020). Evidence soon demonstrated the psychological burden of COVID-19 on individuals and the need to align behaviors with containment measures through science communication, moral decision-making, and leadership, among others (Van Bavel et al., 2020). In France, the CoviPrev survey initiated in March 2020 revealed that one fourth of the population reported being affected by depression, anxiety, dissatisfaction with life, and sleep disturbances, with the highest levels being observed at the beginning of each confinement but falling by up to 5% and 10% points for depression and anxiety, respectively, during the summer period in-between (Verbeke, 2021) (Santé Publique France, 2021).

In the national evaluations, the pandemic's impact on mental health is recognized in several settings, including workplaces and schools (Pittet et al., 2021), as well as in terms of the effects of postponing treatment for various pathologies, such as for cancer and mental conditions (Pittet et al., 2020). Further, the lack of understanding of the full psychological impact of COVID-19 on the entire population, beyond institutional psychiatric care, is acknowledged (Deroche et al., 2020), as well as the challenges in measuring this and making predictions of its consequences, citing the high likelihood of increased depression and anxiety rates in the case of subsequent confinements (Santé Publique France, 2021). A survey on the effect of the confinement under the COCONEL project revealed that the measure was widely supported, but at the cost of increased social inequalities and mental health disorders (Deroche et al., 2020).

A study carried out in April 2020 identified that those in isolation and women are at an increased risk of anxiety, sleep disturbances, concentration problems, and feelings of sadness (Dubost et al., 2020). The student community particularly stood out, with a doubling of depression rates from 13.5% before (23-25 March 2020) to 26.7% after (30 March-1 April 2020) the onset of the pandemic. While heightened anxiety was reported among the student population following the first confinement, the second confinement was characterized by a worsening of depression cases in terms of severity of symptoms, including with suicidal tendencies. Franck (2020) highlights that poor mental wellbeing was also prevalent among individuals with disabilities, farmers, and students. In response to these observations, several behavioral and mental health studies have been launched, including one mandated by the President on January 29th, 2021, to investigate the impact of confinements on the psychological status of citizens.

3.3. Communication

France's early response was characterized by weak communication, in contrast to Germany's success in disseminating measures, such as social distancing and availability of diagnostic tests, aided mainly by cultural and organizational factors (Deroche et al., 2020). Additionally, misinformation and poor access to credible sources of information combined with low literacy rates among the lower-income strata deepened the social divide and contributed to resistance to the timely adoption of measures and the dissemination of preventive practices. The CNS was instrumental in communicating the containment measures to manage the crisis. However, it added to the complexity of gathering and unifying experts, and to the multiple communication channels, which were at times perceived as disharmonious (Deroche et al., 2020). The emergence of a plethora of experts on COVID-19, some self-proclaimed and expressing contradictory opinions, and the important number of related articles flooding social media and news channels naturally drew the public towards engaging in the ongoing scientific and political debates. Consequently, the evolution of public interventions and guidelines were not perceived as adjustment of measures to the new scientific knowledge or other resources that were becoming contemporaneously more available. These were instead perceived as a breach of the guidelines at the time, increasing the level of agitation amongst the public and mistrust towards health authorities. To combat this, the Senate report confirms the necessity of contextualization, clarity and honesty in the communication of the scientific limitations that confine the translation of evidence into reactive and evolving policies.

Science communication strategies have been criticized for their lack of educational elements, lack of focus on the responsibility of citizens, and not targeting young people (Deroche et al., 2020). The rise of conspiracy theories and fake news around COVID-19 obscured the reliability of information even when it originated from credible sources and raised the question on who would benefit from the spread of fake news (Green & Cladi, 2020). Communication efforts at the onset of the vaccination campaign in the first semester of 2021 did little to decrease vaccine hesitancy, which was fueled by a lack of understanding of the factors driving vaccination and a lack of public reassurance by the government (Shah, 2020) (Soullier, 2020). It is at this cultural and behavioral intersection that social scientists can contribute by bringing lessons learnt from previous vaccination campaigns, for example against measles in France or in the Global South, to tailor effective communication practices for the "hard-to-reach" and to overcome vaccine hesitancy and misinformation (Deroche et al., 2020).

3.4. Civil society and community involvement
In France, social work was not given due consideration in the initial phase of the response, in spite of their commendable efforts since the beginning of the pandemic in supporting preventive measures and treatment interventions, but was only considered in a secondary phase, after the closing of community

centers. For example, the Senate report criticized the delivery of meals to COVID-19 positive patients in quarantine, where meals were left outside front doors without offering more direct care, as often the fire brigade was called to open doors where numerous meals had accumulated outside. In such instances, service personnel (i.e., social workers) is identified as key prevention personnel to signal the presence of vulnerable populations to the relevant territorial civil protection authorities.

The lack of involvement of civil society and the missed opportunity to incorporate lessons learnt from the fight against HIV/AIDS into the COVID-19 response are noted. However civil society engagement mechanisms are not identified in the evaluations, despite the example of the Yellow Vests movement ("gilets jaunes") in the Autumn of 2018, which the President addressed by involving associations that could negotiate local solutions with the movement (Deroche et al., 2020). Calling for strengthened health democracy by including social scientists and health system users in the CNS (Pittet et al., 2021), the CNS had advocated for a Citizen and Civil Society Committee ("Comité Citoyen et de la Société Civile") in decision-making, but was not supported, showing that politicians excluded the civil society from politics. Instead, a COVID-19 control-and-liaison committee was established, which however focused on the role of health information systems and digital technologies in the response instead of liaising with civil society (Deroche et al., 2020).

3.5. Inequities

While the differential impact of COVID-19 on certain populations is presented above with respect to basic measures and mental health, evidence is also presented below on its effect in exacerbating inequities, in geographic, social, and economic terms.

Territorial analysis in the suburbs of Lyon and Ile de France showed populations in peripheral or poorer neighborhoods presented more risk factors for COVID-19 (Dubost et al., 2020). Further, higher exposure risk is found in multi-person households, in non-European immigrant populations, and in persons aged between 30-49 years irrespective of living conditions, with almost double the COVID-19 seroprevalence in priority city areas (Quartier Prioritaire de Politique de la Ville – QPV), which represent poverty-concentrated territories (Warszawski et al., 2020). In Marseille, the homeless population living in the same urban area as the general population demonstrated a significantly increased risk of infection (Loubiere et al., 2021). Economic studies which contain the mapping of populations living under precarious conditions in Paris demonstrate the higher risk and vulnerability of households in precarious territorial units that are typically characterized by being overcrowded, large, with many youths facing economic uncertainty and low education levels (Goutte et al., 2020). The rate of infection was double in crowded households (defined as <18m^2 per person) compared to other households, at 9.2% vs. 4.5% respectively. In densely inhabited neighborhoods and households, the lack of an attending doctor was also observed (Deroche et al., 2020). Interestingly, those who were required to remain active during the confinement periods, such as essential workers, were often residing in priority neighborhoods or close-by, where the disease prevalence was higher (Fondation Abbé Pierre, 2021).

Similarly, aggravating factors of social inequities related to confinement such as comorbidities, mental health, material and physical safety, social support, housing and isolation, access to digital technology, and education, may have caused a "double" or "triple hardship" within certain sub-populations (Dubost et al., 2020). For instance, it has been shown that women, in addition to constituting the bulk of the health and social care workforce, experienced an increased load of domestic and parental tasks, suffered increased unemployment, as well as high rates of domestic violence. While COVID-19's impact on mortality in men has been show-cased, its impact on increasing social inequities in women as a risk factor is less visible. COVID-19's greater impact on the poor and the elderly is evidenced by correlating mortality rates to a social and age gradient (Yanez et al., 2020).

Finally, locations such as food distribution centers, hostels, and emergency centers, showed a higher prevalence of COVID-19 infections, with one in two people interviewed having contracted the virus in comparison to the one-in-ten incidence found in the general population. In France, 5.5 million individuals in need of food support benefitted from €1.5 billion of food aid per year, but since April 2020, there has been an increase of 25-30% in demand (Ouest France, 2020). Requests for food aid from the Secours Populaire shot up by 45%, while from the "Restos du Coeur" reached 45% in Seine-Saint-Denis and 30% in Paris. With a big part of their volunteers aged 70 years and over, the FAP, Red-Cross, and Secours Populaire noted fewer human resources to sort, stock, and distribute the goods, due to the confinement restrictions (Birchem, 2020). As per the Ministry of Solidarity and Health, the budget for food aid is projected to increase substantially for the 2021-2027 period, with the figure of people in need of food aid reaching 8 million at the end of 2020 compared to 5.5 million in 2019 (Rey-Lefebvre, 2020). In addition, institutions of care for the elderly (EHPAD) or the handicapped, social residences for children or migrants, and prisons are identified as locations where the risk of infection was highest, with similar mortality rates than in other countries' respective institutions (Pittet et al., 2021). However, no conclusions are inferred regarding the level of care provided for COVID-19 patients in these institutions. This topic will be addressed through a newly created and dedicated platform for health research focusing on populations living in care institutions (Deroche et al., 2020). Further, specialized COVID-19 accommodation centers were opened for those mildly ill, without a home or who could not stay at their home due to limited opportunity for isolation and increased risk of comorbidities. The percentage of COVID-19 positive cases in such accommodation centers in the Ile-de-France during the summer of 2020 was 52% compared to 10% in the rest of the population. Social sciences are essential to address and overcome these inequities, as discussed later, and bridge the gap between the *Solidarity* and *Health* components of the French Ministry of Solidarity and Health.

4. DISCUSSION

4.1. Discussion of results & practical policy recommendations

Our analysis was limited to the period of March 2020-February 2021 and excluded the impact of the preventive vaccination campaign. This was in order to ensure consistency with the data analyzed in the Final report, which was only released and made available in May 2021, and which limited the timing and scope of this case study. Further, due to time limitations, the case-study excluded the analysis of documents such as detailed national plans and strategies, and for the same reason access to key informants as primary sources of information was not possible. The Senate report largely compensates for the latter, given that it includes the opinions on the pandemic response of more than 30 politicians and other experts. However, the subjective nature of the Senate report constitutes a source of bias, as a repository of politicians' opinions and interpretation of evidence. Finally, the case-study provides a wealth of information and perspectives on the measures adopted but less so on their effectiveness, due to the challenges of measuring their individual impact, although this point is included in the Discussion section.

Despite the time limitations of this case-study, the analysis of basic public health measures in the first year of the pandemic presented in this paper is relevant and applicable to the second year, especially as the examined interventions are beneficial to the health and well-being of populations world-wide, even in non-pandemic periods (Muller et al., 2021). NPIs can significantly contain the COVID-19 pandemic, with distancing and the simultaneous implementation of two or more NPIs associated to decreased virus transmission (Bo et al., 2021). Indeed, it is important that the complete chain of measures is observed to effectively combat COVID-19 (Deroche et al., 2020), as demonstrated during the HIV/AIDS pandemic (Piot & Coll Seck, 2001) (UNAIDS, 2010). Compared to highly intrusive options such as curfews and lockdowns, governmental support to vulnerable populations, for example through food assistance, and risk-communication strategies tailored to the local context are strongly recommended, as these measures may also foster higher compliance (Haug et al., 2020). Nonetheless, all prevention measures, backed up by social sciences, need to be results-based with hard indicators and targets that are monitored over the short and medium term. We reported on these trends (Figure 1) but the qualitative studies explaining the changes among vulnerable groups still need to be undertaken as in Germany (Fisher et al., 2020).

Further, given the social and mental health impact of COVID-19 containment measures recognized by the WHO (De Miguel et al., 2021), social sciences merit urgent consideration by expert researchers for the prevention and control of diseases at the local and international levels alike (Green & Cladi, 2020). The interdependency of health, social, ecological, economic, financial, and political parameters (Van Bavel et al., 2020) (Ferreira et al., 2020) must be accounted for to design effective interventions, as exemplified by the BESSI collaboration (Michie & West, 2020) (BESSI, 2021). Designing effective NPIs must thus also take into consideration community-based care, the Primary Health Care (PHC) system, which is characterized by a shortage of staff, general practitioners and nurses, especially in the rural areas and suburbs of big cities, gaps in continuity of care, limited preventive care accessibility to vulnerable populations, and lack of resources. However, the evaluations focused on hospital bottlenecks and deaths at the tertiary level (Pittet et al., 2021), thus missing the opportunity to highlight the importance of strengthening health systems as a whole in order to overcome the social injustice in access to services in the long-term and achieve higher effectiveness of the basic measures against COVID-19, as learnt from the recent Ebola response. In view of the gap between community and state provision, a strengthened community-based approach for social and health care surveillance and delivery is called for, through state partnerships with community-based associations.

Due to the extent and nature of the impact of the pandemic, public health responses must take into account the embedded behaviors, social environments, and structures that were conducive to the emergence and transmission of COVID-19 (Michie & West, 2020). Public health is not limited to the health sector but seeks to coordinate collective efforts, based both on scientific knowledge and citizen and civil society engagement, on the basis of a shared political project. Community engagement, exemplified by Scandinavian countries, thus, lie at the core of public health, which can be reinforced following a multidisciplinary approach and improved training of health professionals (Deroche et al., 2020) (Pittet et al., 2021). Targeting public health messages through trusted community leaders, especially in marginalized communities, building partnerships between public health authorities and organizations that are working directly with them, and disseminating information on recognizing inaccurate sources of information through discussions between the policy community and humanities experts, can help to safeguard the public from misinformation (Shah, 2020). Content must be carved around the collective social responsibility that individual behaviors bear in the fight against the virus (Van Bavel et al., 2020).

In conclusion, the evaluations illustrate the dominance of impact markers for health and the economy, resulting in the formulation of "Propositions" largely overlooking the present and, consequently, future social inequities. In view of better exploiting social sciences and considering these gaps, we propose operational recommendations for each of the five aspects of our analysis (basic measures, mental health, communication, community engagement and inequities) (Supplementary Table S1) for the institutions and agencies involved in the response. We also provide practical applications to complement the "Propositions" formulated in the French evaluations, using four examples (Supplementary Table S2).

4.2. Evaluation as a tool for social justice

According to the literature, vulnerable populations (Van Bavel et al., 2020), (Bajos et al., 2021), (Pittet et al., 2020), (Dubost et al., 2020) include the homeless, those who do not have access to sanitary services or clean water, those living in conditions where physical distancing cannot be observed such as prisons and refugee camps, persons without health insurance and with limited access to health services, or those in occupations that do not allow for remote working such as cleaning, retail, agricultural labor, where employees depend on a daily wage, or who need to use public transport to reach their work. However, due to the lack of a common definition or methodology for their identification, prioritization mechanisms for vulnerable populations have not been established by the Haut Conseil de Santé Publique (HCSP) in France, as opposed to the

USA and the UK. Indeed, the decree dated 29th August 2020 which officially identifies the populations eligible for partial unemployment compensation was criticized by the President of the Scientific Committee as restrictive only to populations vulnerable to COVID-19 (Jacquot, 2020).

In the French evaluation reports, references to targeted interventions for the benefit of vulnerable populations are rare. However, social science research can contribute to the creation of public policies, including adapted health and psychosocial strategies, that ensure that activities are tailored to specific populations, ethnic groups (Gorce, 2021), and geographies. Such activities can be informed by past experiences with HIV/AIDS, or local scale COVID-19 responses, with the example of Nigeria (Irwin et al., 2021), where social sciences were used for targeting measures to tackle inequity instead of imposing general lockdowns. In its concluding remarks, a social science study pointed that it may be too late to work on medical predispositions and pre-existing health conditions that might put a certain group of persons at higher risk, therefore it is wiser to target upstream and downstream mechanisms, like exposure to COVID-19 and access to treatment, respectively (Dubost et al., 2020). This may partially explain why the evaluation reports did not consider addressing inequities as an issue.

Social sciences as well as aspects relating to overcoming inequities were largely under-represented in France's 2020 public policy evaluation processes, despite the World Health Organization's guidelines for Intra Action Reviews (IAR) placing social sciences at the core of public health approaches (WHO, 2020) (Shah, 2020). Illustrative of this is the composition of the team responsible for the design of the evaluation reports (Oct. 2020, May 2021) as well as the Conseil National de Santé (CNS) for COVID-19 which was founded in March 2020 and is the main advisory body to the French Government (Blaize, 2021). As social scientists were largely absent from the evaluations conducted by leading public health bodies in France, intervention measures may not have fully reflected COVID-19's social gradient. Indeed, the attention to the latter is lacking in the national evaluations analyzed in this paper, with "sociology", "anthropology" or "psychology" not mentioned per se and limited only to the provision of an analysis of the crisis's social consequences through meeting key informants involved in the social response and a case-study in a local underprivileged territory (Pittet et al., 2021). The prevention measures introduced in France thus hit a wall when confronted with social inequities, as inequalities in terms of professional circumstances, promiscuity, and differential access to protection measures are deeply embedded in the French society (Dubost et al., 2020).

Further, while trends for basic public health measures were already available in August 2020, they were not included in the Mid-term report for the preliminary analysis and recommendations before France faced its second wave.

The above-mentioned gaps point to the conclusion that evaluations must be more comprehensive, participative, and timely, in order to inform a more effective and equitable response, provided social sciences are included in governance and research activities.

In terms of governance, the lack of involvement by citizen associations in decision-making and solution design is noted as is the poor consideration of social determinants, though singularly documented through the exposure gradient and mortality (Dubost et al., 2020). In response to this, the governing body of the CNS recommended its thematic diversification through expansion to other domains, such as economic and social, in order to be able to conduct comprehensive evaluations of the propositions put forward to the council (Deroche et al., 2020). However, responsibilities between the various layers of advising bodies were unclear and added to the bureaucracy and complexity of final public sector decision-making. This gap between risk evaluation and management is present also in other institutions, like the HCSP, which seems to be a competing or duplicating entity to numerous other existing specialized agencies (Pittet et al., 2020). As a solution, an inter-ministerial crisis cell («une cellule interministérielle de crise») for decision-making chaired by the prime-minister or a minister has been presented, consisting of experts offering their insights but who are not accountable for decision-making (Deroche et al., 2020).

In terms of research, both bio-medical and social domains were challenged by the novelty of the COVID-19 virus, which can partially explain the limitations of the two evaluations and can justify why decisions were not able to be taken based on these. As the continuous evolution of the pandemic constantly defines a new status quo to respond to, certain findings and perspectives are quickly rendered outdated, thus justifying the delays in the formulation and dissemination of the evaluation findings. To combat this, WHO has recommended the use of regular IARs for COVID-19 (WHO, 2020), to which national research bodies like the "Agence Nationale de Recherche Nord & Sud sur le SIDA et les hépatites virales" (ANRS), have considerably modified their procedures to carry out evaluations very quickly (Deroche et al., 2020). Following such an approach, the findings from the evaluations we reviewed could have been rapidly leveraged in the context of the current COVID-19 response while lessons for future pandemics, which eventually became the focus of the evaluation, could have been drawn later. With WHO-Europe not having the authorization to disseminate the IARs from their member states, the blame and shame culture still appears to prevail, rather than learning quickly and collectively with a few countries such as Spain and Sweden now advocating for the internal and independent evaluations of institutions (Garcia-Basteiro et al., 2020) (Swedish Ministry of Health and Social Affairs, 2020).

Some considerations are provided below (Table 1) for the conduct of participative and comprehensive evaluations for decision-making towards addressing social inequalities. These are applicable broadly, including to other country contexts or pandemics.

Table 1: *Recommendations towards addressing social inequalities on the conduct of public health crisis evaluations.*

Evaluation aspect	Recommendations
Design	Engagement of social scientists (social epidemiologists, psychologists, anthropologists, etc.), local and national experts, civil society, communities, and social institutions
	Early identification of vulnerable populations and ethnic groups for inclusion in the design of targeted measures, outreach methods, and their monitoring and evaluation
Scope	Inclusion of behavioral, social and humanitarian aspects of basic measures and other NPIs, as well as mental health and basic measures in the scope of health systems' evaluations
Methods	Social sciences, as per the Final report, to be linked to research in health from the onset of projects and included in pluri-, inter-, and trans-disciplinary approaches
Timeline	Performance of rapid assessments (3-6 month turn over) as per the WHO IARs
Financing	Earmarking a minimal budget for social sciences-supported activities (based on leveraging minimal resources for a health system component, such as the monitoring and evaluation of HIV/AIDS)
Dissemination	Promotion of a learning platform within Europe (by regions, and international) for lessons-learnt exchange per intervention

(i.e., what works or not)
Articulation of social challenges at national and international levels, between policy and civil society actors

5. CONCLUSION

The case-study of France demonstrates that the differential impact of COVID-19 on socially vulnerable populations and argues that a central role that must be played by communities to ensure an inclusive, equitable and effective response. To prevent further infections, measures such as social distancing, hand hygiene and mask wearing must be informed by behavioral psychology research to determine a population's willingness to accept and adopt these measures and anticipate interventions to address potential negligence or resistance and counter risky behaviors such as mask avoidance in public spaces (Green & Cladi, 2020). Indeed, our opinion is that understanding the relationship between evaluation, decision-making and communication can transform evidence into effectively implemented public health measures.

To render the response to COVID-19 and future pandemics more equitable, the social sciences (i.e., sociology, anthropology, psychology) must address a number of questions: Who are the most vulnerable populations where inequities must be addressed? Where are they located? What is the best way to engage and reach vulnerable communities and what should the role of civil society associations, NGOs and local government representatives be? How to formulate messaging and communications to ensure it resonates among these populations? How will the impact of the measures promoted among them be monitored/evaluated and assessed? Considering the G7 leaders' "USD 4.3 billion to finance equitable access to tests, treatments and vaccines in 2021" (G7a, 2021) commitment, it is reasonable to argue that investing in tools specific for addressing the respective social issues is a relatively small cost with a valuable sustainable benefit and impact (G7b, 2021).

The present analysis of France's COVID-19 response could be complemented by further research to improve our understanding of the importance and role of social sciences in pandemic preparedness and response to imminent new waves and future pandemics. Future research efforts should leverage detailed data from secondary sources beyond those used in this analysis, including plans, committee reports, detailed strategies and measures implemented. In addition, primary data from interviews with community leaders, experts, and decision-makers should also be collected. A comprehensive longitudinal observational research study with economic and social endpoints could provide evidence on the long-term impact of public health measures implemented among vulnerable populations in France but also in other countries. With regards to future pandemics, a sociological analysis of governance bodies and how effectively these are organized to take rapid and evidence-based decisions would be beneficial.

In conclusion, the findings presented here provide a first critical review of the importance of including social sciences stakeholders as well as approaches in the development of pandemic response plans from the onset. Social sciences have a role to play in informing decision-making on the design, implementation and adoption of effective NPIs in the short- and long-term to address the COVID-19 pandemic and beyond, in preparing for the emergence or re-emergence of other infectious diseases (Van Bavel et al., 2020). It should also be noted that the current pandemic may evolve into an endemic disease with emerging variants calling for dynamic and tailored responses over time. This has been the case with viruses like influenza or HIV/AIDS for example. Pandemic preparedness and response should include epidemiological surveillance and early detection of outbreaks, establishing rapid responses, producing, and sharing data, knowledge, and technology, in addition to a profound understanding of a community's needs and its acceptance of basic prevention measures, using social sciences. Only then will social justice be manifested in public policies.

Acknowledgements
We thank Stephane Cullati for his contribution to the review of the paper throughout its development and Lucia Brugnara.

Funding information
The authors received no funding for this publication.

Author Contributions
CP conceived the topic. CP and LD co-developed and co-led the case-study. CP and LD conducted the preliminary analyses. CP drafted and wrote the original manuscript, and MV finalized the manuscript. MV and CP critically revised the manuscript until the approval of the final version of the paper.

Conflict of Interest
The authors declare no competing interests.

Consent for the reproduction of Figure 1 was granted by the Service Droits Santé publique France.

Abbreviations

BESSI Behavioural, Environmental, Social and Systems Interventions

COCONEL COronavirus et CONfinement : Enquête Longitudinale

ECDC European Center for Disease Prevention and Control

EHPAD Établissement d'Hébergement pour Personnes Âgées Dépendantes

FAP Fédération des Acteurs de la Prévention

References

Bajos et al. (2021). *Les inégalités sociales au temps du COVID-19.* Institut pour la Recherche en Santé Publique. Retrieved from https://www.iresp.net/wp-content/uploads/2020/10/IReSP_QSP40.web_.pdf.

Berkhout et al. (2021). *The Inequality Virus.* Retrieved from https://www.oxfam.org/en/research/inequality-virus.

BESSI. (2021). *Behavioural, Environmental, Social and Systems.* Retrieved from BESSI: https://www.bessi-collab.net/.

Birchem, N. (2020, July). *La précarité alimentaire va s'aggraver dans les mois qui viennent.* Retrieved from La Croix l'Hebdo.

Blaize, A. (2021). *Conseil Scientifique du Covid : composition, membres, rapport.* Retrieved from Le Journal des femmes: Santé: https://sante.journaldesfemmes.fr/fiches-maladies/2641195-conseil-scientifique-coronavirus-covid-constitution-gouv-conflit-interet-membres-role-avis/.

Bo et al. (2021). Effectiveness of non-pharmaceutical interventions on COVID-19 transmission in 190 countries from 23 January to 13 April 2020. *International Journal of Infectious Diseases, 102.* doi:10.1016/j.ijid.2020.10.066.

De Miguel et al. (2021). Las variantes del virus no son el inicio de otra pandemia. *El Pais.* Retrieved from https://elpais.com/sociedad/2021-02-10/las-variantes-del-virus-no-son-el-inicio-de-otra-pandemia.html.

Deroche et al. (2020). *Rapport No199, Sénat, Session ordinaire de 2020-2021,8 décembre 2020,Rapport fait au nom de la commission d'enquête(1) pour l'évaluation des politiques publiques face aux grandes pandémies à la lumière de la crise sanitaire de la covid-19 et de sa gestion.* Retrieved from Senat http://www.senat.fr/rap/r20-199-2/r20-199-2.html.

Dubost et al. (2020). *Les inégalités sociales face à l'épidémie de Covid-19 État des lieux et perspectives.* Direction de Recherche des Etudes de l'Evaluation et des Statistiques (DREES). Retrieved from https://drees.solidarites-sante.gouv.fr/publications/les-dossiers-de-la-drees/les-inegalites-sociales-face-lepidemie-de-covid-19-etat-des.

Ferreira et al. (2020). The COVID-19 Contagion–Pandemic Dyad: A View from Social Sciences. *Societies, 10*(4). doi:10.3390/soc10040077.

Fisher et al. (2020). Assessing national performance in response to COVID-19. *The Lancet, 396*(10252). Retrieved from https://www.thelancet.com/article/S0140-6736(20)31601-9/fulltext.

Fondation Abbé Pierre. (2021). *26e rapport sur l'état du mal-logement en France 2021.* Retrieved from https://www.fondation-abbe-pierre.fr/documents/pdf/reml2021_rapport_sur_letat_du_mallogement-web.pdf.

Franck, N. (2020). *Covid-19 et détresse psychologiques: 2020, l'odyssée du confinement.* Odile Jacob. Retrieved from https://www.odilejacob.fr/catalogue/psychologie/psychiatrie/covid-19-et-detresse-psychologique_9782738153807.php.

G7a. (2021). *Joint statement of G7 Leaders | 19 February 2021.* Retrieved from G7 UK 2021: https://www.g7uk.org/joint-statement-of-g7-leaders-19-february-2021/.

G7b. (2021). *100 Days Mission to respond to future pandemics.* Retrieved from G7 UK 2021: https://assets.publishing.service.gov.uk/government/uploads/system/uploads/attachment_data/file/992762/100_Days_Mission_to_respond_to_future_pandemic_threats__3_.pdf.

Gaille et al. (2020). *Les sciences humaines et sociales face à la première vague de la pandémie de Covid-19. Enjeux et formes de la recherche.* Centre National de la Recherche Scientifique (CNRS). Retrieved from https://hal.archives-ouvertes.fr/halshs-03036192v1.

Garcia-Basteiro et al. (2020). The need for an independent evaluation of the COVID-19 response in Spain. *The Lancet, 396*. doi:10.1016/S0140-6736(20)31713-X.

Gorce, B. (2021). *Statistiques ethniques, l'impossible débat*. Retrieved from La Croix: https://www.la-croix.com/France/Statistiques-ethniques-limpossible-debat-2021-06-29-1201163962.

Goutte et al. (2020). The role of economic structural factors in determining pandemic mortality rates: Evidence from the COVID-19 outbreak in France. *Research in International Business and Finance, 54*. doi:10.1016/j.ribaf.2020.101281.

Green, S. & Cladi, L. (2020). Behavioural, environmental, social, and systems interventions against covid-19. *BMJ*(370). doi:10.1136/bmj.m2982.

Haug et al. (2020). Ranking the effectiveness of worldwide COVID-19 government interventions. *Nat Hum Behav*(4). doi:10.1038/s41562-020-01009-0.

Irwin et al. (2021). Using data to combat the ongoing crisis, and the next, in Nigeria. Retrieved from https://blogs.worldbank.org/opendata/using-data-combat-ongoing-crisis-and-next-nigeria.

Jacquot, G. (2020). *Populations vulnérables : pour le professeur Delfraissy, le décret du 29 août «tombe très mal»*. Retrieved from Public Senat: https://www.publicsenat.fr/article/parlementaire/populations-vulnerables-pour-le-professeur-delfraissy-le-decret-du-29-aout.

Khalatbari-Soltani et. al. (2020). Importance of collecting data on socioeconomic determinants from the early stage of the COVID-19 outbreak onwards. *J Epidemiol Community Health, 74*(8). doi:10.1136/jech-2020-214297.

Loubiere et al. (2021). Seroprevalence of SARS-CoV-2 antibodies among homeless people living rough, in shelters and squats: A large population-based study in France. *PLoS ONE, 16*(9). doi:10.1371/journal.pone.0255498.

Michie, S. & West, R. (2020). Behavioural, environmental, social, and systems interventions against covid-19. *BMJ* 370. doi:10.1136/bmj.m2982.

Mintzberg, H. (1979). *The Structuring of Organizations*. Retrieved from https://www.nrc.gov/docs/ML0907/ML090710600.pdf.

Muller et al. (2021). Effects of non-pharmaceutical interventions against COVID-19 on the incidence of other diseases. *The Lancet Regional Health, 6.* doi:10.1016/j.lanepe.2021.100139.

Niedzwiedz et al. (2020). Mental health and health behaviours before and during the initial phase of the COVID-19 lockdown: longitudinal analyses of the UK Household Longitudinal Study. *J Epidemiol Community Health, 75*(3). doi:10.1136/jech-2020-215060.

Ouest France. (2020). *Banques alimentaires. Claude Baland élu président de l'association.* Retrieved from Ouest France: https://www.ouest-france.fr/societe/alimentatio/banques-alimentaires-claude-baland-elu-president-de-l-association-6882465.

Phiri et al. (2021). An evaluation of the mental health impact of SARS-CoV-2 on patients, general public and healthcare professionals: A systematic review and meta-analysis. *EClinicalMedicine, 34.* doi:10.1016/j.eclinm.2021.100806.

Piot, P. & Coll Seck, A. M. (2001). International response to the HIV/AIDS epidemic: planning for success. *Policy and Practice, 79*(12). Retrieved from https://www.scielosp.org/article/bwho/2001.v79n12/1106-1112/.

Pittet et al. (2020). *Rapport d' étape: Mission indépendante nationale sur l'évaluation de la gestion de la crise Covid-19 et sur l'anticipation des risques pandémiques.* République Française.

Pittet et al. (2021). *Rapport Final: Mission indépendante nationale sur l'évaluation de la gestion de la crise Covid-19 et sur l'anticipation des risques pandémiques.* République Française.

Rehle et al. (2004). Second-generation HIV surveillance: better data for decision-making. *Bulletin of the World Health Organization*(82). Retrieved from https://www.who.int/bulletin/volumes/82/2/121.pdf.

Rey-Lefebvre, I. (2020). *L'Europe vient à point nommé financer l'aide alimentaire en France.* Retrieved from Le Monde: https://www.lemonde.fr/societe/article/2020/11/02/l-europe-vient-a-point-nomme-financer-l-aide-alimentaire-en-france_6058245_3224.html.

Santé Publique France. (2021). *CoviPrev : une enquête pour suivre l'évolution des comportements et de la santé mentale pendant l'épidémie de COVID-19.* Retrieved from Santé Publique France: https://www.santepubliquefrance.fr/etudes-et-enquetes/coviprev-une-enquete-pour-suivre-l-evolution-des-comportements-et-de-la-sante-mentale-pendant-l-epidemie-de-covid-19#block-242830.

Shah, H. (2020). Global problems need social science. *Nature, 577.* doi:10.1038/d41586-020-00064-x.

Silk, M. J., & Fefferman, N. H. (2021). The role of social structure and dynamics in the maintenance of endemic disease. *Behavioral Ecology and Sociobiology*(75), p. 122. doi:10.1007/s00265-021-03055-8.

Soullier, L. (2020). *« On ne peut pas balayer les antivaccins et les sceptiques en les réduisant au complotisme ».* Retrieved from Le Monde: https://www.lemonde.fr/politique/article/2020/11/17/antivaccins-on-ne-peut-pas-balayer-les-sceptiques-en-les-reduisant-au-complotisme_6059990_823448.html.

Swedish Ministry of Health and Social Affairs. (2020). *Mats Melin to chair COVID-19 inquiry in Sweden.* Retrieved from Government Offices of Sweden: https://www.government.se/press-releases/2020/06/mats-melin-to-chair-covid-19-inquiry-in-sweden.

Tate, A. J., & Happ, M. B. (2018). Qualitative Secondary Analysis: A Case Exemplar. *Journal of Pediatric Health Care, 32*(3). doi:10.1016/j.pedhc.2017.09.007

UNAIDS. (2010). Combination HIV Prevention: Tailoring and Coordinating Biomedical, Behavioural and Structural Strategies to Reduce New HIV Infections. Retrieved from https://files.unaids.org/en/media/unaids/contentassets/documents/unaidspublication/2010/JC2007_Combination_Prevention_paper_en.pdf.

Van Bavel et al. (2020). Using social and behavioural science to support COVID-19 pandemic response. *Nature Human Behaviour, 4.* doi:10.1038/s41562-020-0884-z.

Verbeke, E. (2021). Dépression : les grands chiffres à retenir. Retrieved from Psychologies: https://www.psychologies.com/amp/Actualites/Sante-mentale/Depression-les-grands-chiffres-a-retenir.

Warszawski et al. (2020). *Premiers résultats de l'enquête nationale EpiCov.* Direction de Recherche des Etudes de l'Evaluation et des Statistiques. Retrieved from https://drees.solidarites-sante.gouv.fr/publications/etudes-et-resultats/en-mai-2020-45-de-la-population-vivant-en-france-metropolitaine.

WHO. (2020). *1st WHO Infodemiology Conference*. Retrieved from World Health Organization: https://www.who.int/news-room/events/detail/2020/06/30/default-calendar/1st-who-infodemiology-conference.

WHO. (2020). *Guidance for conducting a country COVID-19 Intra-Action Review (IAR)*. Retrieved from World Health Organization: https://www.who.int/publications-detail-redirect/WHO-2019-nCoV-Country_IAR-2020.1.

WHO. (2021). *Critical preparedness, readiness, and response actions for COVID-19*. Retrieved from World Health Organization: https://www.who.int/publications-detail-redirect/critical-preparedness-readiness-and-response-actions-for-covid-19.

Yanez et al. (2020). COVID-19 mortality risk for older men and women. *BMC Public Health, 20*. doi:10.1186/s12889-020-09826-8.

Yang et al. (2020). Mental health services for older adults in China during the COVID-19 outbreak. *The Lancet Psychiatry, 7*(4). doi:10.1016/S2215-0366(20)30079-1.

Zhou et al. (2020). Mental Health Response to the COVID-19 Outbreak in China. *Am. J. Psychiatry, 177*(7). doi:10.1176/appi.ajp.2020.20030304.

Appendix

S1: Practical policy recommendations for the five aspects analyzed in the paper: basic measures, mental health, inequities, communication, and civil society and community involvement.

Aspect	Practical policy recommendations
Basic Measures	1. Tailor studies to improve the understanding of the basic measures according to different populations and context in-country 2. Further advance the acceptance, access (beyond the stock shortages) and use of the basic measures (i.e., masks) by various populations 3. Establish monitoring and rapid analysis of behavioral indicators for infection and NPIs to identify barriers and groups for targeted strategies 4. Establish roundtables and task forces with social scientists (i.e., anthropologists, sociologists, psychologists) for the exchange and sharing of recommendations with the Government or CNS
Mental Health	1. Include mental health in national plans, strategies, and budget from the onset of a crisis 2. Launch from the onset the monitoring of the impact of confinements on mental health 3. Evaluate the effectiveness of measures for future decision-making regarding the scale-up or design of context-dependent targeted strategies (i.e., students) or innovations (i.e., online support)
Inequities	1. Early identification of vulnerable populations and establishment of monitoring strategies taking into account social and behavioral aspects as well as the long-term effects of the implemented measures to disseminate these to associations and NGOs to inform policy 2. Context-specific tailoring of measures according to the living and basic needs arrangements of vulnerable populations (i.e., elderly homes, schools and universities, prisons, unemployed) or geographical sites (i.e., hot spots, some suburbs)
Communication	1. Development of targeted communication strategies with the support of behavioral scientists, tailored to the needs of diverse populations, particularly the most vulnerable, depending on the pandemic dynamics 2. Delivery of targeted messages to key populations by engaging social scientists through the existing official bodies 3. Monitoring of the "infodemic" through information technology and social media to overcome health misinformation, adapt strategies to the changing needs of the pandemic and disseminate them through infodemiology conferences (WHO, 2020)
Civil Society and Community Involvement	1. Civil society engagement for strengthening the PHC system and involvement of citizen associations' working with vulnerable populations to enhance social justice and access to services, including via evaluation 2. Explore as a solution the set-up of a « Comité Citoyen et de la Société Civile », or other alternative, and assess its effectiveness in involving communities and civil society in the design of local responses

S2: Practical applications of the final report propositions relating to organizational restructuring and responsibilities.

Final report structural propositions	Translation into practical applications
Proposition n° 21: In case of establishment of an independent ad-hoc council for informing decision-making during a health crisis, ensure that it integrates at least: - Representatives of the various disciplines (health, economy, social sciences) - Representatives of existing expert bodies and agencies	Amend the composition of the Haut Conseil Scientifique to include at least 1/3 social scientists, and 1/3 economists, to complement the existing bio-medical lead, with the aim to inform in real-time the government for policy-making in social aspects (rather than retrospectively through a laborious and tardive evaluation, or not at all).
Proposition n° 13: Structuring the research teams of the INSERM and the new ANRS-emerging infectious diseases under one priority program.	Development, in collaboration with the Secrétariat Général de la Défense et de la Sécurité Nationale (SGDSN), of a costed preparedness plan for the activities of the Conseil, public agencies (INSERM, new ANRS), universities, foundations, CSOs, under one priority program. The funding envelope should be substantial in light of the returns/benefits and high present costs of reanimation and treatments (i.e., hospitals), and vaccinations (i.e., research and campaign).
Proposition n° 2: Develop a continued collaboration between the SGDSN and social sciences research institutions specialized in the organizational analysis of crisis management.	An in-depth assessment of the roles, challenges, and achievements of the existing structures (i.e., state actors and public sector committees, academia, CSOs) in investigating the contribution of inequities in the health crisis and addressing them, by using a sociology of organization analysis (Mintzberg, 1979), and proposing structural improvements.
Proposition n° 3: Initiate a continuous work process on human resources for crisis management between the SGDSN and each ministry to map the needs and skills, and deliver training to ensure over time the maintenance of crisis management skills.	

The first eight months of COVID-19 pandemic in three West African countries: leveraging lessons learned from responses to the 2014-2016 Ebola virus disease outbreak

Benido Impouma[1,2*], George Sie Williams[1], Fleury Moussana[1], Franck Mboussou[1], Bridget Farham[1], Caitlin M. Wolfe[1,3], Charles Okot[1], Katrina Downing[1], Claudia Codeço Tores[4], Antoine Flahault[2], Cyril Pervilhac[1], Georges Ki-Zerbo[5], Peter Clement[6], Steven Shongwe[7], Olivia Keiser[2], Ibrahima Socé Fall[8]

1 World Health Organization Regional Office for Africa, Brazzaville, Congo

2 Institute of Global Health, University of Geneva, Geneva, Switzerland

3 College of Public Health, University of South Florida, Tampa, Florida, USA

4 Fundação Oswaldo Cruz, Rio de Janeiro, Brazil

5 World Health Organization Guinea Country Office

6 World Health Organization Liberia Country Office

7 World Health Organization Sierra Leone Country Office

8 World Health Organization Headquarters, Geneva, Switzerland

*Corresponding author

Benido Impouma

impoumab@who.int

Summary

Experience gained from responding to major outbreaks may have influenced the early COVID-19 pandemic response in several countries across Africa. We retrospectively assessed whether Guinea, Liberia, and Sierra Leone, the three West African countries at the epicentre of the 2014-2016 Ebola virus disease outbreak, leveraged the lessons learned in responding to COVID-19 following the World Health Organization's declaration of a public health emergency of international concern (PHEIC). We found relatively lower incidence rates across the three countries compared to many parts of the globe. Time to case reporting and laboratory confirmation also varied, with Guinea and Liberia reporting significant delays compared to Sierra Leone. Most of the selected readiness measures were instituted before confirmation of the first case and response measures were initiated rapidly after the outbreak confirmation. We conclude that the rapid readiness and response measures instituted by the three countries can be attributed to their lessons learned from the devastating Ebola outbreak, although persistent health systems weaknesses and the unique nature of COVID-19 continue to challenge control efforts.

Introduction

The COVID-19 pandemic continues to develop across Africa since the first case was reported on the continent in Egypt in February 2020 (1)(2). As of 1 March 2021, over 3.9 million cases with 104039 deaths have been reported from all 54 countries (3). This represents a small fraction of the over 113 million cases and 2.5 million deaths reported globally (4). However, despite the unique challenges presented by the COVID-19 pandemic, African countries are experienced in responding to outbreaks of emerging and reemerging infectious diseases. The COVID-19 pandemic in many African countries comes in the context of multiple concurrent infectious disease outbreaks, for example Ebola virus disease (EVD), measles and Lassa fever (5) which require robust public health responses to mitigate the adverse impact of these events.

The major outbreak of EVD in West Africa from 2014 to 2016, during which 28652 infections and 11325 deaths were recorded, was unprecedented (6). Three countries, Liberia, Guinea, and Sierra Leone were at the epicenter of this outbreak. At the onset of this EVD outbreak, key pillars required for an effective response, such as coordination, surveillance, case management, infection prevention and control, and community engagement, were inadequate or fractured (7)(8). The inability to rapidly detect, isolate, and treat cases to break the chain of transmission was a direct derivative of these weaknesses, resulting in the large-scale transmission of EVD and the associated high mortality rates.

However, with support from the international community, these countries overcame these challenges and the EVD outbreak was ended. At the same time, the countries gained experience and built improved mechanisms for responding to infectious disease outbreaks (9)(10)(11). A key factor in improving capacity to detect and respond to outbreaks was the revitalization of the Integrated Disease Surveillance and Response (IDSR) strategy (12)(13)(14). The affected countries reported and successfully responded to several outbreaks of other infectious diseases in the aftermath of EVD (15)(16)(17). In addition, joint assessments of the countries' post-EVD capacities to prevent, detect, and respond to public health risks using a multisectoral approach have shown improvements compared to the pre-EVD period, but at the same time have highlighted that health system challenges remain (18)(19)(20).

Although EVD and COVID-19 differ in their mode of transmission and pathogenesis, many facets of preparedness and response for outbreaks of these two diseases overlap, and therefore key lessons learned from the response to EVD outbreak are applicable to the response to COVID-19 (21). An effective response to COVID-19 also requires the capacity for robust surveillance, rapid case detection, disease confirmation, isolation of suspected and confirmed cases, treatment for moderate and severe cases, and a range of other public health measures to limit or prevent onward transmission.

In this study, we assessed whether the capacities and experience gained after the EVD outbreak in the three affected countries have had an impact on the response to COVID-19. In particular, we analysed the timeliness of case reporting and laboratory confirmation, and how readiness and public health response measures have affected the incidence of COVID-19 during the first eight months of the pandemic. The findings from these analyses offer valuable lessons on the relevance of sustainably building capacities and strengthening health systems to meet the challenges posed by emerging disease outbreaks.

Methods

Study design and setting

We conducted a retrospective observational cross-sectional study to determine if the COVID-19 readiness and response measures implemented in Guinea, Liberia, and Sierra Leone, spanning the period 1 February to 30 September 2020, were derived from the health system strengthening measures put in place as a result of lessons learned from the response to EVD outbreaks. We identified and assessed predictors for timely reporting and laboratory confirmation of cases. All three countries are located in West Africa and together have an estimated population of over 26 million (22).

Key readiness capacities and response measures

We selected seven key readiness capacities covering core thematic areas based on lessons learned from the response to the EVD outbreak as well as World Health Organization (WHO) recommendations to countries. An additional seven response measures implemented by the respective countries were also identified. Table 1 outlines these capacities and measures, their relevance or rationale, and the definitions of their key milestone dates. The time to each milestone for readiness capacities was based on the duration (days) from WHO declaration of COVID-19 as a public health emergency of international concern (PHEIC) to the earliest date on which the readiness capacity was achieved or the measure instituted. For the response measures, the time to each milestone measured the duration in days from confirmation of the first COVID-19 case in the respective countries to the earliest date on which response measures were implemented.

Data sources and measurements

Key milestone dates were obtained from official reports and assessments shared by the respective countries with the WHO Regional Office for Africa (AFRO). In instances where the milestone date was missing, we extracted this information from the official government websites of the respective countries. All milestone dates were cross-checked with the official authorities of the respective countries. The population estimates for the respective countries were obtained from the World Bank database (22).

A line list of confirmed COVID-19 cases reported during the studied period was obtained from each country. We consolidated the line lists from all three countries and selected key variables for our analysis on the timeliness of case reporting and laboratory confirmation. The variables selected were country, date of report, age, sex, date of onset, date of confirmation, place of case detection, and outcome (alive or dead). The date of report refers to the earliest date on which a person was notified to the health authorities as being suspected of having COVID-19. The date of onset refers to the earliest known date on which the case was reported to have begun experiencing signs and symptoms associated with COVID-19. The date of confirmation refers to the date on which the earliest laboratory results were released confirming the diagnosis of COVID-19 in each case. We defined the reporting timeliness as the time interval in days from onset of symptoms to case report, while the laboratory confirmation timeliness was defined as the duration from onset of symptoms to laboratory confirmation.

Only confirmed cases were included in our analysis on time to report and confirmation. A confirmed case of COVID-19 was defined as "a person with a positive Nucleic Acid Amplification Test (NAAT) or a person with a positive SARS-CoV-2 Antigen-rapid diagnostic test (Ag-RDT) *and* meeting either the probable case definition or suspected criteria as per the WHO guideline, or an asymptomatic person with a positive SARS-CoV-2 Ag-RDT *and* who was a contact of a probable or confirmed case" (23). We excluded asymptomatic cases, that is, confirmed cases who were reported as not experiencing any sign or symptoms despite being confirmed positive for COVID-19. This was intended to reduce bias because estimating timely reporting among

48

asymptomatic cases may be more complex, without access to data on their likely dates of exposure to their source case and when that case became infectious.

Missing data

Three (0.1%) values were missing for time to report due to missing dates of report, while 133 (3.2%) were missing for time to confirmation due to missing date of confirmation. We performed multiple imputations for the missing data using the Multivariate Imputation by Chained Equations (MICE) package in R (24). We performed five iterations using the country, age, sex, outcome, and place of detection to impute the missing data.

Data analysis

We plotted a timeline of the key readiness and response milestone dates for the respective countries to show when these capacities or measures were first attained or implemented. Using 30 January 2020 as the date of the WHO declaration of PHEIC, we computed the duration in days to each milestone date for readiness. The number of days to each response measure milestone date was the duration from the first confirmed case in the respective countries. We computed the average number of days to each milestone across all three countries.

We also present key COVID-19 epidemiological parameters such as the number of cases and deaths, the case fatality ratio (CFR), which was defined as the proportion of deaths among all confirmed cases, the cumulative incidence per 100000 population, and the mortality rates per one million population in the respective countries. We analysed the burden of infection among health workers, which was calculated as the proportion of health worker cases among the total health workforce in the respective countries. Data on testing are presented as the cumulative number of tests performed per 10000 population.

We computed the median number of days for case reporting and laboratory confirmation for symptomatic cases in the respective countries. The effect of selected covariates on the timeliness of reporting and confirmation were quantified by using two separate multivariable negative binomial regression models. The selected covariates were country, age group, sex, and place of detection. Our initial choice of these covariates was based on trends observed in the surveillance reports, a priori knowledge, literature available on this topic, and the extent to which data were available. Based on the age-associated mortality observed in the surveillance data, we categorized the cases into two age groups, <50 years and ≥50 years. Given the urban nature of the pandemic and the likelihood of access to health services to be skewed towards the capital cities in these countries, we also categorized the place of detection into two groups, those detected in the capital cities and those detected outside the capital cities. The results are presented as an incidence rate ratio (IRR) with a 95% confidence interval (CI). IRR greater than 1 indicates a longer time to detection or confirmation, while less than 1 indicates a shorter time.

Results

The timeline of key milestones for readiness capacities and response measures are presented in Figure 1. The adoption and finalization of a COVID-19 national strategic preparedness and response plan was the earliest readiness measure achieved across the three countries, taking an average of five days (range 3 days in Liberia to 7 days in Sierra Leone) (Table 2). The screening of all travellers at the respective international airports and the launch of a mass public communication campaign were the last readiness measures implemented, taking an average of 37 days each. It took an average of 29 days for the countries to obtain capacity for performing COVID-19 laboratory testing (range 25 days in Sierra Leone to 35 days in Liberia). Table 2 further shows that the activation of a national incidence management system was the earliest public health response measure implemented, which predated the confirmation of the first case by 15 days on average (range 47 days before the first case in Sierra Leone to 2 days after the first case in Guinea). Results for the timeliness of various readiness and response measures in the respective countries are further shown in table 2.

A total of 14227 cases with 220 deaths (CFR 1.5%) was reported from the three countries during the studied period. Guinea was the most affected with the highest case numbers (n=10652) and highest cumulative incidence of 82 per 100000 population (Table 3). Guinea also reported the highest number of health worker cases (n=513), accounting for an estimated 5.0% of infection among the total health workforce in the country. Liberia reported the highest numbers of deaths (n=82), case fatality ratio (6.1%), and mortality of 16 per million population. Other epidemiological results for the respective countries are shown in table 3.

Of 2406 symptomatic cases included in the study, the overall median reporting time was three days [IQR (1 - 6)] while the laboratory confirmation time was five days [IQR (2 - 8)]. When stratified by the respective countries, Liberia had the longest median reporting time of five days, while Sierra Leone had the shortest median reporting time of one day. The median laboratory confirmation time was also shortest in Sierra Leone (Table 4). Results of the negative binomial regression model showed that country (Liberia and Guinea) and age group (≥50years) predictors were significantly (p<0.001) associated with longer reporting and confirmation times compared to Sierra Leone and those below 50 years old respectively. The place of detection (outside a capital city) was found to be significantly associated with shorter reporting time compared to those within a capital city, although with no influence on the laboratory confirmation time. Table 4 further shows that sex had no influence on the reporting or laboratory confirmation timeliness.

Discussion

Our results show that all selected readiness measures were instituted across the three countries within the first two months of declaration of the PHEIC by WHO. We also found very early response measures implemented across the three countries, with at least one response measure predating the confirmation of the first case. While the incidence of COVID-19 remained relatively low compared to most affected countries globally, our study showed a high case fatality ratio, particularly in Liberia and Sierra Leone. Other findings pointed to a high burden of infection among health workers and definite low testing rates compared to many countries globally. The overall median time of three days to report and five days for laboratory confirmation of symptomatic cases, although with variability among the countries, indicated that this delay could potentially be a key contributor to community transmission of the disease among the local population in the respective countries, despite the response measures instituted.

The relatively rapid readiness and response measures implemented could be attributed in part to the experience gained by these countries and the international community from the devastating EVD outbreak of 2014 – 2016 (25). It took several months for these countries and the international community to recognize the potential threat and scale of the EVD outbreak, thereby delaying the institution of cogent control measures at national level, as well as slow mobilization of international assistance (26). Exposure to a previous major epidemic is associated with faster response, an indication that these countries have learned to move into action early (27). Investments made in strengthening IDSR including laboratory capacities helped these countries to quickly adapt their structures in readiness and response to COVID-19. For example, of the four indicators for real-time surveillance assessed during the joint external evaluation on a scale of 1 to 5 (1 being no capacity and 5 being sustainable capacity), Liberia and Sierra Leone scored 4 (demonstrated capacity) and Guinea scored 3 (developed capacity) on three of the indicators (18)(19)(20). National laboratory systems were also found to improve with specimen referral systems scoring 3 (developed capacity) across all three countries and testing capacity for priority diseases scoring 4 (demonstrated capacity) in Sierra Leone, 3 (developed capacity) in Guinea, and 2 (limited capacity) in Liberia although capacities in Liberia improved in the aftermath of the evaluation. These existing capacities were leveraged in response to the COVID-19 pandemic, however, the fact that all three countries scored 2 (limited capacity) for an interoperable, interconnected, electronic real-time reporting system as well as 2 (limited capacity) for an effective modern point-of-care and laboratory-based diagnostic indicated major weaknesses in these areas and the need for additional investments or support to effectively respond to a pandemic such as COVID-19. Additionally, the rapid support from WHO and other partner institutions to African countries including Guinea, Liberia, and Sierra Leone helped bolster readiness capacities for COVID-19 in key areas, such as in the provision of laboratory reagents and other supplies, technical guidance, training, etc (28)(29).

In spite of the rapidity with which measures were taken, it is clear that health systems in these countries remain fragile and underfunded, (30) and these constraints can crucially affect health outcomes in a pandemic of this nature. The high case fatality ratio in Liberia (6.1%) and Sierra-Leone (3.2%) versus 0.6% in Guinea and the high proportion of health worker infections in Liberia (2%), Sierra Leone (3.5%), and Guinea (5%) in the early period of the pandemic could in part be attributed to the fragility of the health systems in these countries. In Liberia and Sierra Leone, the implementation of a policy to test all dead bodies for COVID-19 to improve detection, case investigation, and contact tracing resulted in the identification of a high number of COVID-19 community deaths, indicating limited use of, access to, and quality of health care services in these countries. The relatively lower testing rates across these three countries with an average cumulative test of 71 tests per 10,000 population (45 tests per 10,000 population in Liberia, 52 tests per 10,000 population in Sierra Leone, and 93 tests per 10,000 population in Guinea) compared to wealthy countries such as Denmark (6,741 tests per 10,000 population), United States of America (3,595 tests per 10,000 population), and the United Kingdom (3,310 tests per 10,000 population)*(https://ourworldindata.org/grapher/full-list-cumulative-total-tests-per-thousand-map?time=2020-09-30)* could also be viewed in the context of resource constraints in low-and-middle-income countries to offer mass-based testing to a larger percent of their population.

The reporting and confirmation timeliness were significantly longer in Guinea and Liberia compared to Sierra Leone. While asymptomatic COVID-19 cases may hold similar transmission potential as symptomatic cases (31), the delay in detection (reporting and confirmation) of cases after the onset of symptoms particularly in the early phase of the pandemic in these countries is an incontestable contributor to the transmission dynamics of the disease among the population. Kieran *et al.* found that the viral load of SARS-CoV-2 is highest at or around symptom onset (32). A systematic review and meta-analysis involving 79 studies also showed that people are likely to be highly infectious with the SARS-CoV-2 virus in the first week after the onset of symptoms (33). These findings mean that delay in the initiation of intervention measures (such as isolation and contact tracing) as a result of the delay in reporting and confirming cases would provide ample time for symptomatic cases to continue transmitting the infection.

Delays in reporting and confirmation among cases ≥50 years may have led to delay in initiation of treatment, one of several factors which could have resulted in the high case fatality ratio in this age group. This finding is consistent with several studies that have shown that people in older age group are at higher risk of complications and deaths from COVID-19, especially when life-saving interventions are delayed (34). Also, we found it interesting to note that COVID-19 cases were reported earlier among people outside the capital cities compared to those living within the capital cities. Disease surveillance systems are likely to be quickly overwhelmed in high-density population areas as the rate of transmission increases (35). This could be a result of high population densities in the capital cities of the various countries making surveillance of COVID-19 more challenging. Intense transmission of EVD in the capital cities of the three countries complicated response efforts in the 2014-2016 outbreak (36).

There are a few limitations to our study. First, although we showed how early these readiness and response measures were implemented, we did not assess the efficiency of their implementation. The early implementation of the restriction measures may have resulted in fatigue among the population, who probably also suffered adverse socio-economic effects. Hence, strict adherence to measures such as wearing a face mask would likely wane over time, potentially resulting in resurgence of cases. Second, most COVID-19 cases are asymptomatic; therefore, the analysis of symptomatic cases may not provide a full picture of the speed with which cases are reported and confirmed in the countries. However, given that mass population-based testing had not been implemented and that most asymptomatic cases were only identified after testing contacts of symptomatic cases, analysis of how rapidly symptomatic cases were identified can provide an estimation of the timeliness of case detection. Third, the statistical power, though not effect, of our analysis, may have been lowered due to omissions or recording errors in onset dates in the line list, leading to the exclusion of potential symptomatic cases. Lastly, we did not account for the effect of contact tracing on reporting and confirmation timeliness because such data were not available. High levels of contacts tracing are more likely to lead to early reporting and confirmation due to the regular monitoring (37).

Despite these limitations, our study has shown that these countries took actions early in the form of readiness and response to avert the negative consequences that they had experienced during the Ebola outbreak of 2014 to 2016. Using lessons learned from the EVD outbreak as well as capacities gained in its aftermath, the countries were able to take key readiness and response measures early which may have contributed to the low incidence of COVID-19 in these countries, despite the unique challenges posed by COVID-19 given the role of asymptomatic transmission in the context of low level of COVID-19 testing. Strong technical and operational support from WHO and partners has also helped these countries to continue to respond to the pandemic. However, eventual control of the pandemic will require continued implementation of public health measures, along with vaccination campaigns. It would be interesting for future studies to consider assessing the effectiveness of the various response measures implemented and their impact on the COVID-19 pandemic in these countries.

Acknowledgements

We wish to thank all those who contributed to this study. We are particularly grateful to Kwaukuan Yealue of WHO Liberia Country Office, Robert Musoke of WHO Sierra Leone Country Office, and Mamadou Balde of WHO Guinea Country Office for validating the data on COVID-19 response and readiness milestone dates for the respective countries.

References

1. **Medhat MA, Kassas M El**. COVID-19 in Egypt: Uncovered figures or a different situation? *Journal of Global Health*. 2020; 10: 010368. doi: 10.7189/jogh.10.010368

2. **Rice BL, Annapragada A, Baker RE**, *et al*. Variation in SARS-CoV-2 outbreaks across sub-Saharan Africa. *Nature Medicine* 2021; https://doi.org/10.1038/s41591-021-01234-8

3. **Africa CDC**. Coronavirus Disease 2019 (COVID-19) – Africa CDC. Africa CDC Dashboard. 2020. https://africacdc.org/covid-19/ (accessed 5 March 2021)

4. **World Health organization.** WHO Coronavirus Disease (COVID-19) Dashboard | https://covid19.who.int (accessed 5 March 2021)

5. **WHO Regional Office for Africa**. Weekly Bulletin on Outbreaks and Emergencies. 2020;(August):1–20. https://apps.who.int/iris/bitstream/handle/10665/331023/OEW07-1016022020.pdf (accessed 5 March 2021)

6. **Centers for Disease Control and Prevention.** 2014-2016 Ebola Outbreak in West Africa | https://www.cdc.gov/vhf/ebola/history/2014-2016-outbreak/index.html (accessed 5 March 2021)

7. **Coltart CEM, Lindsey B, Ghinai I,** *et al*. The Ebola outbreak, 2013–2016: Old lessons for new epidemics. *Philosophical Transactions Royal Society B Biological Science*. 2017; 372: 2013–2016. doi: 10.1098/rstb.2016.0297

8. **McNamara LA, Schafer IJ, Nolen LD**, et al. Ebola Surveillance — Guinea, Liberia, and Sierra Leone. *MMWR Supplement* 2016; 65(Suppl-3):

35–43. DOI: http://dx.doi.org/10.15585/mmwr.su6503a6external icon

9. **Vetter P, Dayer JA, Schibler M, Allegranzi B**, *et al.* The 2014-2015 Ebola outbreak in West Africa: Hands On. *Antimicrobial Resistance and Infection Control.* 2016; 5:1–17. http://dx.doi.org/10.1186/s13756-016-0112-9

10. **Mobula LM, Nakao JH, Walia S**, *et al.* A humanitarian response to the West African Ebola virus disease outbreak. *Journal of International Humanitarian Action* 2018; 3. https://doi.org/10.1186/s41018-018-0039-2

11. **Marston BJ, Dokubo EK, Steelandt A Van**, *et al.* Ebola Response Impact on Public Health Programs. *Emerging Infectious Diseases.* 2017; 23: S25-S32. 10.3201/eid2313.170727

12. **Nagbe T, Naiene JD, Rude JM**, *et al.* The implementation of integrated disease surveillance and response in Liberia after Ebola virus disease outbreak 2015-2017. *Pan African Medical Journal.* 2019; 33: 3. doi: 10.11604/pamj.supp.2019.33.2.16820

13. **Njuguna C, Jambai A, Chimbaru A**, *et al.* Revitalization of integrated disease surveillance and response in Sierra Leone post Ebola virus disease outbreak. *BMC Public Health.* 2019; 19: 364. https://doi.org/10.1186/s12889-019-6636-1

14. **Hemingway-Foday J, Souare O, Reynolds E**, *et al.* Improving Integrated Disease Surveillance and Response Capacity in Guinea, 2015-2018. *Online Journal of Public Health Informatics.* 2019; 11: e364 doi: 10.5210/ojphi.v11i1.9837

15. **Rude JM, Kortimai L, Mosoka F**, *et al.* Rapid response to meningococcal disease cluster in Foya district, Lofa County, Liberia January to February 2018. *Pan African Medical Journal.* 2019; 33: 6. doi: 10.11604/pamj.supp.2019.33.2.17095

16. **Suk JE, Jimenez AP, Kourouma M,** *et al.* Post-ebola measles outbreak in lola, Guinea, January-June 2015. *Emerging Infectious Diseases.* 2016; 22: 1106–1108. doi: 10.3201/eid2206.151652

17. **World Health** Organization. Measles outbreak confirmed in northern Sierra Leone _ WHO _ Regional Office for Africa. https://www.afro.who.int/news/measles-outbreak-confirmed-northern-sierra-leone (accessed 5 March 2021)

56

18. **World Health Organization**. Évaluation externe conjointe des principales capacités RSI de la République de Guinée. 2017; 23–8. https://apps.who.int/iris/handle/10665/258726 (Accessed 5 March 2021)

19. **World Health Organization**. Joint External Evaluation of IHR Core Capacities of the Republic of Liberia. Mission report. September 2016 https://apps.who.int/iris/bitstream/handle/10665/255268/WHO-WHE-CPI-2017.23-eng.pdf?sequence=1&isAllowed=y (Accessed 5 March 2021)

20. **World Health Organization**. Joint External Evaluation of IHR Core Capacities of the Republic of Sierra Leone. November 2017. https://apps.who.int/iris/bitstream/handle/10665/254790/WHO-WHE-CPI-2017.16-eng.pdf?sequence=1 (Accessed 5 March 2021)

21. **Mobula LM, Samaha H, Yao M,** *et al.* Recommendations for the COVID-19 response at the national level based on lessons learned from the Ebola Virus disease outbreak in the Democratic Republic of the Congo. *American Journal of Tropical Medicine and Hygiene*. 2020; 103: 12–17. doi: 10.4269/ajtmh.20-0256

22. **The World Bank**. Population estimates and projections | DataBank. The World Bank Data Bank. 2020. https://databank.worldbank.org/source/population-estimates-and-projections# (accessed 5 March 2021)

23. **World Health Organization.** Public Health Surveillance for COVID-19, WHO Interim Guidance. 1 August 2020. https://apps.who.int/iris/handle/10665/333752 (accessed 5 March 2021)

24. **van Buuren S, Groothuis-Oudshoorn K**. mice: Multivariate imputation by chained equations in R. *Journal of Statistical Software*. 2011; 45: 1–67. DOI: 10.18637/jss.v045.i03

25. **Maxmen A**. Ebola prepared these countries for coronavirus – but now even they are floundering. *Nature*. 2020; 583: 667–668. doi: 10.1038/d41586-020-02173-z.

26. **Moon S, Sridhar D, Pate MA,** *et al.* Will Ebola change the game? Ten essential reforms before the next pandemic. the report of the Harvard-LSHTM Independent Panel on the Global Response to Ebola. *Lancet*. 2015; 386: 2204–2221. http://dx.doi.org/10.1016/S0140-6736(15)00946-0

27. **Tsuei SH-T**. How previous epidemics enable timelier COVID-19 responses: an empirical study using organisational memory theory. *BMJ Global Health.* 2020; 5: e003228. doi: 10.1136/bmjgh-2020-003228

28. **World Health** Organization. COVID-19 in Africa: marking six months of response | WHO | Regional Office for Africa. https://www.afro.who.int/covid-19-africa-marking-six-months-response (accessed 5 March 2021)

29. **World Bank**. World Bank's Response to COVID-19 (Coronavirus) in Africa. Factsheet. 2020. https://www.worldbank.org/en/news/factsheet/2020/06/02/world-banks-response-to-covid-19-coronavirus-in-africa (accessed 5 March 2021)

30. **World Bank**. Health Nutrition and Population Statistics | DataBank. World Bank. 2020. https://databank.worldbank.org/source/health-nutrition-and-population-statistics# (accessed 5 March 2021)

31. **Ra SH, Lim JS, Kim G,** *et al.* Upper respiratory viral load in asymptomatic individuals and mildly symptomatic patients with SARS-CoV-2 infection. *Thorax.* 2020;. 76: 61-63 doi: 10.1136/thoraxjnl-2020-215042

32. **K. A Walsh, K. Jordan, B. Clyne,** *et al.* SARS-CoV-2 detection, viral load and infectivity over the course of an infection. *Journal of Infection* 2020; 81: 357-371. doi: 10.1016/j.jinf.2020.06.067

33. **Cevik M, Tate M, Lloyd O,** *et al.* SARS-CoV-2, SARS-CoV-1 and MERS-CoV Viral Load Dynamics, Duration of Viral Shedding and Infectiousness: A Living Systematic Review and Meta-Analysis. *SSRN Electronic Journal.* 2020; 5247: 1–10. http://dx.doi.org/10.1016/S2666-5247(20)30172-5

34. **Starke KR, Pretereit-Haack G, Schubert M**, *et al.* The age-related risk of severe outcomes due to covid-19 infection: A rapid review, meta-analysis, and meta-regression. *International Journal of Environmental Research and Public Health.* 2020; 17: 1–24. doi: 10.3390/ijerph17165974

35. **Lee VJ, Ho M, Kai CW,** *et al.* Epidemic preparedness in urban settings: new challenges and opportunities. *Lancet Infectious Diseases.* 2020; 20: 527–529. http://dx.doi.org/10.1016/S1473-3099(20)30249-8

36. **Campbell L, Adan C, Morgado M**. Ebola Response in cities: responding in the context of quarantine.

https://reliefweb.int/sites/reliefweb.int/files/resources/alnap-urban-2017-ebola-response-in-cities-learning-for-future-public-health-crises.pdf (accessed 5 March 2021)

37. **Keeling MJ, Hollingsworth TD, Read JM**. Efficacy of contact tracing for the containment of the 2019 novel coronavirus (COVID-19). *Journal of Epidemiology and Community Health*. 2020; 74: 861–866. doi:10.1136/jech-2020-214051

Table 1: Selected COVID-19 readiness capacities and response measures, their rational, and definition of key milestone date on which capacities were attained on response measures first implemented

Category	Capacities/measures	Relevance/rationale	Definition of milestone date
	National strategic preparedness and response plan	A strategic preparedness and response plan (SPRP) outlines the public health measures that a country stands ready to implement to prepare for and respond to outbreaks. For a novel disease outbreak, an SPRP is crucial to guide policymakers and public health responders in critical decision-making processes.	Earliest date on which SPRP was finalized and adopted
	Surveillance capacity at health facility level	The ability of health workers to use case definitions to diagnose and report suspected cases of COVID-19 for early case detection.	Earliest date on which 90% of health facilities were covered with staff trained to detect and report suspected cases of COVID-19
	Diagnostic capacity at national level	The ability of the country to test and confirm a case of COVID-19 which is essential to trigger early response actions	Earliest date on which country gained capacity for conducting RT-PCR test for COVID-19
	Capacity for screening at points-of-entry	Useful for early detection of cases given the threat posed by importation of confirmed cases from other parts of the world. The international airports were considered as the place of greatest risk of importation during the early phase of the pandemic.	Earliest date on which screening of travellers began at the international airports
	Capacity for rapid response	A multi-disciplinary team is needed in the early phase of an epidemic for rapid investigation of alerts, quarantine or isolation of cases in order to find cases timely and implement quick public health measures to prevent mortality or interrupt transmission.	Earliest date on which trained national rapid response team was operationalized
Readiness	Capacity for case management	Prompt and optimal care necessary for preventing or reducing mortality.	Earliest date on which a functional treatment unit was made operational for the management of COVID-19 cases

60

	Capacity for risk communication and community engagements	Communicating the risk of the disease early, promoting preventive measures, engaging with the population through influencers to enhance preventive measures and respond early to rumors and misbeliefs	Earliest date on which the country initiated mass communication of COVID-19 messaging
	Activation of incidence management system	Critical to improve communication and information flow as well as to coordinate the public health response	Earliest date on which incidence management system was activated
	Suspension of commercial flights	Implemented to reduce the risk of international importation of cases while the countries study the situation and prepared better to manage international travelers	Earliest date on which international airport was closed
	Closure of schools	Implemented to reduce the risk of COVID-19 transmission among students	Earliest date on which all schools were closed
	Restriction on internal movements	Implemented to reduce the risk of spread of COVID-19 between different parts of the country	Earliest date on which restriction on internal movement started
	Restriction on mass gatherings	Implemented to reduce the risk of transmission of COVID-19 among people in mass gatherings such as concerts, sporting events, religious places, funerals, etc.	Earliest date on which restrictions were implemented
	Mandatory wearing of face mask in public	Implemented to reduce the risk of human-to-human transmission of COVID-19	Earliest date on which wearing of face mask in public became mandatory
Response	Mandatory testing of travellers	Implemented after the resumption of commercial flights to prevent the importation of COVID-19 while also preventing international spread from these countries	Earliest date on which mandatory testing of travelers commenced

61

Table 2: *Duration to attainment or implementation of selected COVID-19 readiness capacities and response measures in Guinea, Liberia, and Sierra Leone, 1 February – 30 September 2020*

Categories	Measures/capacities	Number of days to measures			
		Guinea	Liberia	Sierra Leone	Mean
Readiness measures reference date: 30 January 2020	National preparedness and response plan finalized and adopted	4	3	7	5
	90% of health facilities with staff trained in COVID-19 surveillance	N/A	21	27	-
	Testing capacity available (RT-PCR)	27	35	25	29
	Screening of travellers commenced at international airports	37	22	51	37
	National rapid response team activated	N/A	6	39	-
	Functional treatment unit ready for case management	14	25	53	31
	Mass public communication campaign commenced	31	31	50	37
Response measures reference dates Liberia: 16 March 2020; Guinea: 13 March 2020; Sierra Leone: 31 March 2020	National incidence management system activated	2	1	-47	-15
	Suspension of all commercial flights	8	32	-9	10
	School closure	14	5	0	6
	Restrictions on internal movements commenced	8	23	5	12
	Mandatory wearing of face mask commenced	36	42	22	33
	Mandatory testing of all travellers commenced	22	129	174	88
	Restrictions on mass gatherings commenced	14	25	-15	8

N/A means the date on which the milestone was first achieved was not available or could not be determined to compute the number of days to achievement after the declaration of PHEIC by WHO.

Table 3: *Key epidemiological features of COVID-19 in Guinea, Liberia, and Sierra Leone, 1 February – 30 September 2020*

Category	Variable	Guinea	Liberia	Sierra Leone	Total
Population	[a]Estimated population	13,133,000	5,058,000	7,977,000	26,168,000
	Cases	10,652	1,344	2,231	14,227
	Cumulative incidence per 100,000 pop	82	27	28	54
Cases	Health worker cases	513	214	230	957
	Cases among total health workers (%)	5.0	2.0	3.5	3.5
	Deaths	66	82	72	220
Deaths	CFR (%)	0.6	6.1	3.2	1.5
	Deaths per million population	5	16	9	0.8
	[b]Number of RT-PCR tests	121487	22499	41128	185114
Tests	Test per 10,000 population	93	45	52	71
	[c] Positivity rate (%)	8.8	6.0	5.4	7.7

[a]Population estimates for 2020 sourced from World Bank data; [b]number of tests based on number of persons tested; [c]positivity rate is the proportion of all COVID-19 RT-PCR that tested positive for SARS-CoV-2 infection.

63

Table 4: *Results of negative binomial regression model for reporting and confirmation timeliness of symptomatic COVID-19 cases in Guinea, Liberia, and Sierra Leone, 1 February to 30 September 2020*

Variables	Modalities	Symptomatic cases (n)	Time to report			Time to laboratory confirmation		
			Median (IQR)	[3]IRR (95% CI)	P-value	Median (IQR)	IRR (95% CI)	P-value
	Total	2406	3 (1-6)			5 (2-8)		
Country	Sierra Leone	451	1 (0-4)	Reference		3 (2-6)	Reference	
	Liberia	309	5 (2-8)	1.81 (1.56, 2.09)	<0.001	5 (3-8)	1.42 (1.28, 1.58)	<0.001
	Guinea	1646	3 (1-5)	1.16 (1.03, 1.30)	0.003	5 (3-8)	1.43 (1.31, 1.55)	<0.001
Age group	<50 years	1720	2 (1-5)	Reference		5 (2-8)	Reference	
	≥50 years	686	3 (1-6)	1.16 (1.06, 1.27)	<0.001	5 (3-9)	1.11 (1.05, 1.19)	<0.0001
Sex	Females	838	2 (1-5)	Reference		5 (2-7)	Reference	
	Males	1568	3 (1-6)	1.09 (1.00, 1.18)	0.05	5 (2-8)	1.05 (0.98, 1.12)	0.23
Place of detection	Capital city	1771	3 (1-6)	Reference		5 (3-8)	Reference	
	Outside capital city	635	1 (0-4)	0.68 (0.62, 0.76)	<0.001	4 (2-7)	0.96 (0.89, 1.03)	0.53

3IRR, incidence rate ratio

Monitoring and Evaluation of COVID-19 response in the WHO African Region: challenges and lessons learned

Benido Impouma[1,2*], Caitlin M. Wolfe[1,3], Franck Mboussou[1], Bridget Farham[1], Tessa Saturday[1], Cyril Pervilhac[1], Nsarhaza Bishikwabo[1], Tamayi Mlanda[1], Fleury Moussana[1], Etienne Minkoulou[1], Richard Mihigo[1], Ambrose Talisuna[1], Humphrey Karamagi[1], Olivia Keiser[2], Antoine Flahault[2], Joseph Cabore [1], Matshidiso Moeti[1]

1. World Health Organization, Regional Office for Africa, Brazzaville, Congo

2. Institute of Global Health, University of Geneva, Geneva, Switzerland

3. College of Public Health, University of South Florida, Tampa, Florida, USA

Keywords: COVID-19; monitoring and evaluation; African region; health emergencies

Corresponding author:

impoumab@who.int

Summary

Monitoring and evaluation (M&E) is an essential component of public health emergency response. In the WHO African region (WHO AFRO), over 100 events are detected and responded to annually. Here we discuss the development of the M&E for COVID-19 that established a set of regional and country indicators for tracking the COVID-19 pandemic and response measures. An interdisciplinary task force used the 11 pillars of strategic preparedness and response to define a set of inputs, outputs, outcomes and impact indicators that were used to closely monitor and evaluate progress in the evolving COVID-19 response, with each pillar tailored to specific country needs. M&E data was submitted electronically and informed country profiles, detailed epidemiological reports, and situation reports. Further, 10 selected key performance indicators (KPIs) were tracked to monitor country progress through a bi-weekly progress scoring tool used to identify priority countries in need of additional support from WHO AFRO. Investment in M&E of health emergencies should be an integral part of efforts to strengthen national, regional and global capacities for early detection and response to threats to public health security. The development of an adaptable M&E framework for health emergencies must draw from the lessons learned throughout the COVID-19 response.

Recurring disease outbreaks characterize the 47 countries of the World Health Organization (WHO) African region, along with other public health events that threaten national and regional health security. Over 100 events are detected and responded to annually [1], with more than 348 detected across the region from 2017-2019. Preparedness and response to these events is guided by a set of standard protocols and procedures, which fall under the International Health Regulations (IHR) 2005 [2], informed by both the WHO Emergency Response Framework [3] and the Integrated Disease Surveillance and Response Framework (IDSR) [4]. These protocols require countries to build and maintain a set of core capacities that are essential for early detection and response to acute public health events in order to avoid interference with trade and travel, as was seen in the West African Ebola virus disease outbreak in 2014-2016, and which is now the case with the ongoing COVID-19 pandemic in the region. COVID-19 is unique in that it has affected all 47 countries of the WHO African Region simultaneously, requiring a robust multisectoral response, with the WHO Regional Office for Africa (WHO AFRO) overseeing the regional response.

Previous response to outbreaks has resulted in the development of a number of Strategic Preparedness and Response Plans (SPRP), all of which have contained a monitoring and evaluation (M&E) component, albeit often underdeveloped. WHO AFRO is responsible for providing support to all countries in their implementation of public health and social interventions in order to interrupt transmission, monitor trends and identify areas that require further support. Additionally, WHO AFRO prioritizes interventions and resource allocation across all affected countries. The scale and magnitude of the COVID-19 pandemic in the region required that the M&E component of the COVID-19 SPRP be expanded and transformed into a stand-alone Monitoring and Evaluation Framework for COVID-19 in the WHO African Region [5]. This was closely aligned with the WHO Monitoring and Evaluation Framework [6] and originated from the global 2019 COVID Strategic Preparedness and Response Plan [7], and the Strategic Response Plan for the WHO African Region [8]. The framework was structured to address different audiences from the 47 countries of the region, who all provide data, including the Ministries of Health at the centre of effective M&E processes with support from the WHO Country Offices, WHO AFRO, and international partners.

Here we discuss the processes that led to the development of this framework, its content and implementation, preliminary findings, and challenges and lessons learned. We conclude with forward-looking actions required to strengthen the M&E of COVID-19 and other public health emergencies of potential international concern.

Developing the framework required the following key steps: (i) development of the foundational SPRP for the COVID-19 pandemic; (ii) establishment of a regional multidisciplinary task force responsible for overseeing the development of the M&E framework and its implementation; (iii) development of standard operating procedures and an action plan for implementation of the framework at country level; (iv) development of an electronic information management system to support collection, analysis, interpretation and reporting on progress made in monitoring and evaluating the SPRP; and (v) the overall implementation of the plan of action of the framework. A regional multidisciplinary task force was immediately established as COVID-19 cases were confirmed in the African region, drawn from expertise within and outside WHO AFRO, including representatives from five WHO Country Offices and from each of the 11 pillars of the SPRP ([i] coordination, planning, and monitoring; [ii] risk communication and community engagement; [iii] surveillance, rapid response teams, and case investigation; [iv] points of entry; [v] laboratory services; [vi] infection prevention and control; [vii] case management; [viii] operational logistics and support; [ix] external communication; [x] research, innovation, and vaccines; and [xi] continuity of essential health services), M&E experts with previous experience working with UNAIDS, USAID, Global Fund, GIZ, the World Bank and PEPFAR, experts in strategic planning, and data scientists.

This task force used these 11 SPRP response pillars as the basis for defining a set of inputs, outputs, outcomes, and impact indicators that were used to closely monitor and evaluate progress in COVID-19 response. Each pillar was tailored to specific country needs and built on the three-pronged preparedness and response strategy,[3] (i) coordination and support, (ii) scaling up country readiness and response operations, and (iii) research and innovation. A set of country-specific and regional technical and managerial indicators were developed and critically reviewed to ensure that they provided information that informed action, at the same time creating transparency and accountability.

Criteria outlined by MEASURE Evaluation [9] were applied to crosscheck the robustness of indicators and narrow their scope, based on eight principles: i) relevance, ii) accuracy, iii) importance, iv) usefulness, v) feasibility, vi) credibility, vii) validity, and viii) distinctiveness [9]. The indicators were assessed by the multidisciplinary team on a scale of one, two, or three; three indicating the highest importance.

The selected indicators were further categorized into country-level and regional-level. Country-level indicators cover multisectoral response at the national level (49 indicators across the 11 pillars). The regional-level indicators were used as tools to aid Ministries of Health, WHO Country Offices (WCOs), and WHO Regional Offices (59 indicators across the 11 pillars). Together, these repositories provided comprehensive indicators to enable the intended users to monitor, evaluate, and understand how the COVID-19 outbreak has been managed at national and regional levels.

Given the rapid spread of COVID-19 in the region, the need for reducing the burden of data collection, and accelerating the process of decision making to adjust the needed public health and social measures (PHSM) to interrupt transmission as the pandemic evolves, a set of 31 key performance indicators (KPIs) were derived from the repositories to facilitate daily and weekly monitoring of the evolution of the pandemic at country and regional levels. These standardized KPIs were selected for reporting to WHO AFRO and aligned with the global M&E Framework in response to COVID-19 in the African Region. Further, a traffic light approach was used to assess each KPI over time, with pre-determined thresholds (S1).

Following the finalization of the framework, the M&E task force developed a detailed implementation plan. This covered the implementation of M&E activities through immediate and short-term goals (through the end of 2020), medium-term goals (first quarter 2021), longer term goals (through World Health Assembly [WHA], May 2021), and beyond (through 2021). The roll-out of this implementation plan throughout the 47 countries in the region provided guidance on the elements of M&E, the organization, monitoring, and evaluation dimensions, the prioritization of activities over time, proposed timelines, and estimated resources to support implementation of the COVID-19 M&E framework. At the country level, WHO AFRO supported the establishment and development of multisectoral task forces, along with partners, to track and coordinate response actions to ensure accountability, as the implementation of country-level M&E for COVID-19 required multisectoral support.

An electronic system was developed to track KPIs through an online portal. Initial data submission was through a standardized Microsoft Excel template, which was subsequently replaced by a web-based database build with OpenDataKit (ODK) and Enketo Smart Paper (https://enketo.org/). Data submission, as well as editing and revising submissions with new or corrected information, was at country level through the WHO Country Offices and at regional level through the response pillars. Some regional KPIs were automatically calculated using the country-level data entered, while others required manual entry by each response pillar. The data entry interval was determined by the KPI and could be daily, weekly, monthly and annual at both levels. An online interactive dashboard created with Microsoft Power BI was provided for data entry. This portal is available to the public.

Training was conducted virtually across the region, with six modules introducing the M&E Framework for COVID-19, including full question and answer sessions to solicit feedback from the country offices.

The implementation of this M&E framework provided countries with the structure required to design their own preparedness and response plans early in the COVID-19 pandemic, which were aligned to the global SPRP and thus included an M&E component. As of 8 March 2020, 33 countries had submitted detailed plans to WHO AFRO, with an estimated overall budget of USD 166.6 million, the highest from Ethiopia and lowest from Mauritius. Of the nine pillars identified as priority for the COVID-19 response, logistics required the largest budget, but only 9% of these countries (n=3) submitted plans with budgets that covered all nine pillars. These 33 countries have activated coordination mechanisms and structures to oversee their national pandemic response, including data management and progress reports through daily or weekly situation reports. Twenty-six countries have submitted daily and 15 have submitted weekly situation reports since the start of 2021, while 45 countries submitted regular situation reports through 2020, aligned with guidance provided by WHO AFRO. These, and their associated datasets, are compiled and analyzed at WHO AFRO and provide a regional overview of the pandemic.

Thirty-five countries submitted regular line lists of confirmed cases and aggregated data as of 31 January 2021. Three (Côte d'Ivoire, Sao Tome & Principe and Niger) submitted almost daily; the rest shared weekly or monthly. These line lists were used to compile 31 country profiles, develop detailed epidemiological reports for 28 countries, prepare 108 modelling reports, as well as 34 external situation reports and 14 bi-weekly progress reports on COVID-19 from 5 July to 31 December 2020.

Selected KPIs were used to monitor country progress through a bi-weekly progress scoring tool developed against 10 select KPIs. These KPIs were used to identify priority countries in need of additional support from WHO AFRO. Key indicators included the percent change in new cases over the previous two-week period, the case fatality ratio over the last 14 days, number of deaths over the last 14 days, doubling time, testing capacity, number and percentage of healthcare worker infections, recovery rates, and attack rates. Assessed on a scale of 0-2 (values were assigned using the traffic light system by pre-determined thresholds), the scores for each of the 10 select KPIs to monitor progress were tallied to provide an overall progress score. The situation was classified as improving if the overall score fell between 0-5, stable if the overall score fell between 6-10, and deteriorating if the overall score fell between 11-20. Following scoring, the 10 indicators for each country were assessed to make recommendations to WHO AFRO regarding immediate priorities. Table 1 shows the number of countries in the WHO African region by progress score for three of the selected KPIs used to monitor country progress over time.

Reviewing existing capacities in monitoring and evaluation of outbreaks and other public health emergencies in countries highlighted the challenges confronted by each of the 47 countries and WHO AFRO, not only in rapidly adapting existing strategic information systems, but most importantly in using M&E systems to routinely track the evolution of the COVID-19 pandemic. Additionally, the limited information available to be used to guide decisions on public health and social interventions became clear. While significant investments have been made over the past years in strengthening the monitoring and evaluation of programmes for HIV, TB, and malaria with the support of the Global Fund, World Bank, USAID, PEPFAR and others, the investments in M&E for managing emerging or recurrent outbreaks in the WHO African region were limited. This was clear from the absence of dedicated M&E officers within disease surveillance and response programmes. This likely contributed to the multiplicity of data reporting and requests received from countries, which overburdened WHO Country Offices and may have resulted in inconsistencies within the data that originated from different sources. Further, the massive scale of the COVID-19 pandemic and necessary response overstretched the existing limited workforce.

Despite the limited investment in the monitoring and evaluation of health emergencies, the assessment of IHR core capacities in 44 out of 47 countries, the field presence of WHO working closely with Ministries of Health and in-country partners, the adoption of IDSR, and capacity building of disease surveillance officers have resulted in countries systematically activating epidemic management committees, notifying WHO AFRO of any acute public health events, and sharing situation reports and datasets on new and ongoing public health events. These existing systems and procedures were instrumental in collecting, compiling, analyzing and sharing data on COVID-19 in the region. The use of electronic systems for evidence-based preparedness and response to COVID-19 contributed to close monitoring of the pandemic in each country and in the region [10].

These indicators were also used to report on progress made by each country and by the region in preparing for and responding to COVID-19. Using selected KPIs for bi-weekly monitoring of country progress, such as cumulative incidence, case fatality ratio (CFR), healthcare worker infections, and others, facilitated the categorization and prioritization of countries in need of immediate support from WHO AFRO and partners. For example, countries with a high percentage of healthcare worker (HCW) infections were supported in strengthening infection and prevention control. Table 1 shows select KPIs used for monitoring country progress and reports the scores for these indicators over the last four epidemiological weeks of 2020, where the number of countries with greater than 20% increase in HCW infections declined from 7 to 2 (Table 1). Further, while initial laboratory capacity presented a challenge in effectively testing for SARS-CoV-2, WHO AFRO used the country progress monitoring to identify countries that needed additional assistance in scaling up their testing capacity. By July 2020, 12 of the 47 Member States reached the target threshold of a weekly average of 10 tests conducted per 10000 people. By 21 October 2020 a total of 12351482 SARS-CoV-2 PCR tests had been performed in the region.

Routinely measuring progress made by countries in their national response to COVID-19 remains a challenge for several reasons. First, the urgency of supporting the implementation of response interventions takes precedence over the need for carrying out evaluation of response at national and regional levels. Second, the absence of comprehensive guidance and universal evaluation for COVID-19 national response has led to the proliferation of metrics used to measure progress and evaluate overall response, with less of a focus on subnational assessments. Third, the difficulties in combining public health data with data from other sectors and performing real-time analysis of multiple and often incongruent data has impeded data-driven decision-making processes at different levels.

The importance of a robust M&E framework for COVID-19 cannot be understated. When decision-making during a pandemic needs to be data-driven, M&E plays a crucial role in assessing the continued appropriateness of ongoing response measures and identifying changes that need to be made. Building on the process that led to the development of the framework for the M&E of COVID-19 and its implementation, there is an urgent need for WHO AFRO and the global health community to invest in a versatile M&E framework that can be easily and rapidly adapted to all infectious diseases with a potential for international spread. A comprehensive package of guidelines for M&E of health emergencies that build on the work and lessons learned in dealing with HIV, TB, malaria, Ebola virus disease (EVD), and now COVID-19 is critical, with context- or event-specific indicators based on the type of health emergency. The development of such a versatile M&E framework would allow for a more robust M&E process earlier on in the response to future health emergencies.

The COVID-19 pandemic has also demonstrated the importance of a truly multisectoral response, highlighting the close link between public health and economic outcomes. The lessons learned from the experience of developing and implementing the M&E framework for COVID-19 should build on what has been learned from M&E for infectious disease health emergencies such as HIV and EVD. Specifically, while an ultimate end goal may be publicly available data and information systems that combine public health data and data from other sectors, with customizability depending on location-specific needs, a more immediate working priority is the democratization of data, including the derived analytics and insights. Given the challenges of creating a combined dataset when the required data differs in origin and availability, primary datasets across sectors should be made readily and regularly available to allow for analyses that guide decision-making. Health emergencies such as COVID-19 are rapidly changing, and evidence-based decision-making requires access to up-to-date data.

Additionally, linkage of the M&E systems with research entities focused on areas spanning the multisectoral response will directly inform areas for improved communication and collaboration. A dedicated task force overseeing M&E implementation is critical, as the engagement of national authorities and partners at national and regional levels as part of an all-inclusive process is key to ensuring successful implementation of the framework. Moreover, there is a need for agreement on pandemic performance metrics and indicator selection to standardize M&E assessments across the region, along with a need to build expertise and capacity in data collection, analysis, and interpretation, as this is essential for real-time monitoring and evaluation activities. As the pandemic unfolds there is also a strong need for evaluation capacity and a continued need to document the implementation process. Lastly, investment in M&E of health emergencies should be an integral part of efforts to strengthen national, regional and global capacities for early detection and response to threats to public health security.

In conclusion, one year on from the virus's arrival in the African region [10], the COVID-19 pandemic continues to unfold, as new variants and vaccines have entered the picture, emphasizing the continuous learning opportunities available through monitoring and evaluation. While the WHO African region is adept at responding to simultaneous outbreaks and emergencies, the COVID-19 pandemic represented the first time that all Member States were affected simultaneously by the same emergency, highlighting the need for M&E systems that are easily deployed, easy to use, and informative at the national level. As the M&E Framework for COVID-19 built on the lessons learned from EVD and HIV, the development of an adaptable M&E framework for health emergencies must draw from the lessons learned throughout the COVID-19 response.

Financial support

This research received no specific grant from any funding agency, commercial or not-for-profit sectors

Conflict of interest

The authors have no competing interests to declare.

Author contributions

All authors contributed significantly to the work, and fulfil criteria listed for authorship. BI, CP, FMb conceptualised this project and determined the methodology. TS, CMW, BF and BI, made substantial contributions in writing the initial versions of the manuscript. BI, FMb, TM, FMo and CMW contributed to the data collection, curation, and information synthesis. BI, FMb, BF, TM, CP, CMW, and NB provided key input on the content and structure of the manuscript. All authors (BI, CMW, FMb, BF, TS, CP, NB, TM, FMo, EM, RM, AT, HK, OK, AF, JC, and MM) contributed to the editing and revision process, and reviewed and approved the final version of the manuscript to be published.

Data availability statement

The data that support the findings of this study are available on request from the corresponding author [BI]. Some of the data are publicly available through situation reports produced by Ministries of Health and WHO AFRO on their respective websites, however not all data are publicly available due to confidentiality concerns.

References

1. **Impouma B**, *et al.* Measuring Timeliness of Outbreak Response in the World Health Organization African Region, 2017–2019. *Emerging Infectious Diseases.* 2020; 26(11): 2555-2564. DOI: 10.3201/eid2611.191766.

2. **World Health Organization**. The International Health Regulations (2005) Third Edition. (https://www.who.int/ihr/publications/9789241580496/en/). Accessed 7 January 2021.

3. **World Health Organization**. Emergency Response Framework. (https://www.who.int/hac/about/erf_.pdf). Accessed 7 January 2021.

4. **World Health Organization Regional Office for Africa**. Technical Guidelines for Integrated Disease Surveillance and Response in the African Region: Third edition. (https://www.afro.who.int/publications/technical-guidelines-integrated-disease-surveillance-and-response-african-region-third). Accessed 13 January 2021.

5. **World Health Organization Regional Office for Africa**. Monitoring and evaluation framework for the COVID-19 response in the WHO African Region. (https://www.afro.who.int/publications/monitoring-and-evaluation-framework-covid-19-response-who-african-region). Accessed 3 January 2021.

6. **World Health Organization**. COVID-19 SPRP Monitoring and Evaluation Framework. (https://www.who.int/publications/i/item/monitoring-and-evaluation-framework). Accessed 23 January 2021.

7. **World Health Organization**. 2019 Novel Coronavirus: Strategic Preparedness and Response Plan (4 February 2020).

(https://www.who.int/publications/i/item/strategic-preparedness-and-response-plan-for-the-new-coronavirus). Accessed 10 October 2020.

8. **World Health Organization Regional Office for Africa**. COVID-19 Strategic Response Plan in the African Region (4 May 2020). (https://www.afro.who.int/publications/covid-19-strategic-response-plan-who-african-region). Accessed 10 October 2020.

9. **MEASURE Evaluation**. Selection of Indicators. (https://www.measureevaluation.org/prh/rh_indicators/overview/rationale 2). Accessed 10 October 2020.

10. **Impouma B**, *et al*. Use of electronic tools for evidence-based preparedness and response to the COVID-19 pandemic in the WHO African region. *Lancet Digital Health*. 2020; 2: e500-e502. DOI: 10.1016/S2589-7500(20)30170-9.

Table 1: *Number of countries in the WHO African region by score for three selected KPIs used to monitor country progress over time for the last four epidemiological weeks of 2020.*

Progress indicators for COVID-19 response	Target ranges	Epi week 49	Epi week 50	Epi week 51	Epi week 52	Target
% change in no. new cases compared to previous week (n=46†)	≤-50%	0	7	6	4	A reduction of over 50% during the last 4 weeks corresponds to a sustainable decrease
	-50 to 20%	7	19	22	26	
	>20%	39	20	18	16	
Weekly case fatality rate (CFR) (n=46†)	≤1	27	28	30	29	Target: weekly CFR <1
	1 to 2.5	15	11	12	13	
	>2.5	4	7	4	4	
% change in no. of health worker infections compared to previous week (n=47)	≤-50%	1	3	2	6	A decline of at least 50% in the number of new deaths during the last 3 weeks correspond to a durable drop
	-50 to 20%	39	40	40	39	
	>20%	7	4	5	2	

† Tanzania not assessed.

78

Supplemental Information (SI): List of 31 key performance indicators (KPIs) for the monitoring and evaluation of the response to COVID-19

Coordination & Incident Management
Performance Indicator 1: % of approved national budget utilized to date
Performance Indicator 2: % of WCO response funding utilized to date
Performance Indicator 3: % coverage of IMST staffing need
Performance Indicator 4: % of national staff in IMST
Performance Indicator 5: % of WCO IMST staff deployed to or supporting decentralized IMSTs
Control at point of entries
Performance Indicator 6: % of travelers who tested positive on arrival in the last 7 days
Performance Indicator 7: Percentage of designated points of entry with screening, isolation facilities and referral system for COVID-19
Performance Indicator 8: Mechanism of tracking travelers from affected countries is in place and operational
Surveillance & control of transmission
Performance Indicator 9: % of new confirmed cases among known contacts
Performance Indicator 10: % of alerts investigated within 24 hours during the last 7 days
Performance Indicator 11: % of contacts under follow-up seen during the last 24 hours
Laboratory services: testing strategy in place and applied
Performance Indicator 12: % laboratory results made available within 48 hours
Performance Indicator 13: % increase in lab testing capacity
Laboratory services: diagnostic capacity at decentralized levels established and functioning

Performance Indicator 14: % new tests performed during the current week by labs at decentralized level

Case Management and IPC

Performance Indicator 15: Bed occupancy rate for suspected cases (%) at present

Performance Indicator 16: Percentage of COVID-19 treatment centers functional at sub-national level

Performance Indicator 17: Bed occupancy rate for confirmed cases at present

Performance Indicator 18: Bed occupancy rate for critical and severe COVID-19 cases at present

Performance Indicator 19: Case fatality ratio

Performance Indicator 20: % of confirmed cases among healthcare workers

Performance Indicator 21: % of new confirmed cases among healthcare workers during the last 7 days

Performance Indicator 22: % of districts that have reported at least one confirmed case during the last 7 days

Performance Indicator 23: Case fatality ratio of confirmed cases reported during the last 7 days

Performance Indicator 24: % of new confirmed cases isolated within one day after symptoms onset during the last 7 days

Performance Indicator 25: % of health care workers trained in case management of COVID-19 cases

Risk communication and community engagement

Performance Indicator 26: A rumor management mechanism is in place and operational and evidenced by a report

Safe essential service delivery

Performance Indicator 27: % of change in consultations in selected primary health facilities and prenatal clinics

Performance Indicator 28: % of change in surviving infants receiving third dose of DPT-containing vaccine

Performance Indicator 29: % of change in ODP attendance

Performance Indicator 30: % of change in number of people living with HIV in target area who received ART

Procurement of Critical Supplies

Performance Indicator 31: Has the WCO experienced any stockouts of critical supplies or essential materials in the last week?

Performance Indicator Assessment

Good	90%-100%	<5%
Acceptable	80%-89%	5-10%
Poor	Less than 80%	>10%
	Indicators 7, 9-11, 15, 17, 18, 24	*Indicators 6, 19-21*

Good	60%-100%	> 40%
Acceptable	40%-60%	20%-40%
Poor	Less than 40%	Less than 20%
	Indicators 12, 13	*Indicators 14, 16*

Good	>= 0%	No
Acceptable	(-1%)-(-5%)	--
Poor	Less than (-5%)	Yes
	Indicators 27-30	*Indicator 31*

81

Quality Improvement of Health Systems in an Epidemic Context: A Framework based on Lessons from the Ebola Virus Disease Outbreak in West Africa

Authors

Lucia Brugnara, Cyril Pervilhac, François Kohler, Mohamed Lamine Dramé, Sylvia Sax, Michael Marx (MM *Corresponding author*, evaplan at the University Hospital, Ringstr. 19b, 69115 Heidelberg, Germany, michael.marx@urz.uni-heidelberg.de)

Institutional affiliation

Lucia Brugnara, Heidelberg Institute of Global Health, University of Heidelberg, Germany

Cyril Pervilhac, Global Health Institute, University of Geneva, Switzerland

François Kohler, NGO Les Enfants de l'Aïr, et Faculté de Médecine de l'Université de Lorraine, France

Mohamed Lamine Dramé, Belgium Development Agency, CTB, Bénin

Sylvia Sax, Heidelberg Institute of Global Health, University of Heidelberg, Germany

Michael Marx*, Heidelberg Institute of Global Health, University of Heidelberg, and evaplan at the University Hospital, Heidelberg, Germany

*corresponding author, michael.marx@urz.uni-heidelberg.de, Ringstr.19b 69115 Heidelberg Germany Tel: +49(0)6221-138230

Acknowledgements

We like to express our sincere thanks of gratitude to Joost Butenop (KfW), Alexia Zurkuhlen (HealthRegion CologneBonn), Etienne Guillard (SOLTHIS), Lyne Souci (Global Fund), and Shawn M. D'Andrea (Harvard Humanitarian Initiative/ HHI) for their support and input to this paper.

Conflict of Interest

Authors declare that they have no competing interests.

The content of this publication does not reflect the official opinion of the various institutions engaged. Responsibility for the information and views expressed therein lies entirely with the authors.

Funding

No external funding was received

Abstract

Quality improvement (QI) in health generally focuses on the provision of health services with the aim of improving service delivery. Yet, QI can be applied not only to health services but also to health systems overall. This is of growing relevance considering that due to deficiencies in health systems, the main countries affected by Ebola Virus Disease (EVD) outbreak in West Africa (2014-2016) were insufficiently prepared for the epidemic, and, according to the WHO, epidemics are increasingly becoming a threat to global health. Our objective was to analyze QI constraints in health systems during this EVD epidemic and to propose a practical framework for QI in health systems for epidemics in developing countries. We applied a Framework Analysis using experiences shared at the "Second International Quality Forum" organized by the University of Heidelberg and partners in July 2015, and information gather from a systematic literature review. Empirical results revealed multiple deficiencies in the health systems. We systemized these shortfalls as well as the QI measures taken as a response during the epidemic. Based on these findings, we developed six specific "Priority Intervention Areas" which ultimately resulted in the synthesis of a practical QI framework. We deem that this framework which integrates the "Priority Intervention Areas" with the WHO building blocks is suitable to improve, monitor and evaluate health system performance in epidemic contexts in developing countries.

Keyword: *Ebola Virus Disease, Ebola, West Africa, Quality Improvement, Health Systems, Epidemic, Outbreak*

Introduction

Quality Improvement (QI) in health is the "pursuit of continuous performance improvement"[1], or "actions taken to ensure that interventions established to be efficacious are implemented effectively every time they are needed[2]". It should focus on closing the gap between current and potentially feasible health system performance, underpinned by the human right of "enjoyment of the highest attainable standard of health"[3]. QI mechanisms have been described in different settings, mostly in developed countries[4,5]. In the context of developing countries, QI can "optimize the use of limited resources and improve the achievement of health outcomes" [1,6]. Mechanisms such as standardization of norms and guidelines, prioritization of actions, cost-effectiveness approaches, and integration and harmonization of existent initiatives are some activities related to quality improvement.

The health system building blocks presented by the WHO in 2007[7] have been widely used to analyze, design and implement actions to strength the performance of health systems and, consequently, to improve their quality in different settings. Although it is a valuable tool, criticism has been raised regarding its practical use. For example, the interconnection between the different blocks are often insufficiently taken into account due to a "silo thinking"[8,9].

Epidemics create additional strain on health systems, especially in developing countries. The World Health Organization (WHO) considers that pandemics and epidemics will become serious security threats in the 21st century and that health systems need to be strengthened for their prevention and combat[10]. The Ebola Virus Disease (EVD) outbreak in West Africa, which began in 2014 and lasted until June 2016, was the first in the sub-region and the largest ever recorded. More than 28,616 people worldwide suffered from EVD in that epidemic. About 40,6 % (11.310) of them died[11]. The health systems in this context were hardly prepared to cope with the outbreak[12] due to inadequate and limited curative strategies, massive underfunding, inefficiency and chronic shortage of skilled workforce, especially in rural areas. The deficiencies of the health system and QI measures were identified as one of the major aggravating factors that impeded an effective response to EVD. There is urgent need for further research and development to improve future preparedness and response[10,13].

Objective

Our objectives are to synthetize constraints of quality improvement in health systems during the West Africa EVD epidemic and to propose a practical framework for establishing QI in health systems to improve preparedness for and response to epidemics in developing countries.

Methodology

This paper uses a Framework Analysis based on the discussions and experiences shared at the "2nd International Quality Forum" organized by the University of Heidelberg and partners in July 2015[14] and a systematic literature review. One of the forum themes was disease outbreaks with a focus on EVD and linkages to QI measures with case studies and discussions of different actors´ experiences in the EVD West Africa outbreak. During the forum, we gather the information of six representatives of different agencies that worked in the field in Guinea, Sierra Leone and Liberia during the epidemic (key respondents).

For the literature review, we searched for articles using the terms "quality improvement", "delivery of health care", or "health services", matching to "Ebola virus" in the PubMed (MeSH Terms) and Cochrane databases (Key Terms), as well as in Google Scholar (Key terms, first 100 articles). Additionally, we used a snowball strategy to include further publications which were referred to by the search engines as related articles. Besides, relevant literature previously known by the authors of this paper were included. Only papers published between January 2007 and November 2018 that fulfilled the criteria of health policy system research per Gilson [15] were considered. Articles on basic research, specific technologies or treatments, papers based on epidemic models or about a national context outside Africa were excluded. Our review focused on empirical data on the West Africa EVD outbreak, but also considered national policies of the affected countries and recommendations based on former EVD outbreaks experiences in Africa. Aspects related to the health system financing, although essential for its performance, were not considered here as this would have exceeded the scope of the study.

We carried out the Framework Analysis[16] to systematically arrange the identified constraints during the West Africa Ebola epidemic and quality improvement measures taken. In a first round of analysis of the gathered material, we identified six recurrent key areas where constraints occurred and measures were taken. These, we call "Priority Intervention Areas" (PIAs). We then used these PIAs as an index for a second round of data analysis and for building up a systematic framework. We reviewed again the information presented at the Forum, the selected articles and policy papers and arranged the information in a spreadsheet. We reviewed more than 200 documents out of which in the final round we used three policy papers, 45 publications, and the information from the six key respondents.

Finally, we combined the identified PIAs of our Framework Analysis with the WHO health system building blocks[7] to establish a practical framework for Quality Improvement of health systems in epidemic contexts.

Results

Empirical results

The three countries mostly affected by the West Africa EVD epidemic, Guinea, Sierra Leone and Liberia, are fragile post-conflict countries, and their health systems were unprepared for the challenges of an epidemic of such magnitude[17]. Their health services were mostly limited to curative approaches, massively underfunded, inefficient in technical and allocative terms, and with chronic shortages of skilled workforce especially in rural areas.

In our Framework Analysis we could map the main constrains and quality improvement measures during the EVD outbreak in West Africa according to six Priority Intervention Areas (PIAs): *i) surveillance; ii) basic infrastructure and WASH; iii) infection control, patient and staff safety; iv) case management; v) maintenance of routine services;* and *vi) cultural aspect and community engagement.* A resume of our finding is presented in table 1, the complete Framework Analysis table is presented in Annex 1.

We found that a key constraint in the three main affected countries was a week *surveillance* system[18–22]. For example, in Liberia, cases were initially reported on paper to the central level, and staff in Morovia, Liberia´s capital, had to enter this information manually into the electronic system. The growing number of cases caused a backlog of information, compromising the outbreak response[19]. Problems with case documentation were also reported during the Heidelberg Forum (Shaw D`Andrea, personal communication). Besides, staff was not trained in case recognition or contact tracing[22]. Different strategies to improve the quality of the surveillance systems were implemented[19,23–36], such as training in active surveillance, documentation of cases, laboratory capacity, and even e-health mechanisms[36]. Also the experiences from other African countries showed the importance to improve and strength the surveillance system to control the EVD epidemic[37–39].

Already before the epidemic, the International Monetary Fund (IMF) described general weaknesses of essential components of the health sector in the region, like gaps in the quality of care in rural areas and lack of *basic health infrastructure* (including Water, Sanitation and Hygiene - *WASH* - facilities)[40]. Other authors and policy papers also reported the lack of running water, sanitation facilities, and problems on the energy supply[18,31–33,41–45]. Even the supply of soap was a problem[22]. During the Heidelberg Forum, the importance of improvement measures for basic health and WASH infrastructure was discussed (François Kohler, personal communication), and confirmed by different authors[33,38,41].

All six key respondents who were working for different agencies active in the field during the epidemic stressed that among the biggest challenges for an adequate response were deficiencies in *infection control, patient and staff safety*. Lack or insufficient trained staff, lack of infection prevention control (IPC) measures and personal protective equipment (PPE), inadequate or absence of guidelines, lack of culture of quality of care and inadequate hygiene behavior were confirmed as critical issues in the literature[18,19,21,22,29,31–33,41,43–51]. This increased the risk of infection among health workers[52]. At the beginning of the outbreak, their infection risk was 21 to 32 times higher than the general adult population[53]. Quality improvement measures in these areas were carried out by different agencies, like training of health workforce (Francois Kohler and Shaw D´Andrea, personal communication), performance management, PPE distribution, standardization of infection control measures, and creation of isolation units at community level[23,38,46,47,54]. As a result, the incidence rate of health staff infected among all cases of EVD dropped from 16% in March 2014 to 4% in March 2015[53].

Furthermore, shortcomings related to *case management* were stressed, including the lack of trained workforce on treatment and support measures, quality of care and performance monitoring, proper guidelines, misallocation of resources, inadequate or insufficient material for patient care, problems with safe patient transport and lack of care facilities. These were described during the Forum and in the literature [18–22,29,31,33,41,42,44,45,47,51,55,56]. For instance, Joost Butennop from KfW reported that guidelines for case management existed, but staff in the field did not apply them. Similarly, essential materials like catheters and fluids for simple hypovolemic treatment were available in some cases, but patients in need didn´t receive it in time[55]. Complicated and costly laboratory tests to quantify the viral load were done in some very remote areas, while at the same time, there was lack of basic and simple biochemical or hematological tests needed for the diagnosis of easily treatable metabolic abnormalities. Some of these and other challenges in case management were suitably addressed[21,25,26,29,31–

[33,39,41,42,47,54,55,57,58], for example through relevant staff training in case management[33], reformulation and/or sharing of guidelines[29,39], and the construction of treatment yards in remotes areas[25,31].

There were several reasons which in addition lead to a ***disruption of other health services***, including mother and child care or HIV, malaria and TB services[18,20,21,23,29,32,33,41,43,44,47,51,52,59–62]. First, people were reluctant to visit health facilities because they were afraid of being contaminated there; second, part of the health staff was also afraid or even suffered from contamination, thus did not regularly stay on duty; and third, there was an overload of work in general. For example, in Guinea, even in regions not affected by the EVD, the number of malaria treatments and ante-natal attendance dropped[59]. Policy makers suggested the reinforcement of basic services[41,47]. Health staff[52] and communities[32] were included in decision-making process, and different donor initiatives were integrated (François Kohler and Lyne Souci, personal communication). The Global Fund mitigated the impact of EVD epidemic by allocating US\$ 1,6 million from its emergency fund for the purchase of approximately 440,000 additional long-lasting insecticidal nets (LLIN) in Liberia. In Sierra Leone, the Global Fund provided the same amount to finance Artemisinin-based Combination Therapy (ACT) for Mass Drug Administration, an intervention proposed by the Ministry of Health and supported by many partners.

Finally, important obstacles were identified related to ***cultural aspects and community engagement.*** Burial traditions where relatives and friends are to wash, touch or even kiss the deceased, distrust of population towards health services and politics, lack of solidarity among neighbors in urban areas, reluctancy to report cases seriously hampered the epidemic control[18–21,23,32–34,41,42,44,47,51,52,54,55,63,64]. An extreme case occurred in a remote area of Guinea at the beginning of the outbreak where eight officials and journalists were killed by a mob due to fear and distrust of the local population[65]. Measures to improve the outbreak response considering the cultural context were implemented by agencies and described by different authors, such as safe burial trainings, cooperation with local leaders, adaptation of measures to local and socio-cultural contexts and integration of communities[23,25,30–33,38,39,42,43,47,54,66,67].

Priority Intervention Areas	Most relevant shortcomings and challenges during the EVD outbreak	QI measures applied as response to the EVD outbreak
Surveillance	- Weak surveillance system and case documentation - reluctance of community to report - lack of trained staff and overload of work - lack of reliable information - low laboratory capacity	- Strengthening self-surveillance - triage at community level - Involving local health staff - increasing laboratory capacity - improving information systems - doing active surveillance - training - use of e-health and social media strategies - laboratories' network
Basic infrastructures and WASH	- Weak infrastructure - lack of water and electricity - lack of soap - inadequate hygiene behavior	- Improving water and energy supply, and basic infrastructure at community health facilities - training and campaigns on hand washing
Patient and Staff Safety, infection control	- Unprotected contact with patients - unsafe triage - lack of IPC measures and material and PPE - lack of training - guidelines not applied - inadequate hygiene behavior - insufficient health staff - weak culture of quality of care	- Standardizing infection control measures - producing guidelines - training of health personnel in hygiene and infection control standards (including peer-to-peer) and performance management - availability of IPC material and PPC equipment, quarantine, - training on transport of bodies and patients - isolation units at community level, - institutionalizing infection control policy
Case management	- lack of proper guidelines and their use - no or ineffective training of health staff - no monitoring of health staff performance	- introducing, improving and adapting guidelines (including local experience) - training, mentoring and monitoring of staff

	Challenges	Responses
	▪ insufficient hospital beds ▪ lack of culture of quality of care and outcome monitoring ▪ low mobility, difficulties to transport patients ▪ inadequate material ▪ inadequate care	▪ mainstreaming guidelines in existing programs ▪ early case recognition ▪ isolation and early treatment ▪ improving case management (e.g. supportive care) ▪ increasing number of hospital beds and yards (including isolation units in community settings) ▪ improving distribution of supplies
Maintenance of other routine services	▪ Overload of health system with EVD response lead to disruption in other routine services ▪ Weak routine service provision already before the outbreak ▪ fear of contamination	▪ Strengthening key basic services like mother-child health, vaccination, malaria, HIV/ AIDS ▪ reinforcing routine services ▪ staff participation in decision making ▪ including public health priorities of different donors
Cultural aspects and community engagement	▪ burial traditions ▪ unprotected contact with infected bodies ▪ people´s distrust in public service ▪ people´s reluctancy to support contact tracing activities ▪ communication and cultural barriers ▪ social stigma and fear ▪ lack of solidarity among people in urban areas	▪ strategies to increase community engagement (e.g. local committees, training of local health staff), ▪ recognizing women as main care-takers ▪ training community in hygiene, care, safe burials and quarantine ▪ cooperating with local leaders ▪ adapting measures to local socio-cultural context ▪ increasing cultural awareness

Conceptual result

As part of the Framework Analysis and based on the empirical results, Priority Intervention Areas (PIAs) have been synthesized. The integration of the PIA with the WHO health system building blocks, then, led to a conceptual result in form of a practical framework, a tool for QI in epidemic contexts with key outputs and outcomes for improving preparedness and response in an epidemic context (see Table 2). We excluded the WHO building block "health financing" from the scope of the present research.

Tabel 2: QI-PIA framework – combining the WHO health system building blocks with priority intervention areas for epidemic contexts

PIA / WHO building blocks	Surveillance	Basic infrastructure, water and sanitation (WASH)	Patient and Staff Safety	Case management	Provision of other routine services	Cultural aspects and community engagement
Health Services and facilities						
Outcome:	Patients enjoy safe and quality services					
Outputs:	Health services are prepared for epidemics while ensuring continuation of routine services					
	▪ Health services, facilities and laboratories are prepared for surveillance ▪ Mechanisms and procedures for passive and active surveillance are in place	▪ Basic facilities are equipped with water, sanitation and electricity	▪ Facilities adapted for infection and control safety measures	▪ Effective services for epidemic case management are provided ▪ Sufficient numbers of beds and isolation units	▪ Safe (alternative) sites for other health services are available ▪ Effective services are provided	▪ Health facilities and services accessible for local communities ▪ Services adapted to the social-cultural context and accepted by community
Health Workforce						
Outcome:	Sufficient number of competent, motivated, and compensated staff					
Outputs:	HR systems and training programs build capacities and competencies for epidemics					
	▪ HW are trained and properly perform surveillance tasks	▪ HW demonstrate awareness and apply strict hygiene measures	▪ HW are competent and observe safety and infection control procedures	▪ HW are skilled in diagnosis and appropriate case management	▪ Sufficient qualified staff allocated to routine services	▪ Community health workers and community members are receive training and mentoring

Medical products	Outcome:	Supply of medical products is ensured also under stress / during an epidemic			
	Outputs:	Supply chains for products relevant in an epidemic are set up			
		▪ Surveillance products (e.g. laboratory products and chemicals) are readily available	▪ WASH products and medical waste disposal equipment (e.g. incinerators) available	▪ Personal protection material and infection control products are available	▪ Medical products and drugs for treatment of epidemic are readily available	▪ Medical products and equipment for routine services are available	▪ Medical products adapted/ accepted by local culture
Information	Outcome:	Population and health staff have high levels of awareness how to react in an epidemic			
	Outputs:	Communication strategy for epidemics prepared; information management is up-to-date			
		▪ IT based information system for surveillance is functional ▪ Surveillance data is constantly updated ▪ Modern communication strategies in use (e.g. e-health, social media)	▪ Communication campaigns on hygiene are implemented (e.g. on hand washing or contact with infected bodies)	▪ Information and experiences are shared between stakeholders ▪ Guidelines for patient and staff safety, infection control are spread	▪ Information on up-to-date case management is provided to health staff	▪ Data on other services are available for analysis and for adjustment of strategies	▪ Communication strategy is adapted to local context ▪ Mass media campaigns with culturally adapted messages
Governance	Outcome:	Governance structure strengthened with multi-stakeholder coordination and community engagement			
	Outputs:	Government policies on continuous QI in health systems are in place			

93

▪ Population and stakeholders are aware and support surveillance ▪ Decision makers apply evidence-based policies	▪ Sector plan for health and WASH infrastructure ▪ Commitment to provide basic infrastructure and WASH	▪ Clinical protocols and guidelines are endorsed ▪ Advocacy and institutionalization of infection control	▪ Multi-stakeholder coordination for effective case management	▪ Strategies and coordination mechanisms for basic packages (e.g. mother-child, malaria, vaccination, HIV) are in place	▪ Community leaders, community health workers, and local population are engaged ▪ Trust building measures between health services and local population are implemented

94

Surveillance

It is important to strengthen the surveillance system namely by improving laboratory capacity, equipment availability and maintenance, as well as awareness and training of the health workforce for the control of epidemics. Information systems need to be operational and effective to produce and efficiently process data for evidence-based decision making and to monitor the epidemic spread as well as the performance of the system. For example, information through mobile devices can be useful to estimate the extension of the epidemic and needs related[68].

Basic infrastructure and WASH facilities

Basic infrastructure in health, especially water, sanitation, and electricity are essential for a good performance of health systems, even more in an outbreak context with extraordinary strain. Basic facilities need to be available in a timely manner to be operational and fit to cope with extraordinary stress. This includes availability of essential medical materials for hygiene and waste disposal as well as trained staff and communication strategies on hygiene adapted to the local context.

Patient and Staff safety and case management

Standardization and application of QI within health workforce education and on-the-job training including local management skills[69], infection prevention control (IPC) and use of personnel protection equipment (PPE) should be top priorities to improve preparedness and response to epidemics[70-72]. Guidelines [73,74] should be available and, if needed, adapted according to the situation. The application of guidelines needs to be instructed and closely monitored. PPE and other medical products should be available and maintained at all levels of health services, as well as the adaptation of facilities for infection control and effective case management.

Maintenance of routine services

Priority areas of services and packages of basic health services should be identified, with strategies to assure effective services, including health staff's assignments, medical products provision and safe sites for service provision. Vaccination services, mother and child care, malaria and HIV treatment and control and provision of non-communicable disease support such as diabetes and mental health services should be considered.

Community engagement

Health emergencies are "as much a social as a health phenomenon"[67] even more in poor settings. Therefore, one of the steps necessary to improve an outbreak response is the local population's involvement including local healers, religious authorities, community health workers and community leaders[23,28,71,75]. Medical products and services should be adapted and/or accepted by local culture. Markers of the health system response could be the increased acceptance of services, community leaders' active participation, communication strategies and plans with messages and outbreak strategies adapted to the local culture.

Discussion

Quality Improvement and Priority Intervention Areas (QI-PIA) in Health Systems in an Epidemic Context

There were different factors that lead to the EVD epidemic in West Africa, from human environment alteration and contact with wild animals, bushmeat consumption to human mobility [64]. Yet, as most authors agree, a main reason for the magnitude of the epidemic was the unpreparedness of the health systems to cope with the situation [17,76,77].

Guinea, Sierra Leone and Liberia made efforts to control the epidemic by addressing and overcoming the deficiencies encountered in the health systems. Though they did not explicitly use the term "quality improvement", they introduced relevant measures like training of health workforce on patient safety, issuing or adapting treatment guidelines, or improving sanitarian and hygiene infrastructure in health centers. The short-term resilience plans developed by countries during the epidemics and the local response measures taken have shown that QI can generally be employed in any country during an outbreak[78–80]. These efforts along with international support could finally contain the epidemic. However, it was difficult to translate knowledge into action, and to develop concrete, executable solutions underpinned by system-level understanding[81]. The approach to control EVD was "enhanced, but not transformed" [11], and the low levels of preparedness and gaps in the response came at a high humanitarian cost.

Various authors synthetized the experiences from the EVD epidemic in West Africa in different frameworks[82–84]. The particularity of our approach was to first explore the constraints and relevant measures from empirical evidence, and then on this empirical basis to introduce Priority Intervention Areas as cross-cutting themes for QI in health systems (QI-PIA). This allowed us to not only identify areas described by many authors, like the gaps in human resources and infection control, but also important areas that didn't received much attention in the literature, namely, issues of basic infrastructure or hygiene as well as cultural aspects and community engagement. The importance of addressing such aspects is becoming apparent again in the current EVD outbreak in Central Republic of Congo [85,86] that started mid-2018.

Use of WHO Building Blocks for a QI Framework in an Epidemic Context

The WHO building blocks are widely recognized as an important framework for strengthening health systems. Though, there is also criticism some of which refer to a lack of interrelation between the different blocks ("silo-thinking")[8,9], *or* insufficient analyses within certain blocks. For example, the "leadership/governance" block is commonly used to describe administration and political matters, while other critical governance issues like social aspects and community engagement especially in rural and poor regions are underrated or absent[2]. Outcome monitoring is well addressed in some building blocks (e.g. measuring essential health services), while more needs to be done in others (e.g. information, monitoring of health workforce performance, or governance). Finally, challenges that arise particularly in epidemic contexts are not explicitly addressed by the WHO building blocks.

The results of this study suggest that the integration of the Priority Intervention Areas (QI-PIA) with the WHO building blocks can contribute to overcoming these shortcomings, leading to a practical framework particularly for epidemic contexts. Moreover, as it has the format of a results framework with key outputs and outcomes, it may be applied as a general management tool for designing baseline assessments, planning and budgeting of quality improvement at any level of the health care pyramid and for monitoring progress over time.

Adaptation of "Priority Intervention Areas" for a QI Framework in different Epidemic Contexts

Outbreaks and epidemics have certain challenges and response requirements in common like expected surveillance and information outcomes, while other challenges are disease specific like person-to-person or vector transmission. Therefore, the QI-PIAs Framework needs to be adapted to the specific situation, disease and country. For example, in the case of a Zika or Chikungunya outbreaks, the issues of Patient and Staff Safety would not be as important as in an EVD, but additional aspects of vector control would be necessary. When developing or adapting the framework, new scientific knowledge and tools, like e.g. the progressing development of an Ebola vaccine[87] should be taken into account.

Study limitations

In our literature review we used specific criteria and key terms to search for documents related to quality improvement and EVD epidemic in West Africa. We may have missed relevant documents on quality improvement in the West Africa EVD epidemic that didn´t used the terminology we searched for. Yet, our intention was not to quantify the experiences, but to arrange them in broad, applicable categories to identify the Priority Intervention Areas. The Framework Analysis, although being a method that systematizes findings, is a qualitative method, with its intrinsic limitations[88]. It´s function is to provide insights and explanations in an attempt to build up new theories[16], not to validate hypotheses.

Finally, although the QI-PIA framework described above has been developed based on empirical data, it is still a theoretical framework. Its practicality and effectiveness would still need to be further tested and researched under real conditions.

Conclusion

The main reason for the magnitude of the EVD epidemic in West Africa was the unpreparedness of the health systems, which claimed many lives. The affected countries achieved to apply certain responsive measures, despite of weak capacities, limited resources and the immense stress. However, the measures were not systematic and comprehensive enough.

Hence, a systematic approach to QI is critical to improve preparedness and responsiveness. QI should become a continuous process that not only focuses on clinical care or service provision, but also at the health system level overall, especially in resource poor settings of low-income countries. If the goal is to improve the performance of the whole system, quality improvement methods need to focus on all critical aspects including local governance or information and communication systems adapted to the local culture. This is even more relevant in light of the WHO´s concern that epidemics are increasingly becoming a threat to global health.

For this, derived from our Framework Analysis, we suggest a practical framework that combines key Priority Intervention Areas specific to an epidemic context with the WHO health system building blocks. Such a framework should be applied not only during an outbreak. Rather, it should become part of a health policy for continuous QI. We also suggest engaging the various stakeholders in its development and application, e.g. by bringing together national and international policy makers and experts, international and national NGOs, as well as the civil society and community-based organizations.

Finally, we point at further research needs to advance the discussion and to generate additional evidence, namely around following topics: i) verification and consolidation of the QI-PIA framework in other contexts (other countries, different outbreak scenarios), ii) expansion of the framework including the WHO building block of finance, and iii) study of the feasibility and effectiveness of applying the QI-PIA framework under real conditions.

References

1. Leatherman S, Ferris TG, Berwick D, Omaswa F, Cris N. The role of quality improvement in strengthening health systems in developing countries. *Int J Qual Heal Care.* 2010;22(4):237-243. doi:10.1093/intqhc/mzq028.

2. Massoud MR, Barry D, Murphy A, Albrecht Y, Sax S, Parchman M. How do we learn about improving health care: A call for a new epistemological paradigm. *Int J Qual Heal Care.* 2016:1-5. doi:10.1093/intqhc/mzw039.

3. World Health Organization. Health and human rights. WHO. http://www.who.int/mediacentre/factsheets/fs323/en/. Published 2016. Accessed May 7, 2017.

4. Schouten LMT, Hulscher MEJL, van Everdingen JJE, Huijsman R, Grol RPTM. Evidence for the impact of quality improvement collaboratives: systematic review. *BMJ.* 2008;336(7659):1491-1494. doi:10.1136/bmj.39570.749884.BE.

5. Øvretveit J, Bate P, Cleary P, et al. Quality collaboratives: lessons from research. *Qual Saf Heal Care.* 2002;11:345-351.

doi:10.1136/qhc.11.4.345.

6.   Prytherch H, Nafula M, Kandie C, et al. Quality management: where is the evidence? Developing an indicator-based approach in Kenya. *Int J Qual Heal Care*. 2016:1-7. doi:10.1093/intqhc/mzw147.

7.   World Health Organization. *Everybody's Business: Strengthening Health Systems to Improve Health Outcomes: WHO's Framework for Action.* Geneva: WHO Document Production Services; 2007. http://www.who.int/healthsystems/strategy/everybodys_business.pdf. Accessed April 1, 2017.

8.   Mounier-Jack S, Griffiths UK, Closser S, Burchett H, Marchal B. Measuring the health systems impact of disease control programmes: a critical reflection on the WHO building blocks framework. *BMC Public Health*. 2014;14(278):1-8. doi:10.1186/1471-2458-14-278.

9.   Adam T, Hsu J, De Savigny D, Lavis JN, Rottingen JA, Bennett S. Evaluating health systems strengthening interventions in low-income and middle-income countries: Are we asking the right questions? *Health Policy Plan*. 2012;27:iv9-iv19. doi:10.1093/heapol/czs086.

10. Kieny M, Evans DB, Schmets G, Kadandale S. Health--system resilience: reflections on the Ebola crisis in western Africa. *Bull World Health Organ*. 2014;92(850). doi:10.2471/BLT.14.149278.

11. WHO Ebola Response Team. After Ebola in West Africa — Unpredictable Risks, Preventable Epidemics. *N Engl J Med*. 2016;375(6):587-596. doi:10.1056/NEJMsr1513109.

12. Flessa S, Michael Marx B. Ebola fever epidemic 2014: a call for sustainable health and development policies. *Eur J Heal Econ*. 2015;17:1-4. doi:10.1007/s10198-015-0710-0.

13. McKey B. West Africa Struggles to Rebuild its Ravaged Health-Care System. *Wall Street Journal*. https://www.wsj.com/articles/africa-struggles-to-rebuild-its-ravaged-health-care-system-1433457230. Published June 4, 2015.

14. Second Quality Improvement QI Forum 2015. Quality Improvement Mechanisms in Health System Strengthening: Where is the Evidence? http://s572455629.online.de/2nd-qi-forum-2015. Accessed May 6, 2017.

15. Gilson L (ed. . *Health Policy and Systems Research: A Methodology Reader.* Geneva; 2012. http://www.who.int/alliance-

hpsr/alliancehpsr_reader.pdf. Accessed March 31, 2017.

16. Ritchie J, Spencer L. Qualitative Data Analysis for Applied Policy Research. In: Huberman AM, Miles MB, eds. *The Qualitative Researcher's Companion*. First edit. Thousend Oaks: Sage Publications; 2002:305-329.

17. Barbiero VK. It's not Ebola … it's the systems. *Glob Heal Sci Pract*. 2014;2(4):374-375. doi:10.9745/GHSP-D-14-00186.

18. Ministère de la Santé (République de Guinée). Plan de relance du Système de Santé de la Guinée. 2015.

19. McNamara LA, Schafer IJ, Nolen LD, et al. Ebola surveillance - Guinea, Liberia, and Sierra Leone. *Morb Mortal Wkly Rep*. 2016;65(3).

20. Elston JWT, Cartwright C, Ndumbi P, Wright J. The health impact of the 2014–15 Ebola outbreak. *Public Health*. 2017;143:60-70. doi:10.1016/j.puhe.2016.10.020.

21. Arwady MA, Bawo L, Hunter JC, et al. Evolution of ebola virus disease from exotic infection to global health priority, Liberia, mid-2014. *Emerg Infect Dis*. 2015;21(4):578-584. doi:10.3201/eid2104.141940.

22. Forrester JD, Pillai SK, Beer KD, et al. Assessment of Ebola Virus Disease, Health Care Infrastructure, and Preparedness — Four Counties, Southeastern Liberia, August 2014. *Morb Mortal Wkly Rep*. 2014;63(40):891-893. doi:mm6340a3 [pii].

23. Abramowitz SA, McLean KE, McKune SL, et al. Community-Centered Responses to Ebola in Urban Liberia: The View from Below. *PLoS Negl Trop Dis*. 2015;9(4). doi:10.1371/journal.pntd.0003706.

24. Naidoo D, Durski K, Formenty P. Laboratory response to the West African Ebloa outbreak 2014-2015. *Wekly Epidemiol Rec*. 2015;90:393-408. doi:10.1016/j.actatropica.2012.04.013.

25. Nyenswah T, Fahnbulleh M, Massaquoi M, et al. Ebola epidemic-Liberia, March-October 2014. *MMWR Morb Mortal Wkly Rep*. 2014;63(46):1082-1086. http://www.ncbi.nlm.nih.gov/pubmed/25412068. Accessed November 19, 2018.

26. Moll R, Reece S, Cosford P, Kessel A. The Ebola epidemic and public health response. *Br Med Bull*. 2016;117:15-23. doi:10.1093/bmb/ldw007.

27. Crowe S, Hertz D, Maenner M, Ratnayake R, Baker P, Lash RR. A plan

101

for community event-based surveillance to reduce ebola transmission - Sierra Leone, 2014-15. *Morb Mortal Wkly Rep.* 2015:70-73. http://www.who.int/csr/disease/ebola/ebola-6-months/sierra-leone/en. Accessed December 10, 2018.

28. Olu OO, Lamunu M, Nanyunja M, et al. Contact tracing during an outbreak of Ebola Virus Disease in the Western Area Districts of Sierra Leone: Lessons for future Ebola outbreak response. *Front Public Heal.* 2016;4(4):130. doi:10.3389/fpubh.2016.00130.

29. Cooper C, Fisher D, Gupta N, MaCauley R, Pessoa-Silva CL. Infection prevention and control of the Ebola outbreak in Liberia, 2014-2015: Key challenges and successes. *BMC Med.* 2016;14(2). doi:10.1186/s12916-015-0548-4.

30. Nyenswah T, Westercamp M, Kamali AA, et al. Evidence for Declining Numbers of Ebola Cases — Montserrado County, Liberia, June–October 2014. *Morb Mortal Wkly Rep.* 2014;63(46). https://www.cdc.gov/mmwr/pdf/wk/mm6346.pdf. Accessed May 7, 2017.

31. World Health Organization. Liberia: a country – and its capital – are overwhelmed with Ebola cases. World Health Organization. http://www.who.int/csr/disease/ebola/one-year-report/liberia/en/. Published 2015.

32. Vetter P, Dayer JA, Schibler M, et al. The 2014-2015 Ebola outbreak in West Africa: Hands On. *Antimicrob Resist Infect Control.* 2016;5(17). doi:10.1186/s13756-016-0112-9.

33. Cancedda C, Davis SM, DIerberg KL, et al. Strengthening Health Systems while Responding to a Health Crisis: Lessons Learned by a Nongovernmental Organization during the Ebola Virus Disease Epidemic in Sierra Leone. *J Infect Dis.* 2016;214(S3):S153-63. doi:10.1093/infdis/jiw345.

34. Stehling-Ariza T, Rosewell A, Moiba SA, et al. The impact of active surveillance and health education on an Ebola virus disease cluster-Kono District, Sierra Leone, 2014-2015. *BMC Infect Dis.* 2016;16(1):661. doi:10.1186/s12879-016-1941-0.

35. Burki T. *Are We Learning the Lessons of the Ebola Outbreak?*; 2016. doi:10.1016/S1473-3099(16)00080-3.

36. Sacks JA, Zehe E, Redick C, et al. Introduction of Mobile Health Tools to

Support Ebola Surveillance and Contact Tracing in Guinea. *Glob Heal Sci Pract*. 2015;3(4):646-659. www.ghspjournal.org. Accessed November 15, 2018.

37. Oleribe O, Oladipo O, Nwachukwu C, Abimbola A, Nwanyanwu O. The Complicated and Complex Ebola Viral Disease (EVD) in West Africa. *Am Assoc Sci Technol*. 2014;1(3).

38. Oleribe OO, Salako, Babatunde L, Ka MM, et al. Ebola virus disease epidemic in West Africa: lessons learned and issues arising from West African countries. *Int Clin Med*. 2015;15(1):54-57.

39. World Health Organization. Ebola response: What needs to happen in 2015. WHO. https://www.who.int/csr/disease/ebola/one-year-report/response-in-2015/en/. Published 2015. Accessed January 28, 2019.

40. Permanent Secretariat for Poverty Reduction Strategy, Republic of Guinea, International Monetary Fund. *Guinea: Poverty Reduction Strategy Paper*.; 2013. https://www.imf.org/external/pubs/ft/scr/2013/cr13191.pdf. Accessed May 8, 2017.

41. Ministry of Health, Republic of Liberia. Investment plan for building a resilient Health System in Liberia. 2015. https://au.int/web/sites/default/files/newsevents/workingdocuments/27027-wd-liberia-_investment_plan_for_building_a_resilient_health_system.pdf. Accessed May 7, 2017.

42. World Health Organization. Guinea: The Ebola virus shows its tenacity. World Health Organization. http://www.who.int/csr/disease/ebola/one-year-report/guinea/en/. Published 2015. Accessed May 6, 2017.

43. Government of Sierra Leone. National Ebola Recovery Strategy for Sierra Leone. *Gov Sierra Leone*. 2015:1-58. https://ebolaresponse.un.org/sites/default/files/sierra_leone_recovery_strat egy_en.pdf. Accessed December 5, 2018.

44. Buseh AG, Stevens PE, Bromberg M, Kelber ST. The Ebola epidemic in West Africa: Challenges, opportunities, and policy priority areas. *Nurs Outlook*. 2015;63(1):30-40. doi:10.1016/j.outlook.2014.12.013.

45. Pathmanathan I, O'connor KA, Adams ML, et al. Morbidity and Mortality Weekly Report Rapid Assessment of Ebola Infection Prevention and Control Needs-Six Districts, Sierra Leone, October 2014. *Morb Mortal Wkly Rep* . 2014;63(49):1172-1174. http://www.cdc.gov/mmwr. Accessed

December 10, 2018.

46. Nyarko Y, Goldfrank L, Ogedegbe G, Soghoian S. Preparing for Ebola Virus Disease in West African countries not yet affected: perspectives from Ghanaian health professionals. *Global Health.* 2012;11(7). doi:10.1186/s12992-015-0094-z.

47. Ministry of Health and Sanitation, Government of Sierra Leone. Health Sector Recovery Plan (2015-2020). 2015.

48. Hageman JC, Hazim C, Wilson K, et al. Infection Prevention and Control for Ebola in Health Care Settings — West Africa and United States. *Morb Mortal Wkly Rep.* 2016;63(3 Suppl):50-56. http://www.cdc.gov/vhf/ebola/outbreaks/2014-west-africa/partners.html. Accessed November 28, 2018.

49. Alvarez RA, Micha G, Harris L. Leading Hospitals and Experts in the German-speaking World General Consultation. www.health-excellence.com.

50. Dunn AC, Walker TA, Redd J, et al. Nosocomial transmission of Ebola virus disease on pediatric and maternity wards: Bombali and Tonkolili, Sierra Leone, 2014. *Am J Infect Control.* 2016;44(3):269-272. doi:10.1016/j.ajic.2015.09.016.

51. Gostin LO, Friedman EA. A retrospective and prospective analysis of the west African Ebola virus disease epidemic: Robust national health systems at the foundation and an empowered WHO at the apex. *Lancet.* 2015;385(9980):1902-1909. doi:10.1016/S0140-6736(15)60644-4.

52. Jones S, Sam B, Bull F, et al. 'Even when you are afraid, you stay': Provision of maternity care during the Ebola virus epidemic: A qualitative study. *Midwifery.* 2017;52:19-26. doi:10.1016/j.midw.2017.05.009.

53. World Health Organization. *Health Worker Ebola Infections in Guinea, Liberia and Sierra Leone.* Geneve; 2015. https://apps.who.int/iris/bitstream/handle/10665/171823/WHO_EVD_SDS _REPORT_2015.1_eng.pdf?sequence=1. Accessed February 11, 2019.

54. Okware SI, Omaswa F, Talisuna A, et al. Managing ebola from rural to urban slum settings: Experiences from Uganda. *Afr Health Sci.* 2015;15(1):312-321. doi:10.4314/ahs.v15i1.45.

55. Lamontagne F, Clément C, Fletcher T, Jacob ST, Fischer WA, Fowler RA. Doing Today's Work Superbly Well — Treating Ebola with Current

Tools. *N Engl J Med.* 2014;371(17):1565-1566. doi:10.1056/NEJMp1411310.

56. Boozary A, Farmer P, Jha A k. The Ebola Outbreak , Fragile Health Systems , and Quality as a Cure. *Jama.* 2014;312(18):1859-1860. doi:10.1056/NEJMp1411310.6.

57. World Health Organization. Ebola Situation Report - 22 July 2015 | Ebola. http://apps.who.int/ebola/current-situation/ebola-situation-report-22-july-2015. Published 2015. Accessed May 7, 2017.

58. Vogt F, Fitzpatrick G, Patten G, et al. Assessment of the MSF triage system, separating patients into different wards pending ebola virus laboratory confirmation, Kailahun, Sierra Leone, July to September 2014. *Eurosurveillance.* 2015;20(50). doi:10.2807/1560-7917.ES.2015.20.50.30097.

59. Plucinski MM, Guilavogui T, Sidikiba S, et al. Effect of the Ebola-virus-disease epidemic on malaria case management in Guinea, 2014: A cross-sectional survey of health facilities. *Lancet Infect Dis.* 2015;15(9):1017-1023. doi:10.1016/S1473-3099(15)00061-4.

60. Delamou A, Ayadi AM El, Sidibe S, et al. Effect of Ebola virus disease on maternal and child health services in Guinea: a retrospective observational cohort study. *Lancet Glob Heal.* 2017;5:e448-e457. doi:10.1016/S2214-109X(17)30078-5.

61. Moisan F, Traore A, Zoumanigui D, et al. Public health structures attendance during the Ebola outbreak in Guéckédou, Guinea. *Epidemiol Infect .* 2016;144:2338-2344. doi:10.1017/S0950268816000728.

62. Camara BS, Delamou A, Diro E, et al. Effect of the 2014/2015 Ebola outbreak on reproductive health services in a rural district of Guinea: An ecological study. *Trans R Soc Trop Med Hyg.* 2017;111(1):22-29. doi:10.1093/trstmh/trx009.

63. Southall HG, DeYoung SE, Harris CA. Lack of cultural competency in international aid responses: the ebola outbreak in Liberia. *Front Public Heal.* 2017;5(55):3389-5. doi:10.3389/fpubh.2017.00005.

64. Alexander KA, Sanderson CE, Marathe M, et al. What factors might have led to the emergence of ebola in West Africa? *PLoS Negl Trop Dis.* 2015;9(6). doi:10.1371/journal.pntd.0003652.

65. Callimachi R. Fear of Ebola Drives Mob to Kill Officials in Guinea. *The*

New York Times. https://www.nytimes.com/2014/09/19/world/africa/fear-of-ebola-drives-mob-to-kill-officials-in-guinea.html. Published September 18, 2014.

66. World Health Organization. How Liberia reached zero cases of Ebola virus disease. *Wkly Epidemiol Rec* . 2015;90(21):259-260. www.who.int/wer. Accessed January 12, 2019.

67. Gillespie AM, Obregon R, El Asawi R, et al. Social mobilization and community engagement central to the Ebola response in West Africa: lessons for future public health emergencies. TT -. *Glob Heal Sci Pract*. 2016;4(4):626-646. doi:http://dx.doi.org/10.9745/GHSP-D-16-00226.

68. Flahault A, Geissbuhler A, Guessous I, et al. Precision global health in the digital age. *Swiss Med Wkly*. 2017;147(w14423). doi:10.4414/smw.2017.14423.

69. Scott V, Crawford-Browne S, Sanders D. Critiquing the response to the Ebola epidemic through a Primary Health Care Approach. *BMC Public Health*. 2016;16(410). doi:10.1186/s12889-016-3071-4.

70. Wiwanitkit V, Tambo E, Ugwu EC, Ngogang JY, Zhou X-N. Are surveillance response systems enough to effectively combat and contain the Ebola outbreak? *Infect Dis poverty*. 2015;4(7). doi:10.1186/2049-9957-4-7.

71. Ghazanfar H, Orooj F, Abdullah MA, Ghazanfar A. Ebola, the killer virus. *Infect Dis poverty*. 2015;4(15). doi:10.1186/s40249-015-0048-y.

72. GBD 2015 SDG Collaborators. Measuring the health-related Sustainable Development Goals in 188 countries: a baseline analysis from the Global Burden of Disease Study 2015. *Lancet*. 2016;388:1813-1850. doi:10.1016/S0140-6736(16)31467-2.

73. Sterk E (Médecins SF. Filovirus haemorrrhagic fever guideline. 2008. http://www.slamviweb.org/es/ebola/FHFfinal.pdf. Accessed May 9, 2017.

74. World Health Organization. *Clinical Management of Patient with Viral Haemorrhagic Fever: A Pocket Guide for Front-Line Health Workers*. Geneva; 2016. http://apps.who.int/iris/bitstream/10665/205570/1/9789241549608_eng.pdf. Accessed May 9, 2017.

75. Hewlett BS, Amola RP. Cultural context of Ebola in Northern Uganda. *Emerg Infect Dis*. 2003;9(10):1242-1248.

https://www.ncbi.nlm.nih.gov/pmc/articles/PMC3033100/pdf/02-0493.pdf. Accessed May 11, 2017.

76. Sanders D, Sengupta A, Scott V. Ebola epidemic exposes the pathology of the global economic and political system. *Int J Health Sci (Qassim)*. 2015;45(4):643-656. doi:10.1177/0020731415606554.

77. Flahault A, de Castaneda RR. Ebola : Vaincre ensemble ! - University of Geneva | Coursera. 2014. https://www.coursera.org/learn/ebola-vaincre-ensemble. Accessed May 8, 2017.

78. Ministère de la Santé, République de Guineé. Guide d´Elaboration des Plans d´Action Operationels des Districts Sanitaires. 2015.

79. Ministère de la Santé, République de Guinée. Guide d'Elaboration des Plans d'Action Operationels des Directions Regionales de la Santé. 2015.

80. Ministère de la Santé, Guinée R de. Guide d´Elaboration des Plans d´Action Operationels des Hospitaux Publics. 2015.

81. Kreindler SA. What if implementation is not the problem? Exploring the missing links between knowledge and action. *Int J Health Plann Manage*. 2016;31(2):208-226. doi:10.1002/hpm.2277.

82. Jacobsen KH, Aguirre AA, Bailey CL, et al. Lessons from the Ebola Outbreak: Action Items for Emerging Infectious Disease Preparedness and Response. 2016. doi:10.1007/s10393-016-1100-5.

83. Shoman H, Karafillakis E, Rawaf S. The link between the West African Ebola outbreak and health systems in Guinea, Liberia and Sierra Leone: A systematic review. *Global Health*. 2017;13(1). doi:10.1186/s12992-016-0224-2.

84. Heymann DL, Chen L, Takemi K, et al. Global health security: The wider lessons from the west African Ebola virus disease epidemic. *Lancet*. 2015;385(9980):1884-1901. doi:10.1016/S0140-6736(15)60858-3.

85. Ahmadou B, Ahuka-Mundeke S, Ahmed YA, et al. Outbreak of Ebola virus disease in the Democratic Republic of the Congo, April-May, 2018: an epidemiological study. *Lancet (London, England)*. 2018;392(10143):213-221. doi:10.1016/S0140-6736(18)31387-4.

86. World Health Organization. Attacks in the Democratic Republic of the Congo. WHO News. https://www.who.int/news-room/detail/17-11-2018-who-statement-on-latest-attacks-in-the-democratic-republic-of-the-congo.

Published 2018. Accessed February 11, 2019.

87. Henao-Restrepo AM, Camacho A, Longini IM, et al. Efficacy and effectiveness of an rVSV-vectored vaccine in preventing Ebola virus disease: final results from the Guinea ring vaccination, open-label, cluster-randomised trial (Ebola Ça Suffit!). *www.thelancet.com*. 2017;389(10068):505-518. doi:10.1016/S0140-6736(16)32621-6.

88. Maxwell JA. Understanding and Validity in Qualitative Research. In: Huberman AM, Miles MB, eds. *The Qualitative Researcher's Companion*. Thousand Oaks, California: Sage Publications; 2002:37-64.

Using HIV surveillance data: recent experiences and avenues for the future

Cyril Pervilhac[1], John Stover[2], Elizabeth Pisani[3], Tim Brown[4], Ruben Mayorga[5], Owen Mugurungi[6], Mohammed Shaukat[7], Lv Fan[8], Peter D Ghys[9]

[1]World Health Organisation, Switzerland; [2]Futures Group, USA; [3]Family Health International, Indonesia; [4]The East-West Center/Thai Red Cross Society Collaboration on HIV/AIDS Modelling, Analysis & Policy, Thailand; [5]Organización de Apoyo a una Sexualidad Integral frente al SIDA (OASIS), Guatemala; [6]Ministry of Health, Zimbabwe; [7]National AIDS Control Organisation, India; [8]China Center for Disease Control and Prevention, Beijing, China; [9]UNAIDS, Switzerland.

Abstract

HIV surveillance systems provide information that is crucial to our understanding of epidemic dynamics among different populations in different settings. Surveillance data are also used for advocacy, to inform policies and programming, and for monitoring. Multiple data sources may be used and will expand in the future as service statistics from treatment programs become available.

Important and new priorities in HIV surveillance data use at the national and local levels can build on past experience with surveillance reports, national estimates, advocacy materials, and communications to the media.

A new framework, integrated analysis of data from expanded surveillance systems and other sources, is proposed to inform improved programming. The approach allows making effective program choices, based on the analysis of biological and behavioural data and the coverage of interventions in an integrated fashion. The comparison of surveillance data with financial data provides added insights in the adequacy of the response.

These findings and experiences set a new agenda for technical and structural directions to improve data use in countries.

2005 Lippincott Williams & Wilkins

AIDS 2005, 19 (suppl 2):S53–S58

Keywords: *HIV surveillance, monitoring, programme, data use, policies*

1. Introduction

Within the framework of Second Generation HIV Surveillance (1) there are multiple sources of surveillance data, including HIV, STI and AIDS case reporting, HIV serosurveys, STI surveys, behavioural surveys, vital registration, and mortality data from censuses and surveys. In the near future there may be an expansion of these sources with the use of service data from Prevention of Mother to Child Transmission (PMTCT), Voluntary Counselling and Testing (VCT) and ART and tuberculosis treatment programmes. Beyond understanding the dynamics of the epidemics in different settings and among different populations, the use of the information generated by Second Generation Surveillance systems by different audiences is the ultimate purpose of collecting and analysing HIV surveillance data, and is bound by ethical obligations. This information is required for advocacy, for policy formulation, planning and monitoring and evaluation of specific programmes and the national response.

Global advocacy based on HIV surveillance data has been successful in mobilizing increased resources. These new resources from large international initiatives and bi-lateral funding for scaling-up prevention and care efforts across the world also put new demands on surveillance systems. The role of surveillance in guiding the allocation of these new resources and monitoring their impact is under increased scrutiny. In addition, the use of the information generated by surveillance systems needs to be tailored to specific circumstances and needs in each country.

In this paper, we review important and new priorities in the use of data based on recent experiences in countries with epidemics that have different magnitudes and dynamics, both at the national and local levels. We also suggest a new framework for integrated data analysis that makes use of all relevant data to better inform policies and programmes.

2. Experiences with traditional uses of HIV surveillance data

Many countries have developed a variety of effective approaches for analysis and dissemination that enhance the use of information for advocacy, and national policy and planning decisions.

2.1. Surveillance reports

Most countries now produce annual surveillance reports that describe the methodology, sites and results. Those serve as an official source of surveillance information and can be very effective in communicating results to other government organizations, the news media, donor organizations, and other interested parties. These reports provide details of surveillance site selection, protocols for selecting participants, types of tests used, quality control procedures, sample sizes and results. Where such reports do not exist there is often confusion about the official results and people do not know where to go to get the latest information. Very often, behavioural surveillance data is published in separate reports with a similar format. Some of these reports have a slant towards serving the academic realm rather than the applied programmatic or policy end users. Some countries have recently broken this mould, preferring to bring behavioural and biological information together into a single volume that aims to draw attention to the implications of the data by highlighting important findings and trends written in non-technical language and making liberal use of graphics and dynamic headlines (e.g. 2).

2.2. National HIV/AIDS estimates

Estimates provide planners and advocates with interpreted results which avoids potential mis-use and mis-understanding of the surveillance data. Among the most common problems are:

• Estimates of the number of HIV-infected people in the country made by multiplying adult prevalence by the total population rather than the adult population

• Presentation of the number of people who are infected with HIV as equivalent to the number of AIDS cases

• Claims that since prevalence has stopped rising the epidemic is over.

• Claims that a lower estimate of prevalence this year than in previous years is necessarily an indicator of the success of the national prevention program.

Methods and tools for making estimates have recently been further developed and disseminated (3-6). In some countries new national estimates are prepared whenever new surveillance results become available. These estimates are prepared by an expert group that reviews all the surveillance data available in the country. The power and usefulness of advocacy efforts built on surveillance data is related to the perceived validity of the information and degree of consensus around the key messages (7-10). In China, a renewed focus on estimates has allowed policy-makers to better understand the epidemic while contributing to improve surveillance activities (11). In 2003 the new estimates led to a better understanding of the distribution of transmission groups. The estimates process included prevalence data, data on high-risk groups and their partners, geographic data and the population size of high-risk groups with national estimates for 2003.

2.3. Advocacy materials

Many countries also prepare advocacy documents on a regular basis to communicate surveillance findings and the consequences of those findings. This has provided a consistency to figures on the extent and impact of the epidemic and helped focus the national debate on what needs to be done. The AIM booklets (e.g. 12 for Kenya) have sections describing the current epidemiological situation in the country, projections for the future, the impacts of AIDS on social and economic development, the status of programs to address the epidemic, and recommendations and conclusions about the way forward. Some countries have also produced shorter brochures or wall charts that can be printed in larger numbers and distributed even more widely (13).

In India, surveillance data and estimates have been used to help generate public response and to help target prevention activities and plan resources (14). Recently the National AIDS Control Organisation has shifted its emphasis to include strong political advocacy, decentralization and state ownership of programs, focusing on care and support of persons living with HIV and AIDS and mainstreaming HIV and AIDS care in the health system, focusing on vulnerable groups, promotion of behavioral change, involvement of the non-health sector, and enlisting participation of non-governmental organizations and communities. In addition, surveillance data in India contributed to redesign program activities to target interventions for sex workers, to drive policy for PMTCT, and to bring a new focus on the role of STIs in HIV transmission in low-prevalence states.

2.4. Communications to the media

It is important to carefully consider the key messages that need to be disseminated to the media in press releases and press conferences and to put them in appropriate formats to avoid any misinterpretation. For example, if surveillance data indicate that prevalence has remained constant for the past several years, some might interpret that as a sign of success or even a sign that prevention efforts are working. In fact, it may simply be due to the fact that prevalence has reached a natural plateau where new infections are balanced by AIDS deaths. In some cases a new estimate of prevalence may be lower than previous estimates. It may be statistically insignificant or it may be due to the expansion of surveillance sites to rural areas, or due to small samples. To help interpretation, the estimate can be compared to revised estimates of previous years and ranges can be provided (15). In either case the lower estimate does not mean that prevalence is declining, but, of course, this will be the first interpretation of most people if the estimates are provided without further explanation. In Malawi, after the preparation of the recent national prevalence estimate, the expert team worked with the communications officer at the National AIDS Commission to prepare a press release and conduct press conferences to ensure that the proper information and messages were disseminated. In Zimbabwe, communicating the change in estimates was important. The Minister of Health and Child Welfare released the estimates. The initial debate focused on whether there was a real decline in adult HIV prevalence from 33.7% in 2001 to 24.9% in 2003. In reality, there was no decline, and close scrutiny of the data indicated that prevalence had been overestimated in 2001 for a variety of reasons, including false positive HIV serology tests. As a result, the Ministry of Health informed, based on the current estimates methods with the prevalence rates, that there was evidence of a leveling off but no decline in HIV prevalence with the details clarified above (9).

3. A framework for the future: integrated analysis of data from expanded surveillance systems and other sources

3.1. What is integrated analysis?

Although there is a lot of HIV sentinel surveillance trend data from many countries and behavioral surveillance trends in a few countries, there has been only limited success in linking biological and behavioral data. Integrating data analysis is a new way to address country needs for advocacy materials to influence policy.

The links between biomarkers and behavior are present at the level of the individual, and prospective cohort studies show strong links between behavior and biological outcomes. However, to see these links at the population level temporal dynamics need to be included, that is, it is *past* trends in behaviors, HIV and STIs, and responses that determine *current* HIV prevalence levels. This leads to a need for models as well as for data. The main reason that these links are not being seen is that while a lot of data are being collected, often no one is charged with putting together the "big picture". That is, existing information on past and present responses, on the epidemiology of HIV and STI and behavioral data, are not being analyzed in an integrated fashion with appropriate attention to the influence of the past on the present, and the effects of responses are not incorporated into most analyses.

Integrated analysis and advocacy is a process which can be summarized in seven steps:
1. Systematic collection and synthesis of biological, behavioral, programmatic and policy, resource allocation and coverage information
2. Extraction of key trends in HIV, STIs, behavior and responses over time
3. As a central part of this process, identification and planning to fill data gaps
4. Use of tools to build locally relevant models and projections, e.g., Workbook approach (5), incidence spreadsheets (16), EPP (4), the Asian Epidemic Model (17) and Spectrum (6)
5. Analysis of past and current responses for relevance and effectiveness
6. Use of models to evaluate effectiveness of and estimate costs of alternative prevention and care strategies for the future
7. Proactive advocacy and active support for the use of existing data and strategy analyses to make the most effective program choices and mobilize adequate resources to contain the epidemic.

3.2. An example from Indonesia

In Indonesia donors have contributed large amounts of funding towards HIV prevention programs since 1996. Surveillance data are contributing to reorient HIV prevention policies and resource allocation. In 2001, at a time of very low HIV prevalence and little available behavioral data, programs had a strong focus on information, education and counseling especially among female sex workers.

They were geographically limited, centered on Non-Governmental Organizations (NGOs), with very limited government buy in.

Despite the early strategy of prevention, condom use in Jakarta remained low at 10.3% to 11.7% among female sex workers and 4.1% among their clients, while HIV prevalence among sex workers in Jakarta quadrupled to 6.7% among massage parlor-based sex workers and 2.7% among brothel-based sex workers by 2003. Behavioural surveillance showed that the major reason that condoms were not being used was clients' reluctance.

From HIV data it was apparent that there had been rapid rises in prevalence in three populations, *waria* or transvestite CSWs, prisoners and IDUs. By 2002 the prevalence in *waria* was 21.7% and in prisoners 24.5%. However, the largest increase was among IDUs, who rose from 0% in 1997 to 47% and 48% in two separate surveys in 2003 (Figure 1).

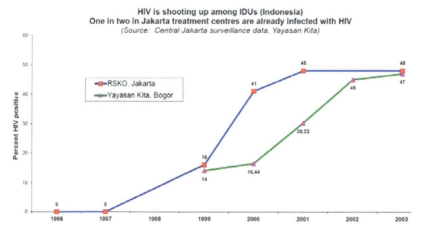

Simple spreadsheet models for estimations suggested that the risk of incident HIV infection was approaching 100% in one year in IDUs and 40% in prisoners. About 55% of IDUs were found to be sexually active, few used condoms regularly and 53% of those who were sexually active had more than one sexual partner. Modeling three separate prevention strategies allowed to calculate that between 16,000 and 26,000 HIV infections could be averted in Jakarta by 2010. The largest contribution would be from eliminating unprotected sex between IDUs and their partners. In more sophisticated models by 2010 about one-third of infections would have occurred in IDUs and the other two-thirds in other risk groups, with a large contribution from sexual partners of injectors. If the epidemic among IDUs had been prevented, there would have been virtually no HIV epidemic in Jakarta by 2010.

The triangulation of these data has led to a complete rethinking of program priorities. IDUs and prisoners have emerged as major priority populations, and programs for IDUs must stress safe sex. In addition, programs for high-risk sex must focus more on clients. It was also recognized that impact on the course of the epidemic can only be achieved through high coverage of prevention programmes, and that the government is the best partner to achieve this. This rethinking has led to a realignment between 2001 and 2003 respectively of prevention funding with a decrease from 71% to 23% for female sex workers, and an increase from 11% to 53% for high-risk men and from nothing to 17% for IDUs, and 10% for prisoners.

3.3. An example from Thailand

A model, created with the Asian Epidemic Model, incorporating the key transmission modes was built and correctly reproduced ten years of epidemiological surveillance trends (18). The relative contribution of different transmission modes to new infections was calculated (19). As can be seen in Figure 2, injecting drug use dominated the early epidemic, but was quickly overtaken by sex work infections. As Thailand's effective national programs took hold in the early 1990s (20, 21), however, new infections in sex work fell rapidly, husband-to-wife transmission increased to half of new infections and injecting drug use became again an important mode of transmission. These results demonstrate that prevention efforts can have a major impact on transmission, but that national responses must continuously adapt as the epidemic evolves over time.

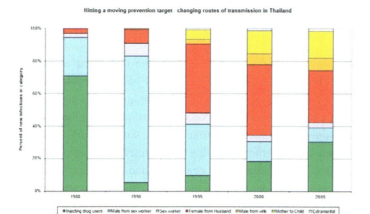

Hitting a moving prevention target   changing routes of transmission in Thailand

Similar exercises using both AEM and EPP are currently underway in Bangladesh, Cambodia, China, Indonesia and Vietnam.

3.4. An example from Latin America and the Caribbean (LAC): comparison of surveillance data with resource allocation data

Surveillance and financial data are being used by epidemiologists and economists to develop estimates for resource requirements to address HIV/AIDS prevention and care. They applied country-specific knowledge in 10 LAC countries to re-estimate the costs, coverage, and capacity of the health and education systems to expand HIV/AIDS interventions by 2005. A discrepancy of US$ 173 million existed between the model estimates and those of country specialists, largely due to the estimated future price of highly ART with estimates of the model reflecting efficiency gains that could result from purchasing arrangements that lead LAC countries to lower prices for antiretroviral drugs (22).

Additional specific use of combined surveillance and financial data are currently being developed in the region by the Regional Initiative against AIDS in the LAC (SIDALAC) to identify the resource allocation priorities in relation to programmatic areas (e.g. Information Education and Communication, Condoms, STI, IDU, Prevention of vertical transmission, blood banks), and the vulnerable populations (23). In complement, NGOs, NGO networks, and cooperation agencies use the model to advocate further for reallocation of program support where towards the new transmission sub-groups. For example, in many countries in Central America, HIV prevalence is higher among men who have sex with men (MSM) than among female sex workers. Moreover

MSM represent a larger population than female sex workers. In Guatemala these comparisons of surveillance data with data on prevention spending and a political mapping exercise have contributed to devise policy strategies and a variety of activities to increase prevention funding for MSM, including through a proposal approved by the Global Fund to Fight AIDS, Tuberculosis and Malaria.

4. The way forward: improving data use

First of all, data analysis and use should be appropriately budgeted for. Relatively simple improvements in data processing, coding, analysis and presentation can greatly increase the utility of existing data. A closer connection between HIV programme staff and data analysis staff is critical; this cannot be achieved unless both epidemiology and HIV programme managers agree to dedicate staff time to improved data analysis on an on-going basis

Simple logistical obstacles, e.g. the lack of standardised sampling procedures in the field, poor data recording and storage systems, high turnover of staff, can be overcome through better oversight and quality assurance, as well as routine training of technical staff. WHO and UNAIDS have recently developed guidelines for use of surveillance data that can be used in formal and hands-on training for programme managers and surveillance professionals (24).

An important reason for the disconnect between data availability and data use lies in the fact that the people charged with the data analysis rarely have a close connection with the people who are actually involved in planning HIV prevention and care services. The consequence is that surveillance reports, and especially behavioural surveillance reports, either stick to the "core indicators", or run frequency distributions on every item in the questionnaire. Modelling should be seen as a regular surveillance effort, rather than a specialised activity. Modelling that incorporates coverage data and comparisons with financial data can be very powerful as indicated above. To support informed data analysis and integrated analysis, an appropriately organized structure need to be set up, both to perform the analyses and to ensure translation and messaging targeted at policy makers. A strategy for the marketing of surveillance data to the various audiences should be developed as part of the national plan for surveillance and monitoring and evaluation, with the support of a technical working group on data analysis.

Clearly, the types of analyses described above are relevant at different levels of programme planning and management. Modelling exercises focusing on transmission patterns are most useful in shaping the national level response – for deciding which behaviours should be prioritised in the national response to maximise the impact of prevention programmes, and which sub-populations are most in need of care and support. More detailed analyses of exposure to interventions and behaviour change is critical in the planning, monitoring and evaluation of prevention and care at a local level. This is especially true in the increasing numbers of countries which are decentralising their health systems. Yet the capacity to undertake such analysis is often limited even at the national level, and is rarely available at the local level. National level public health authorities must therefore assume the responsibility either for creating analytic capacity at the local level, or for performing locally appropriate analyses at the centre, and developing formal systems for discussing them at the provincial or district level.

Finally, capacity should be built through institutionalising training in existing training institutions (e.g. over twenty years of Field Epidemiology Training Programme in Thailand). New training materials and modules addressing the country needs (based on training needs assessments) should be developed and regional networks should be supported to help exchange information and experiences.

Acknowledgements

This paper is based on the presentations made in the "New Strategies for HIV/AIDS Surveillance in Resource-Constrained Countries", Addis Ababa, Ethiopia, 26-29 January 2004, and discussions in the working group whom we gratefully acknowledge. We also thank George Schmid (WHO) for critical comments on the paper.

References

1. UNAIDS/WHO. *Guidelines for Second Generation HIV Surveillance.* Geneva: UNAIDS/WHO Working Group on global HIV/AIDS and STI surveillance; 2000.

2. National AIDS/STD Programme, Directorate General of Health Services, Ministry of Health and Family Welfare. *HIV in Bangladesh: is time running out?* Background document for the dissemination of the fourth round (2002) of national HIV and behavioural surveillance. Dhaka; 2003.

3. The UNAIDS Reference Group on Estimates, Modelling and Projections. Improved methods and assumptions for estimation of HIV/AIDS epidemic and its impact: recommendations of the UNAIDS Reference Group on Estimates, Modelling and Projection. *AIDS* 2002; **16**:W1–W14.

4. Ghys PD, Brown T, Grassly NC, Garnett G, Stanecki KA, Stover J, *et al.* The UNAIDS Estimation and Projection Package: A software package to estimate and project national epidemics. *Sex Transm Inf* 2004; **80(Suppl 1): i5-i9.**

5. Walker N, Stover J, Stanecki K, Zaniewski AE, Grassly NC, Garcia-Calleja JM, *et al.* The Workbook approach to making estimates and projecting future scenarios of HIV/AIDS in countries with low-level and concentrated epidemics. *Sex Transm Inf* 2004; **80(Suppl 1): i10-i13.**

6. Stover J. Projecting the demographic consequences of adult HIV prevalence trends: The Spectrum projection package. *Sex Transm Inf* 2004; **80(Suppl 1): i14–i18.**

7. NASCOP. *"National HIV Prevalence in Kenya" The National AIDS and STDs Control Programme.* Nairobi: National AIDS Commission; March 2003.

8. National AIDS Commission. *"Estimating National HIV Prevalence in Malawi from Sentinel Surveillance Data: Technical Report".* Lilongwe: National AIDS Commission; October 2003.

9. AIDS and TB Programme. *Zimbabwe National HIV and AIDS Estimates 2003*, Health Information and Surveillance Unit, Department of Disease Prevention and Control. Harare: AIDS and TB Programme; 2003.

10. Department of Health. *National HIV and Syphilis Sero-Prevalence Survey of Women Attending Public Antenatal Clinics in South Africa.* Pretoria: Department of Health; 2002.

11. Fan Lv. *Impact of improved estimates process on surveillance activities in China.* "New Strategies for HIV/AIDS surveillance in resource-constrained countries" Conference. Addis Ababa, Ethiopia; 26-29 January 2004.

12. NASCOP and National AIDS Commission. *AIDS in Kenya: Background, Epidemiology, Impact, Interventions.* Nairobi: NASCOP; 2002.

13. National AIDS and STD Control Programme. *HIV/AIDS in Nigeria: Overview of the Epidemic: 2002.* Abuja: Federal Ministry of Health; 2002.

14. Shaukat M. *India presentation.* "New Strategies for HIV/AIDS surveillance in resource-constrained countries" Conference. Addis Ababa, Ethiopia; 26-29 January 2004.

15. Grassly NC, Morgan M, Walker N, Garnett G, Stanecki KA, Stover J, et al. Uncertainty in estimates of HIV/AIDS: the estimation and application of plausibility bounds. *Sex Transm Infect* 2004; **80(Suppl 1): i31-i38.**

16. Pisani E, Garnett GP, Grassly NC, Brown T, Stover J, Hankins C, *et al.* Back to basics in HIV prevention: focus on exposure. *BMJ* 2003; **326**:1384-7.

17. Brown T, Peerapatanapokin W. The Asian Epidemic Model: a process model for exploring HIV policy and program alternatives in Asia. *Sex Transm Infect* 2004; **80(Suppl 1): :i19–i24.**

18. Thai Working Group on HIV/AIDS Projection. *Projections for HIV/AIDS in Thailand: 2000-2020.* Bangkok: Division of AIDS, Ministry of Public Health; 2001.

19. Saidel TJ, Des Jarlais D, Peerapatanapokin W, Dorabjee J, Singh S, Brown T. Potential impact of HIV among IDUs on heterosexual transmission in Asian settings: scenarios from the Asian Epidemic Model. *International Journal of Drug Policy* 2003; **14**:63-74.

20. Nelson KE, Celentano DD, Eiumtrakol S, Hoover DR, Beyrer C, Suprasert S, *et al.* Changes in sexual behavior and a decline in HIV infection among young men in Thailand [see comments]. *N Engl J Med* 1996; **335**(5):297-303.

21. Phoolcharoen W, Ungchusak K, Sittitrai W, Brown T. Thailand: Lessons from a strong national response to HIV/AIDS. *AIDS* 1998; **12(Suppl B)**:S123-35.

22. Opuni M, Bertozzi S, Bollinger L, Gutierrez JP, Massiah E, McGreevey W, *et al.* Resource requirements to fight HIV/AIDS in Latin America and the Caribbean. In: *AIDS* 2002; **16(Suppl 3)**: 58-65.

23. Valladares Cardona R, Izazola-Licea J. *Financiamiento y gasto en respuesta al VIH/SIDA.* Banco Interamericano de Desarrollo: Departamento de Desarrollo Sostenible. (SIDALAC: http://www.sidalac.org.mx) 2004.

24. UNAIDS/WHO. *Guidelines for effective use of data from HIV surveillance systems.* Geneva: WHO; 2004.

Improving the Local Responses to HIV/Aids in Africa: Gaoua District, a Case Study of Burkina Faso

Thesis submitted to the University of Bielefeld in fulfilment of

the requirement for the degree of Doctor of Public Health (Dr. PH.)

in the Bielefeld School of Public Health

Department of Public Health Medicine

Submitted by:

Cyril Pervilhac

Bonn

August 2000

Thesis Director:

Prof. Dr. Alexander Krämer, M.D., Ph.D.

ABSTRACT

This thesis reports on a process of developing a new approach called the "Local Responses to HIV/Aids" undertaken in Gaoua District, Burkina Faso, between 1997 and 2000. It focuses on how communities, and organisations from the public and other sectors (voluntary, non and for profit, Churches) can develop more effective responses to HIV/Aids in their settings.

The study described in this thesis aims: first, to improve the knowledge and gaps (under the form of research conclusions) of how to plan and implement HIV/Aids strategies in rural settings in Africa by testing an approach called the Local Responses; second, to document critically a three years process, including some early results.

The research objectives were fourfold:

- first, to develop a rapid appraisal method which can be a resource for district and communities to circumscribe their needs in relation to HIV/Aids,
- second, to carry out situation analyses at the community and district levels,
- third, to apply the findings to improve responses, and
- finally, to assess the results, including the lessons learnt from using this approach for national and international implications.

The method used is based on health systems research with a pre-experimental before and after prospective intervention study.

The study gives evidence of the importance of carrying out situation analyses for HIV/Aids (baseline, 1997) both at the community and district levels. Based on the findings of the analyses a consensus-building was reached on a common vision to address the epidemic with all key partners from the District, including community representatives. In complement to the existing prevention strategies, the much needed care and counselling and psycho-social support components were identified as neglected up to now, and future priority areas. Under UNAIDS guidance, the partners developed their activities using a strategic planning approach and as a consequence, were able to mobilise their own and external resources too. I document the development of a new organisational tool called the Rapid Organisational Review (ROR). Finally, despite the strengths of this approach, the applications and limitations are presented using the case of migrants as a specific vulnerable group.

Six months of implementation of the Local Responses (2nd semester 1999) are sufficient to document already substantial results:

- The partnerships of non-health public sectors (i.e. Education, Agriculture etc.) and non-governmental partners (i.e. Churches, traditional authorities), and local Associations (Community-Based Organisations of different nature) have increased tremendously.
- Some vulnerable groups (e.g. youth, prisoners) are now addressed specifically.
- Geographic coverage has increased in the District, both in towns and rural areas.
- A massive number of agents of change have been trained for some in HIV prevention from the different local Associations, and others in care and counselling (particularly in the health sector).
- The District of Gaoua and Poni Province have now a locally owned Technical Committee and Provincial Committee who co-ordinate the process locally.

The study reports on some of the national and international positive direct benefits of the "Local Responses" as well.

The study concludes that despite its positive overall outcomes, and its potential in the decades ahead, many issues related to the development of Local Responses still need to be addressed in order for this approach to become more broadly known, credible, and sustainable. Those are related to the methods used for Local Responses, to the policies, and to the research.

LIST OF FIGURES AND TABLES

LIST OF APPENDICES

GLOSSARY

Aids	Acquired Immune Deficiency Syndrome
BMZ	Bundesministerium für wirtschaftliche Zusammenarbeit und Entwicklung (Federal Ministry for Economic Cooperation and Development, F.R. Germany)
CBO	Community-Based Organisation
CDC	The Centers for Disease Control
CDD	Control of Diarrhoea Disease
DH(M)T	District Health (Management) Team
DRI	District expanded Response Initiative
EPI	Expanded Program on Immunisation
HAART	Highly Active Anti-Retroviral Therapy
HIV	Human Immunodeficiency Virus
IEC	Information, Education and Communication
FAO	Food and Agriculture Organization
GDP	Gross Development Product
GPA	WHO Global Programme on AIDS
GTZ	Gesellschaft für Technische Zusammenarbeit (German Agency for Technical Cooperation of the BMZ)
KfW	Kreditanstalt für Wiederaufbau (German Financial Cooperation of the BMZ)
L.R.	Local Responses
MoH	Ministry of Health
NACP	National AIDS Control Programme
NGO	Non-Governmental Organisation
PHC	Primary Health Care
PLWHA	People Living with HIV/Aids
PRA	Participatory Rural Appraisal
RRA	Rapid Rural Appraisal
ROR	Rapid Organisational Review
SMC	Social Marketing of Condoms

STD	Sexually Transmitted Diseases
STI	Sexually Transmitted Infections
TB	Tuberculosis
USAID	United Stated Agency for International Development
UNAIDS	Joint United Nations Programme on HIV/AIDS
WHO	World Health Organization
ZOPP	Zielorientierte Projektplanung (Goal-Oriented Project Planning)

ACKNOWLEDGEMENTS

Because of the new development of the Local Responses to HIV/Aids over the past three years, this research has been a collaborative effort of many people. They have been involved at some point with this study, from the design to the implementation and results, and the discussion of future perspectives. To all of them I owe many thanks for their insights and support.

I owe much to Lucy Gilson through her Thesis on "Value for Money: the Efficiency of Primary Health Units in Tanzania" submitted at the Health Policy Unit, London School of Hygiene and Tropical Medicine (August 1992), and shared during my work with the National Institute for Medical Research (NIMR), Tanzania. It inspired the structure of the present systems research thesis.

Ulrich Vogel, Team Leader HIV/AIDS, GTZ Headquarters, and George Dorros, WHO, Department of Organization of Health Services Delivery, and Carol Larivée, Department of Policy, Strategy and Research, UNAIDS, and all their different teams were instrumental in discussing and stimulating some of the approaches and generic framework which inspired this work in early 1997.

In Burkina Faso, particular thanks are given to Ms. Pascaline Sebgo, Reproductive Health Training Co-ordinator, AIDS/IEC, GTZ, Burkina Faso who participated to the situation analyses, and to the entire GTZ Burkina Faso team who provided support for the field studies. For the community situation analysis, the local Non-Governmental Organisation, Population Santé Développement (PSD), Ouagadougou, were instrumental in carrying out the interviews in the local languages and preliminary community data analysis, and I am grateful for their commitment and perseverance in their work. As an on-going action research, the key local partners are too numerous to cite here but I am most grateful to all of them, from the communities to the District of Gaoua, and Poni Province. I am particularly grateful to Ms. Karidia Kyère, Director of Social Affairs, Gaoua, and member of the Gaoua Technical Committee on AIDS who provided me mid-2000 with the latest development of the Gaoua Local Responses in a Technical Meeting on "Measuring Progress of Local Responses to HIV/AIDS" (Mwanza, Tanzania, 5-7 June 2000).

The success story would not have been possible without the careful steering of Dr. Kékoura Kourouma, the national CPA, UNAIDS, Burkina Faso, and the inputs of Dr. Pierre M'Pelé, UNAIDS "country broker" for Gaoua who made the process to move into strategic planning and implementation from mid-1998 to late 1999. I owe them many thanks to all I have learned from them.

Finally, without the overall stimulation from Jean-Louis Lamboray, Local Responses team, the Department of Policy, Strategy and Research, UNAIDS, the Local Responses could not have become a reality for a whole continent, from a mere three years case-study carried out in Gaoua, Burkina Faso. I owe much thanks for his support and stimulus and to his team as well particularly in the last phase of the study.

Many thanks for the advice and constructive support in the last stages of this thesis, to Dr. J. Chabot and Dr. R. Kerkhoven. Particular thanks to Dr. Y.K. Baruani who gave me thorough insights by reading the thesis from the beginning to the end.

Particular thanks to Professor Alexander Krämer, and Professor Ulrich Laaser, and the participants of the International Journal Club, and the International Working Group, of Bielefeld School of Public Health, from various professional and academic background, and who stimulated discussions and encouragement throughout the different stages of this study.

Finally, I thank my wife, Tina, who suffered as much as I did along this ordeal, and supported me on the front line (most of the time) wholeheartedly throughout this long journey. She wishes wholeheartedly as well that I do not push my limits to the "*Habilitation*".

The situation analyses in 1997 were supported by a research grant from the Federal Ministry of Economic Co-operation and Development (BMZ) Bonn, Germany, via the German Technical Co-operation (GTZ) Regional AIDS Programme (RAP) Office, Abidjan, Côte d'Ivoire, as well as the early stages of consensus-building and planning workshop which took place in early 1998. The different stages described afterwards, the implementation and follow-up work from mid-1998 on were financed by UNAIDS. This includes the documentation compiled mid-2000 of the UNAIDS *Best Practice* Collection Case-Study on "Gaoua District Local Responses: The Burkina Faso approach" I am currently writing and summarised in the Results section (Chapter VII).

We hope the present thesis provides a useful documentation of the innovative approach and an encouraging description of a three years process developed by the communities and district, in partnership with their international partners, to tackle the HIV/Aids epidemic in resources poor setting, efforts which are often either undocumented or part of the grey literature only.

Cyril Pervilhac

Bonn, July 2000

PREFACE

This research stems from a team of different actors from UNAIDS, WHO, and GTZ who in 1996 expressed the need to join hands to develop an innovative way to tackle the epidemics at a local level, starting as an entry point with the Districts. This explains the name of origins to this effort called the "District expanded Response Initiative" for the five case-studies in 1997 which were carried out in five different countries in the Africa region, including Burkina-Faso, described in this thesis.

Local Responses have been over the past three years moving along with different political agendas as reflected in its successive titles. It started as the "District expanded Response Initiative" in early 1997. Then it was called "Health Sector Reform and the Expanded Response" (to move away from the idea that the District was were the solution was lying instead of communities) in 1998. The new name became the "Local Response" (but it became clear that there could be multiple solutions or responses) in early 1999, and, finally, in late 1999 and 2000 it became officially the "Local Responses".

The author was involved for several years in the early to mid-eighties as a program manager in the Africa region in Primary Health Care programs, and so-called vertical programs, encompassing interventions related to communicable diseases which can be prevented by immunisation, Diarrhoea diseases, and Malaria control. He co-ordinated several courses in the late eighties to strengthen management at District level summarised in a recent publication (C. Pervilhac, W. Seidel eds. "Training for better District Health Management" Berlin 1996), with the German Foundation for International Development (DSE Berlin), and organised the European Tropical Epidemiology Course held in Berlin (1989). He was further stimulated in the early nineties to carry out health research (systems and bio-medical) in the Ifakara Research Centre, National Institute of Medical Research, as co-ordinator for research activities.

Upon his return, from his journey in Tanzania, the opportunity to embark in the present HIV/Aids research at the district and community levels was a new challenge to put into practice this experience.

Broadly, this research illustrates how new innovative approaches to tackle the HIV/Aids epidemic, under the umbrella of Local Responses, are feasible. They can create hope among communities, partners, and countries that this epidemic will be controlled in the coming decades in the Africa region, just like in North America and Europe.

CHAPTER ONE:
BACKGROUND AND INTRODUCTION

This chapter introduces first the present research (1.1) by reference to the programmatic context set up to respond to the epidemics of HIV reported for the past ten years, particularly since the late 1980s, in the sub-Saharan Africa Region. The recent developments, originating from UNAIDS and WHO in the late 1990s, to test with five country case studies the present innovative "Local Responses"[46] in the context of Health Sector Reform, are then outlined. Burkina Faso where the present research takes place is one of the case study with a process which took place over a three years period and has been documented separately, including the personal contribution (Appendix 1A Chronological Benchmarks of the Local Responses: General and Research Contributions). The chronology illustrates the nature of this study and its process that has been on-going over a three years period (May 1997- June 2000).

The literature review (1.2) provides details about background information to understand the context of the Local Responses. Namely, it reviews first, the Primary Health Care (PHC) approach, including the types of selective and comprehensive programs; second, the health sector reform context; third, the numerous existing HIV/Aids strategies and interventions. The framework of analysis used in the research and in the presentation of findings is then outlined (1.3). Finally, the thesis is outlined briefly (1.4).

1.1 Research background

The Responses to HIV/Aids in the eighties and early nineties
Ten years after the WHO Global Program on Aids was launched, the HIV/Aids multifaceted and devastating pandemic is still disproportionately impacting on the developing world, as reported in an updated situation of each region in the world (Proceedings of the XI International Conference on AIDS, Vancouver, 1996). This picture describes the situation in the year that preceded this research.

The global responses to AIDS through the WHO Global Program on AIDS, (GPA) in the mid-eighties, was described in more details elsewhere (PANOS Dossier 1988). GPA since then has now being disbanded, and in 1996 the Joint United Nations Program on HIV/Aids (UNAIDS) was created. GPA activities

---

[46] Often referred in the study as "Local Responses" or as originally labelled "District Responses Initiative" (DRI) because of the nature of the local responses at the District level

can now be contrasted to the recent UNAIDS 1996 "Expanded Response to HIV/Aids at local level" activities, (UNAIDS 1996), and summarised as follow:

- sensitising the Governments to Aids (GPA) vs. sensitising individuals and communities, (UNAIDS)

- developing national mid-term plans steered by the Ministries of Health vs. implementing planning and management of Aids at the district level across sectors,

- using a top-down approach, with a vertical program, using the health sector alone vs. using a bottom-up approach, with a horizontal program, using multisectoral approaches,

- a centralised vs. a decentralised decision-making process, in the context of sector reforms,

- adapting a short term view, individual centred responses with the hope that drugs and/ or vaccines will be soon available, vs. a long term view, permanent self-financed responses with prevention interventions, emphasising individual and community behaviours risk reduction measures.

These rapid changes of policies and approaches are not fortuitous but driven by the National AIDS programs, and international agencies concern about the sustainability of HIV/Aids prevention and care programs.

The epidemiology, facilitators and impact of HIV/Aids
Reviewing briefly the epidemiology of HIV/Aids justifies why this study focuses in the Africa region, and west Africa sub-region in particular with the particularities of the epidemics in that region. A review of Aids in the developing world can be referred to elsewhere (Silva Saavedra M 1996).

The epidemiology of HIV infection and Aids is complex as described in a typical natural history of adult HIV infection, with the severity of infectivity and clinical manifestations that vary in severity over a decade. The epidemiology, combined with the different natures of transmission, and the poor prognosis for those infected, make the selection of the correct mix of both prevention and care/ support measures difficult to choose or to deliver effectively.

Despite over a decade of combating the HIV/Aids epidemic, the HIV epidemic continues to spread rapidly with limited effects of prevention measures. In addition, the needs for care, support, and impact have been growing dramatically, and are far from being addressed correctly either (Gilks, Floyd et

138

al. 1998). The following epidemiological HIV/Aids data illustrate the extent and impact of the epidemic world wide and then focuses in Africa, and West Africa, and finally, in Burkina Faso where this study is located.

Based on the 1997 epidemiological data when the present study started, the global burden of HIV world wide is evident. At the end of the year, over 30 million people were living with HIV/Aids, about 40% of whom were women, and 10% children. In addition, more than 11 million people had died because of Aids since the beginning of the epidemic, leaving over 8 million Aids orphans[47] (UNAIDS 1997). The more recent report for 1999 estimates that 18.8 million people around the world have died of AIDS, 3.8 million of them children. Nearly twice that many -34.3 million- are now living with HIV, almost three fourths of those (71%) in sub-Saharan Africa. (UNAIDS 2000). These huge numbers are difficult to grasp in terms of their magnitude, but the 4.0 million of new infections in the Africa region during 1999 represents half a million more than the whole population of Berlin infected yearly, and little over the whole population of the former German Democratic Republic states wiped out in less than twenty years!

As pinpointed in this report, the increasing number of new infections every year provokes an acceleration effect of long-standing epidemics: *„as the rate of HIV infection in the general population rises, the same patterns of sexual risk result in more new infections simply because the chances of encountering an infected partner become higher"* (op. cit. p. 8). The proportion is expected to continue to rise in theses countries *„where poverty, poor health systems and limited resources for prevention and care fuel the spread of the virus"* (MAP (Monitoring the AIDS Pandemic Network) 2000).

Specific major facilitators of the heterosexual HIV epidemic in sub-Saharan Africa have been identified as:

- *"Ignorance of the population,*
- *Poverty including poor health care systems and facilities,*
- *Low socio-economic status especially of women compared to men,*
- *Social demographic and cultural conditions in communities with predominance of one sex such as in the military, migratory work such as in mines, fishing villages and among long distance truck drivers...,*

---

[47] defined as HIV-negative children who lost their mother or both parents to AIDS when they were under the age of 15

- *Highly prevalent infections including sexually transmitted diseases and tuberculosis which facilitate HIV transmission and/ or increase replication of HIV...,*
- *Biological necessity of heterosexual intercourse for procreation,*
- *Mystification of sexuality and denial of existence of sexual life among youths and adolescents..."* (Mhalu 2000).

The infection rates in young African women are far higher than those in young men. The victims are largely women and children. Women because the epidemiology of HIV/Aids in women, combined with socio-economic and political factors, increase their risk (Bererr and Ray 1993). Children as well with "Aids being foremost a disease of the young", because the combination of poor nutrition, poor health services, and widespread infectious diseases make children particularly vulnerable (UNAIDS 1997). In 1997, it was estimated that 5.8 million people were newly infected, and 2.3 million had died with AIDS (UNAIDS 1997). In the year of the present study, the 1997 World AIDS Campaign aimed to "children living in a world of Aids."

Projections into decades ahead further justify both immediate and future action. In 1990, HIV ranked twenty-eighth only among the disease burden measured in Disability-Adjusted Life Years (DALYs), but will move to rank tenth in 2020 (Murray and Lopez 1996). If HIV was still a minor cause of deaths from infectious diseases among adults in the developing world (8.6%) in 1990, it will account for over one third (37.1%) of the share in 2020 (The World Bank 1997).

The overwhelming majority of HIV-infected people -about 95%- live in the developing world, and most of these do not know that they are infected. The incidence of HIV infection in poorer countries (750 per 100,000 people) is more than ten times that of industrial countries. Sub-Saharan Africa is one of the region in the world with the poorest population as documented in the Human Poverty Index (HPI)[48] ranking for developing countries. Poverty offers a fertile breeding ground for the epidemic's spread, which sets off in turn a cascade of economic and social disintegration and impoverishment (UNDP 1997).

In sub-Saharan Africa, the epidemic due mainly to heterosexual transmission has already reached in 1997 an unprecedented high level of 7.4% adult prevalence rate.[49] New infections are thought to be levelling off in that region as

---

[48] composite index of three essential dimensions of human life: longevity (vulnerability to death at a relatively early age), knowledge (illiteracy) and a decent standard of living (access to safe water, to health services, and moderately and severely underweight children under five).

[49] the proportion of adults living with HIV/ AIDS in the adult population (15 to 49 years of age)

a whole, but military conflict epidemic and civil unrest may be spreading the epidemic further in some sub-regions (The World Bank 1997). Different or "interwoven" (Piot P. et al. 1990) epidemics take place in that region of the world which are spread unevenly with its own distinct characteristics that depend on geography, the specific populations affected (e.g. mobility, societal factors), the frequencies of risk behaviours and practices, and the temporal introduction of the virus. In addition, biological factors such as the presence of Sexually Transmitted Diseases (STDs), of Tuberculosis (TB), male circumcision, and the viral characteristics of both HIV-1 and HIV-2,[50] may influence the spread of the epidemic by increasing or decreasing the susceptibility to the virus, altering the infectiousness of those with HIV, and hastening the progression of infection to disease and death (Cohen and Trussell 1996).

For the West Africa sub-region, the most recent UNAIDS report notes that while it is relatively less affected by the HIV infection than East or South Africa, the prevalence rates in some large countries such as Côte d'Ivoire, or Nigeria, are creeping up. In Burkina Faso, a relatively small country in comparison to those, the estimated HIV prevalence rate in young people (15-24) ranged for females between the low and high estimates of 4.07 to 7.51, and for males of 1.28 to 3.33 (UNAIDS 2000). Prevalence estimates in Gaoua District fall in the higher range.

Infant and child mortality is in turn increasing, and consequently reversing gains in infant and child survival gained over the past twenty years. By the year 2010, if the spread of HIV is not contained, Aids may increase infant mortality by as much as 75% and under-five mortality by more than 100% in worst-affected sub-Saharan regions (UNAIDS 1997). The devastating impact of Aids has been well documented elsewhere (Carael and Schwartlander 1998). The victims are predominantly the very poorest, particularly exposed because of the lack of education, information and access to social and health services (UNDP 1997).

Burkina Faso is one among four countries in West Africa (Côte d'Ivoire, Benin and Guinea-Bissau) with a generalised epidemic[51] located mostly in eastern and southern Africa, and concerning approximately half of the countries in the Africa region. Another approximately half of the countries in sub-Saharan

---

[50] HIV-2 is primarily found in west Africa (with the likelihood of transmission of HIV-1 through heterosexual intercourse to be estimated to be about 3 times higher per exposure than for HIV-2, and significant lower perinatal transmission rates of HIV-2 (4%), in comparison to HIV-1 (25-35%) (AIDSCAP, The Francois Xavier Bagnoud Center for Health and Human Rights of the Harvard School of Public Health et al. 1996)
[51] generalised epidemic: prevalence among women attending urban ante-natal clinics is 5% or more; HIV has spread far beyond the original sub-populations with high-risk behaviour, which are now heavily infected

Africa suffer from a concentrated epidemic,[52] and half a dozen from a nascent epidemic[53] (The World Bank 1997). Life expectancy at birth, a common indicator of the health and well-being of a population, has taken a major blow in many countries. In Burkina Faso, life expectancy is now a mere 46 years, or 11 years shorter than it would have been in the absence of Aids (The World Bank 1997). In 2010, the projections put life expectancy at 35 years (UNDP 1997).

Arguments for a research on Local Responses to HIV/Aids

Five key arguments justify a need for research such as the present Local Responses[54] in Sub-Saharan Africa, as outlined next.

First, the unequal regional distribution of the pandemic in sub-Saharan Africa, or disproportionate epidemics, as just described, explains why prevention efforts are being concentrated in that region of the world. The testing of the Local Responses in Burkina Faso is one of the five case study countries[55] selected for this research. The total financial support of global efforts is nevertheless dismal in comparison to the needs. In the third world where 90 percent of the HIV infected live, the countries receive less than 10 percent of finances for prevention and care; prevention programs must be considerably expanded to contain the spread of HIV (Mann and Tarantola 1998).

Second, besides these epidemiological arguments justifying immediate action in the sub-Saharan region, national prevention programs have been less successful than at first hoped, using traditional health education about HIV/Aids to induce widespread behaviour change (Cohen and Trussell 1996). Despite large increase of knowledge of the HIV infection and its causes, positive changes in sexual behaviours are still lagging behind.

A number of interrelated factors affects the final choices of people: their perception of how HIV infection would affect them personally and of how much their own behaviour is risky, the skills they have to negotiate safer behaviours with partners, and the social environment enabling or constraining behaviour (The World Bank 1997).

---

[52] prevalence among women attending urban ante-natal clinics is still less than 5%. HIV prevalence has surpassed 5% in one or more sub-populations presumed to practice high-risk behaviour
[53] HIV prevalence is less than 5% in all known sub-populations presumed to practice high-risk behaviour for which information is available
[54] the local responses carried out originally in 1997-98 in 5 countries in Africa was labelled the District expanded Responses Initiative (DRI) due to its administrative and geographical location, district-based
[55] Zambia, Tanzania, Ghana, Uganda, and Burkina-Faso

Third, HIV/Aids is having a tremendous negative impact on the agricultural production among populations who are for the majority living of this essential sector (up to 90% in most of the countries). This affects the nutrition, survival, and means of earning an income for households in that region of the world. Experts in agriculture (Sayagues 1999) draw attention to the rain-fed, maize-based cropping systems of West and Southern Africa where Aids spells a disaster. If terminal sickness and burial coincide with certain tasks like weeding and harvesting, the crop is compromised. Some solutions to cope with the impact of Aids on rural situation is to introduce in small-holder agriculture farming techniques that require less labour, such as zero tillage, and less expensive inputs, including natural pest control (Mutangadura, Jackson et al. 1999). In addition, high direct costs for taking care of patients and high indirect costs on the loss of labour and impact on families are well-documented in recent studies of the agricultural sector in West Africa (Baier 1997; FAO 1997; FAO 1997), and case-studies in various countries of the Africa region (Topouzis and Guerny 1999). Estimates of the direct cost of the disease in Africa, or lifetime costs per patient for medical care, vary widely from US $ 64 to US $ 11,800. The indirect costs to families are huge with AIDS killing people in their most productive years, leaving behind multiple dependants (Cohen and Trussell 1996).

Fourth, following the original first decade and strong support of external agencies to give financial support and technical guidance to newly created national AIDS control program in Africa, the approach of the late nineties is changing to a bottom-up one. The present research is therefore grounded and directed from the communities and District levels to the national level. As documented in the present research, the countries and their international partners are still lagging behind in understanding and mastering tools to expand the Responses at the local level, a much more daunting and challenging task than to produce a sound national plan.[56]

Fifth, the HIV/Aids epidemic is placing a heavy toll on health services that are already suffering from a lack of human or material resources. Health sector reforms, a key element to the Local Responses, are attempting not only to increase the efficiency use of resources and produce more effective health care (Gilks, Floyd et al. 1998), but to increase the effectiveness of preventive health as well.

---

[56] countries follow short- and medium-term plans to fight the epidemic

Current global country and institution strategies and the responses

Official publications draw heavily as an example for the way forward to respond to the HIV/Aids pandemic upon the successes of the activities in Thailand and Uganda. In addition, Botswana and China have been given as examples of countries that have successfully begun to expand their responses beyond the health sector (Piot 1997). The political leadership, empowering communities, mobilising employers, and addressing socio-economic issues were, beyond the medical field, developmental approaches instrumental in decreasing the rates of infection by avoiding high-risk behaviours (Cohen and Trussell 1996). Unfortunately, the experience of Uganda in stabilising its epidemic trends is still documented in a piecemeal fashion and does not allow to identify the exact causes of this success. In contrast, Thailand benefits from a comprehensive set of unpublished (Tanbanjong, Piyanat et al. 1998) and recently published data (UNAIDS 1998) (UNAIDS 2000) which have already been used extensively[57] to document in a convincing way to different audiences the origins and justifications of the Local Responses. It was in particular used to introduce and stimulate the discussion about the Local Responses during the Pre-Planning and Consensus Workshop (Section 4.3.1) held in March 1998 (Appendix 1A).

"Expanding the global responses to HIV/Aids through focused action Reducing risk and vulnerability: definitions, rationale and pathways" (UNAIDS 1998) which was published following the first year of the present research constitutes the core philosophy and principles of the Local Responses. It was adapted and used to give the rationale and clarify the nature of the present study on several occasions.[58] This conceptual framework, used for the sake of our research as the general definition of the Local Responses suggests pathways to take action to combat the complex epidemic with a multi-dimensional and dynamic responses encompassing:

- the improvement of the quality and scope of short and long-term risk reduction strategies, and addressing vulnerability factors
- the expansion of the partnerships (public and private sectors, including communities) in the design, implementation and evaluation of HIV/Aids related policies and programmes
- the increase in the population coverage geographically, and for the under-serviced communities both in urban and rural areas, women and men in most vulnerable age groups, marginalised populations, and mobile populations

---

[57] J.L. Lamboray's presentations: Technical Workshop (Dar-es-Salaam, May 1998), Health Reform and HIV Workshop (Geneva, June 1998), Health Sector Reform and the Expanded Responses (Eschborn, January 1999)
[58] C. Pervilhac's presentations: Consensus and Planning Workshop (Gaoua, March 1998), and DRI Meeting, GTZ RAP (Accra, March 1998) and Health Reform and HIV Workshop (Geneva, June 1998)

- the involvement of all relevant socio-economic development actors, integrating HIV/Aids prevention and care in other human development initiatives (poverty alleviation, Agriculture, Education sectors etc.)
- the mobilisation of resources (human, institutional, financial) at all levels (local, national and international)
- the enhancement of the sustainability of HIV/Aids programs by strengthening the local and national self-reliance in the design and implementation phases.

As a common denominator to expand the responses, the following three key principles are underlined: the analysis of risk and vulnerability factors for focused strategies, the expansion of the quality and scope of HIV/ AIDS strategies, the enhancement of the responses to include those strategies addressing vulnerability through short-and long-term measures (reaching vulnerable populations, complementing and reinforcing interventions and services, introducing evidence-based strategies).

The present approach recommended to combat HIV/Aids fits narrowly and overlaps the recent WHO Jakarta Declaration on health promotion which identified the need for:

"new responses" with *"new and diverse networks to achieve inter-sectoral collaboration..."* in order to *"unlock the potential for health promotion inherent in many sectors of society, among local communities, and within families. There is a clear need to break through traditional boundaries within government sectors, between governmental and non-governmental organisations, and between the public and private sectors. Co-operation is essential. This requires the creation of partnerships for health on an equal footing, between the different sectors of governance in societies."* (WHO/ HRP/ HEP/41 CHP/BR/97.4)

The Local Responses within UNAIDS Department of Policy, Strategy and Research

The Local Responses to HIV/AIDS was defined recently by UNAIDS/PSR as:

> „As people's decisions in their private lives determine the final outcome of the battle against AIDS, the response is primarily local. With local we mean: involving people where they live –their homes, neighbourhoods and work places... Since there are limits to what people can do on their own, there is a need for local partnerships (between service providers, key social groups, and facilitators/ catalysts)...The local responses approach uses a four-pronged approach: the first is human resource and systems development... the second is policy development... the third is mobilisation of local and external resources... the fourth is learning from action and interaction between stakeholders..."

The "Local Responses to HIV/AIDS: The Global Agenda" (Key Note June 2000), accompanied by the "Strategic approach towards an AIDS-competent society" (Technical Note Number 1) were recently issued from the Local Responses team from UNAIDS Department of Policy, Strategy and Research (Appendix 1B). They summarise in more details successively the recent concept of Local Responses, and the nine steps recommended in order to implement the approach.

The Local Responses: a personal view

The present research, or the development of successful responses, needs to overcome the dual challenge best illustrated and compared with the following piece of modern art exhibited in a gallery: *The cough syrup transport system* [59] (Fig. 1.1).

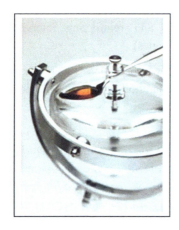

Fig. 1.1 *Cough Syrup Transport System*, 1998

Andreas Slominski, Deutsche Guggenheim Berlin

In order to deliver prevention and care strategies effectively (with the spoon), we are attempting here to develop the best mix of an ingredient, the "syrup," which looks simple in its composition and balance but is not. In addition, we need further to adapt or create a simple and appropriate technologies or tools for an expanded responses, the "transport system" or Local Responses, in order to improve our understanding of the environment and be able to deliver these strategies effectively. The "transport system" (tools and technologies) is still

---

[59] Andreas Slominski, 1998, Detail of the exhibit, at the Deutsche Guggenheim Berlin (20. Feb.-9. Mai 1999)

disproportionately complicated and awkward, or inefficient in the preliminary stages of this research process, in comparison to the 'syrup" (better known and tested strategies).

1.2 HIV/Aids Programme in the Field and Local Responses

To understand better the context in which the Local Responses are striving, it is important to have an understanding of the field in which those are taking place. A review of relevant literature aims to give the necessary background information to understand on what this approach is based and the difficulties of implementation.

First, the Primary Health Care (PHC) District Approach to Program Delivery clarifies the PHC philosophy and the importance of focusing on the local or district level. The issues of comprehensive and selective approaches are revisited, and explain in turn how much the local responses match the original comprehensive PHC approach.

Second, we explain in turn what is the Health Sector Reform and how it can benefit the local responses, and reciprocally how the local responses can benefit the implementation of a successful reform.

Third, in order to have the local responses succeed, strategies and interventions need to be pursued which are reviewed in this section, as well as the issue of focused interventions. In

complement to these three points, throughout the review specific references are made about the present development of the Local Responses approach as well which supports the evidence of a field in full expansion.[60]

1.2.1 Primary Health Care District Approach and Local Responses

The World Health Organization conference held in Alma-Ata in 1978 has been the main governing force in the policies of countries related to delivering comprehensive health care, and was formulated originally as the following goal, with the eight components:

> "the attainment by all people of the world by the year 2000 of a
> level of health that will permit them to lead a socially and
> economically productive life. Primary health care includes at least:

---

[60] At least half of the references of the literature review are dating from the year of the research, i.e. 1997, or more recent

[61] *education concerning prevailing health problems and the methods of preventing and controlling them; promotion of food supply and proper nutrition, an adequate supply of safe water and basic sanitation; maternal and child health care, including family planning; immunization against major infectious diseases; prevention and control of locally endemic diseases; appropriate treatment of common diseases and injuries; and provision of essential drugs" (WHO 1978).*

Twenty years later, following the failures and lessons learnt from PHC, some of the original concerns brought up by experts in the field are still valid: more attention should be paid to the support of village health workers and their training and financial incentives instead of hasty, large, and non-sustainable coverage[62] (Chabot 1984). The Local Responses and Health Sector Reform can be seen as a revisit or a second birth of the Primary Health Care (PHC) approach applied to HIV/Aids. This is reflected in a closer analysis of the PHC concept based on the following Primary Health Care (PHC) definition. The Local Responses approach overlaps and fits well into the PHC principles based on the concepts stated next of equity and services to more at risks or vulnerable groups, of community participation, of prevention and promotion aspects, of technology, and of poverty alleviation:

"... the PHC approach advocates the provision of front-line, first contact services within the framework of the five principles of:

a) health services must be more equally accessible, not neglecting rural and isolated populations or peri-urban dwellers,

b) active participation by the community in their own health decisions is essential,

c) preventive and promotive services rather than curative services should be the focus of health care,

d) the methods and materials used in the health system should be acceptable and relevant, appropriate technology -not synonymous with primitive or poor technology,

---

[61] Next, the 8 PHC components
[62] the polemic on the strategies and approaches used to carry out PHC schemes should not be underestimated: WHO rejected the publication of this open critique of PHC implementation which was submitted and accepted in The Lancet (personal communication with the author, June 1999)

e) health must be seen as only part of total care -nutrition, education, water supplies and shelter are also all essential minimum requirements to well-being"(Walt and Vaughan 1981).

In the late eighties, these PHC principles and the rationale for comprehensiveness were reformulated and acknowledged (Grodos and Xavier de Bethune 1988) as an attempt for PHC to give a 'global' responses to health problems (beyond the strict medical aim to address the ambitious social aim as well), and address issues related to equity, participation, and cost effectiveness. The authors identified four levels that drove the PHC implementation which match in turn the local responses approach as well:

- first, a level of care close to and accessible by the communities and the District level;
- second, an action program for the eight PHC components[63] based on the communities' needs and demands, the populations at risks, and responses to those;
- third, a strategy of organisation of services (hospitals, community participation…) with scientific literature pointing to the need for integrating family planning, STD, and Aids (Ching-Bunge 1995) (Stein 1996) , and of the need for intersectoral collaboration with challenges to overcome the numerous and complex constraints to work within the health sector between programs (Mayhew 1996). The "Ten steps towards an integrated district health system" (WHO 1996) support in details the pathways of the local responses described earlier (1.1) explaining in turn how the local responses for HIV/Aids can tackle the issues of integration of health care delivery. The discovery of the potential roles of other sectors in responses to HIV/Aids such as agriculture (FAO 1997) (Baier 1997) (Hemrich G. et al. 1997), and education (Oulai D. et al. 1993) are only recent developments. Consequently, the methods to analyse and involve these various sectors still need to be more elaborated upon.
- fourth, a general philosophy of the health system (local responsibilities, other development priorities, equity, global health and socio-economic-cultural environment).

---

[63] Ref. above PHC Alta-Ata proceedings

Why the District or local Level?

The operational level of responses and focus at the district level, rather than the regional or national level, on which the local responses is based, comes from its recognition as *"the key level for the management of primary health care (PHC)... It is the most peripheral unit of local government and administration that has comprehensive powers and responsibilities"* (Vaughan and Morrow 1989). The local politicians and civil servants of the government sectors are co-ordinated and linked at the most peripheral administrative level in the District (Mills 1994). This justifies further the focus for the local responses at the District and community levels, the pillar of the PHC approach, in the present democratisation process and empowerment of the local authorities, and civil society. This explains the numerous efforts to work in the eighties and nineties to strengthen that level of the health systems, and to invest into district human resources training as well, despite the known limitations (Pervilhac and Seidel 1995) (Pervilhac 1998). HIV Prevention and AIDS care in Africa. A District Level Approach (Ng'weshemi, Boerma et al. 1997) documents practical issues and approaches for district managers related to organisation, monitoring, behavioural interventions, health interventions, and financing at that critical level of the health care system.

In addition, district health services have recently become the focus for initiating new ways of working and moving toward a "sector-wide approach..." At this level, the "dialogue between governments and donors shifts up a level, from the planning and management of projects, to the overall policy, institutional, and financial framework within which health care is provided" (Cassels A. et al. 1998).

Which specific approach to use to fulfil the PHC goal?

Two schools of thoughts, with opposite views on which approach to pursue, have fuelled an extensive debate and created clashes in the eighties, as documented in a comprehensive and provocative issue of Social Science and Medicine on "Selective or Comprehensive Primary Health Care?" (Rifkin and Walt 1988). The issue of comprehensive vs. vertical approaches for PHC has had repercussions on the origins, present approach, support, and future of large public health programs in the nineties, including the present local responses to combat HIV/Aids.

In 1985, in Antwerp, some leading scientists took a stand against selective care (Barker and Turshen 1986). The dispute originated largely from two different programmatic experiences and views: first, the failure of the Malaria Eradication program which triggered indirectly PHC and a comprehensive approach one hand (Newell 1988). Second, the success of the Smallpox eradication in 1977 combined with other factors (believes in effective and cost-efficient medical interventions, and scarce resources due to the economic crisis which accentuated in the early eighties) led, on the other hand, towards a selective approach to PHC which has been largely supported (Walsh and Warren 1979; Walsh 1988) (Warren 1988) (Warren 1988). It was justified on the following basis:

> *The PHC approach is too idealistic to be implemented by most governments. Instead it was more realistic to target scarce resources to control specific diseases which accounted for the highest mortality and morbidity; which had available low cost technologies for prevention and treatment; and which had techniques that were cost-effective. This approach was called the selective Primary Health Care*" (Rifkin and Walt 1988).

The latter selective approach was mainly driven by international agencies (the Rockefeller Foundation, the World Bank,[64] UNICEF[65], USAID, CDC[66]...), and critical reviews of methods and results have been largely documented elsewhere (Unger and Killingsworth 1986; Newell 1988) (Wisner 1988). The Burkina Faso "vaccination commandos" of the mid-eighties were used as a model of successful top-down approach only ten years ago,[67] and contrasts with the present local responses bottom-up approach. This may explain why at the community level some of the old "sages" (older key informants) in our study still pointed to and expected an outside intervention to tackle the Aids problem. Even within WHO, "Selected Primary Health Care Interventions" (WHO 1980) were discussed in the early eighties among different programs. Vertical programs are the epitome of selective programs; Yaws, Dracunculiasis, and Measles were considered nevertheless to become part of "the eradication in the context of Primary Health Care" in the mid-eighties already (Taylor 1987). D. A. Henderson, an internationally known public health figure, has led as a Director the WHO's successful campaign to eradicate Smallpox; he is still up to

---

[64] Basic Package

[65] GOBI-FFF focused on Growth chart, Oral rehydration, Breast-feeding, Immunization- Family planning, Food supplementation, Female status (promotion)

[66] USAID/ CDC CCCD-ACSI focused on the Combating Childhood Communicable Diseases-African Child Survival Initiative with Immunisation, Diarrhoeal Diseases, and Malaria (the author launched this program as a Technical Officer for CDC Atlanta in Burundi in the mid-eighties)

[67] the researcher was a guest of UNICEF Burkina Faso in the mid-eighties to learn from that model

151

today recognised for his work.[68] This program has influenced up to the turn of the century in turn indirectly international policies, and continues to stimulate the eradication programs, for example Poliomyelitis by year 2000, or Dracunculiasis (or Guinea Worm), or Onchocerciasis.

The original program thrust to combat Aids from the mid-eighties to the mid-nineties was largely driven by the WHO Global *l* Program on AIDS (GPA) which was characterised by a selective approach, although never referred to as such. It aimed to respond to a much feared and unknown epidemic with large resources, world-wide and quickly. It was largely centrally-driven, vertical, top-down, health sector exclusive,[69] and relied essentially on the reduction in risk-taking behaviour through targeting individuals and groups, as the single spearheading strategy. HIV/Aids interventions as vertical and top-down "selective" programs have shown their limitations over a decade after the inception of the Global Aids Strategy (UNAIDS 1998), as mentioned in more details previously (ref. Section 1.1).

The present UNAIDS mandate that started in 1996 states *"the need for a broader/based, expanded responses to the epidemic in sectors ranging from health to economic development... (because) AIDS is not simply a health crisis, but a social and economic crisis..."* *(UNAIDS 1998)* In contrast to the past GPA, the present local responses is locally-driven (district and communities), horizontal, bottom-up, multi-sectoral, and uses a mix of prevention and care and support strategies (ref. next para.) to combat HIV/Aids.

The local responses joins therefore the present trends of the majority of health care programs moving into horizontal and bottom-up "comprehensive" approaches, in the original spirit of PHC.

In addition, the interaction of the HIV infection with other diseases (e.g. STD and TB) necessitates integration at the operational levels, and not independent programs.

With the clearer picture in mind of the larger public health context in which the local responses is grounded and evolving, the forces playing for and against the local responses become more visible. Senior decision-makers and policy-makers have their positions and views that automatically bias their choices either in

---

[68] the researcher attended D.A. Henderson's lecture on "Bioterrorism: Myths and Realities" (current issue of the destruction of all Smallpox virus stocks or not) for the Frank A. Calderone Medal and Award which Henderson received at The Joseph L. Mailman School of Public Health Columbia University, New York, on April 5, 1999
[69] the central National AIDS Programs (NAP) of the Ministries of Health were powerful, often independent sections from the MOH, with large financial and human resources. They were driven by Strategic or Medium Term Plans (MTP).

favour of the local responses or make them hesitant to join the new band. The younger generations of program managers operating in the field are often unaware of the obscure forces at work and do not master the full picture of that complex game.

In conclusion, the local responses approach, overlapping so closely with the PHC and comprehensive approaches, makes it an attractive and praiseworthy agenda. But it can quickly meet some of its limitations as well: too broad, too ambitious, too vague, insufficient tools, in danger of being "recuperated" by some of the failures (Taylor 1987) of PHC schemes (e.g. revamping the old PHC village health workers schemes), functioning beyond the mandate of the health sector therefore, out of control. As a consequence, the local responses may not be such an appealing approach for donors and agencies to control HIV/Aids, particularly after the present unachieved original goal formulated twenty years ago by WHO of *"Health for All by the Year 2000."* In addition, the policy-makers and program managers who come from the selective approach thinking may by default avoid to become involved and be trapped into the local responses. They will prefer to concentrate instead on a few strategies, even if not perfect, particularly in the case of HIV and Aids which already suffer from having so many strategies and interventions (ref. Section 1.2.3), with clearer outputs.

1.2.2 Health Sector Reform and Local Responses

The "Local Responses and Health Sector Reform" was labelled originally in 1997 without even any mention of "Health Sector Reform." The rationale for the approach, though, did mention "sector reforms" among different justifications for the Local Responses multi country case studies. The original generic framework encompassed the need to improve the understanding at the district level of existing structures, both governmental and civil society, and the current trends in public sector reform. Policy tools and approaches were recommended to be used in the situation analysis to that effect.

Health Sector Reform has gained more weight with time in playing a central role to the local responses process with the turning point being the "Health Reform and HIV Workshop: an Agenda for Health Reform and HIV" (Geneva, June 1998). The importance for the UNAIDS partners and cosponsors, particularly the World Bank with early discussion and an important agenda on Health Sector Reform (The World Bank 1993), explains in part this recent emphasis. More central to this refocus, and towards contributing to a successful responses, may be the key importance of political leadership and local partnerships, combined with the effective organisation of health-care provision.

Although often health professionals do not like, in general, to mingle into policies and politics, Health Sector Reform needs, nevertheless, to be perceived by these actors as one of the important enabling structural factors to succeed in expanding the Responses to HIV/Aids. Additionally, one of the lessons learnt from Primary Health Care is that implementing program activities do not fall into a vacuum and that the institutional context in which those take place can either facilitate the success of plans, or constrain those.

We reviewed two essential background materials on "Health Sector Reform: Key Issues in Less Developed Countries" (Cassels 1995) and "Health Sector Reform" in a recent Occasional Paper (Gilks, Floyd et al. 1998). Those were instrumental to help us next to clarify the important questions related to the rationale of the Health Sector Reform, the content and benefits, the tools used, and limitations of the Health Sector Reform.

Why Health Sector Reform?

This has been summarised for and formulated to the various partners under the question: *"Do Health Reforms pass the HIV test?"* [70] In other words, is Health Sector Reform setting an environment which enables the development of effective HIV/ Aids strategies and consequent positive outputs, or not?

Institutional or structural changes of the Health Sector Reform address the necessary organisational structures and management systems improvements that allow strategies to be effective.

Recently, a call was made to have the *"advocates of health reforms... to consider carefully HIV/Aids especially in high-prevalence regions,*[71] (Gilks, Floyd et al. 1998), to resolve important pending issues, for example:[72]

how to link HIV-prevention activities to care and support in ways that promote prevention?

---

[70] J. L. Lamboray's "Health Reform and HIV" presentations, Geneva, June 1998, and Eschborn, January 1999
[71] Gaoua District where the case study took place is of high prevalence
[72] adapted from Gilks et al.

- what is the role of the private sector?
- what are the health staff's attitudes towards HIV and how does it affect the efficiency of services?
- how can district health teams focus efforts on improving quality, efficiency and equity of services for HIV/Aids with scarce resources?
- what are the new needs due to the additional burden that HIV places upon health-service infrastructures (drugs, beds, well-trained and experienced staff for in- and outreach-services)?

The reasons why programs or interventions must go in hand with health sector reforms were crystallised recently in the current state of advances and challenges of HIV Prevention. The answer for success of HIV prevention be it in the richer countries of the North, or the "resource-poor environments of the South" lies in "...*implementing the right combination of interventions and policy initiatives at the correct time*" (Piot 1998) based on evidence from Uganda, Senegal, Tanzania and Thailand.

What is Health Sector Reform and what are the benefits?

"*Health sector reform is concerned with defining priorities, refining policies and reforming the institutions through which those policies are implemented*" (Janovsky 1996). The original definition of health sector reform identified it as a "*sustained process of fundamental change in policy and institutional arrangements, guided by government, designed to improve the functioning and performance of the health sector and ultimately the health status of the population*" (WHO 1995). This major change is often perceived as a threat to the main actors, and can in turn be a factor of resistance to the implementation of reform. We argue, as a possible other facet of the way policies are implemented as well (Walt 1994), that Health Sector Reform appears to be more of a gradual, or incremental or evolutionary process. This coincides with the etymology of "reform",[73] even if the final result of Health Sector Reform may be a fundamental change. The reforms take place over a long period of time through sustained processes instead of a one-off brutal and quick change. Despite the original definition of reforms guided by governments, those are often pushed from the outside, hence creating some scepticism and resistance on the part of the local providers.

---

[73] *re*- again + *formare*- to form: to form again, to restore to a better condition

"*Health Sector Reform is a political process, and recent experience in Europe and North America give evidence that health reform is a highly political and fiercely contested process*" (Cassels 1995). It will never be in everyone's interest and cannot be advanced by technical analysis alone. Stakeholders either on the providers (those involved in service delivery) or purchasers (those concerned about using the service) of health care, all have different interests which need to be determined (Gilks, Floyd et al. 1998), and taken into consideration.

Cassels identifies the reforms of institutions in the health sector to be central to the process of health sector reform, based primarily on practical experiences rather than research. However, it is "*a means to an and, and it is necessary to keep sight of the policy objectives -improved efficiency, equity, more responsive services and, ultimately, better health outcomes, that institutional reforms is designed to achieve*" (Cassels 1995).

It aims to improve the functioning of public bureaucracies, and often in parallel with, and sometimes in responses to, other aspects of institutional reform, such as increasing the role of private providers and increasing the autonomy of provider institutions (Cassels 1995). Ultimately, health reforms aim "*to improve the quality and effectiveness of the services delivered*" (Gilks, Floyd et al. 1998).

The components of health sector reforms programs that are applicable for the local responses are the following:[74]

- improving the performance of the civil service (public sector)
- decentralization
- improving the functioning of the local ministries of health and their links with regional and national levels, including integrated planning and execution
- introducing health financing schemes and broadening the options
- improved partnership between the public and private sectors
- comprehensive plan for HIV/Aids in responses to local needs which integrates the
  prevention and care services.

---

[74] adapted from Cassels and Gilks et al.

The present research was stronger in analysing the last two points issues than the others due to the priorities of the research which needed to focus on partnerships, and plans for action, combined with the fact that the other issues had in turn been studied already earlier in details (Foltz A.-M. et al. 1996). The focus in the present case study is more on the health care systems reform and not so much on health reform in the general sense.

Frenk identifies four levels of the health reform process: systemic with equity issues, programmatic with efficiency and cost-effective issues, organisational with productivity and quality issues, and instrumental with information for action (Frenk 1994).

In summary, the aim of Health Sector Reform is broad and complex, and can be interpreted quite differently depending of the people involved or institutions mandating the work. It needs time to bring about changes. The political nature of the process can make it a difficult venture to embark upon or succeed into. Finally, the scope of assessment and execution necessitate different background and expertise.

What are the tools for Health Sector Reform?
"The process of reform and difficulty of implementing policy and institutional change has been relatively neglected in comparison to the debate about the content of the reform." (Walt and Gilson 1994)

The present status of development of tools for the health sector reform suffers from a number of caveats as identified by Cassels: *"The development of policy and institutional analysis in the health sector lags far behind epidemiological, demographic and economic research. There is no consistently-applied, universal package of measures that constitutes health sector reform"* (Cassels 1995).

"There is limited experience in monitoring institutional change as compared, say, to looking at health outcomes in categorical disease control programs." For example projects seldom have any indicators related to health sector reforms in their planning by objectives frameworks, or any baseline related to this area. Medical planners or epidemiologists are ill-prepared for this task. In addition, *"there is a need for the development of methods which will enable planners to analyze the effects of different approaches to policy and institutional change, as well as to develop better systems and methods for monitoring policy implementation."*

A closer look to the case of the "Decentralization and Health Systems Change: Burkina Faso Case Study" (Foltz A.-M. et al. 1996), based on an original framework to analyse decentralisation and health systems change (WHO 1995), illustrates the complexity of such an approach, far from being a tool which can be replicated by a non-policy specialist. The policy environment found in Burkina Faso is analysed separately (para. 4.2.3).

The various local responses case studies experienced the conceptual and methodological weaknesses with wide interpretations about how to go about assessing Health Sector Reform in each country studied, and with one of the best analysis coming from the most knowledgeable group in the subject.[75] Donors and agencies, including program managers that are under pressure to show results and outputs are obviously hesitant to embark on such an agenda with the present incomplete and status of the tool development still in the experimental stages.

What are the barriers to and limitations of the Health Sector Reform?

Donor agencies express reluctance to support governments *"to address systemic as opposed to programmatic issues"* (Cassels 1995). The reasons vary widely: by lack of clear objectives, because of the complexity of the issues, by lack of tools or expertise. In addition, other reasons are: the limited opportunities to implement changes due to weak stability of systems of governance, the limited political support for fundamental change, the preferred investment in safer private partners (Non-Governmental Organisations, community organisations...).

In addition, Health Sector Reform is often equated to address a *"particular set of prescriptions"* (Cassels 1995) only based on the donors' interests and priorities, or the biases of the expertise (such as user charges, reducing the size of the public sector, cost-effective packages of services and privatization).

The health sector is often isolated to the overall process of decentralisation, as identified recently (Gilks, Floyd et al. 1998) --one of the last bastion of decentralisation in the country administration-- and lacks either the management capacity or political support to direct the process. In the short term, performance may well deteriorate because the capacity to manage, rather than simply administer health care is not widely available. *"There is not yet any clear direct evidence that health reforms lead to better health services. However, successful*

---

[75] Ghana DRI Case study, JSA Consultants Ltd.

efforts to improve the quality and efficiency of services, especially those for HIV-related diseases, will benefit all users" (Gilks, Floyd et al. 1998).

Some of the more pertinent issues in which health sector reforms still need to prove whether it can meet the challenge of HIV/Aids are related to (Gilks, Floyd et al. 1998): the integration of HIV/Aids and STI services into district health plans; the prioritisation and financing of HIV/Aids care and prevention activities relative to other pressing public health and treatment priorities in the district; where does the treatment of HIV/Aids fit within the framework for essential care packages; how do more vulnerable and poorer households can care for their infected and affected by HIV/ AIDS relatives; are there policy guidelines or action plans for additional staff turnover, ill health and death related to HIV/Aids?

The present case study experienced some of these limitations and barriers to various degrees.

In conclusion, the chance for the Health Sector in the nineties is that it is benefiting from, and in turn is influenced by reforms in the area of governance and the public sector in general. The final purpose of reform being to bring government and decision-making to the community level fits well the PHC ideals. Reforms are taking place concurrently in other sectors as well, such as in education and agriculture. Health Sector Reforms are indeed part of broader reform processes taking place in each country. The economic and political reforms in countries are improving the overall administrative and technical structures. For example, the democratization processes are a direct stimulus to the decentralization of activities by empowering more the communities to select their local political leaders, and to take decisions and manage their own revenues. The four different types of processes[76] which constitute decentralization need to be assessed locally, and the limitations of local professional cadre in sub-Saharan Africa to support the process considered carefully (Moore 1996).

As a consequence, health actors need to be pro-active and constructive and not reactive or defensive to such new developments, despite the present above mentioned broad interpretations, and limitations of know-how on how to conduct the full process. The "Local Responses and Health Sector Reform" is a deliberate step to try to have the HIV/Aids strategies take advantage and benefit

---

[76] Deconcentration, delegation, devolution, transfer

from the Health Sector Reform process, and the same time be a catalyst towards successful reforms.

The Local Responses and Health Sector Reform Approach

Ten years into the epidemic, studies pointed already to the importance of the societal context in influencing and conditioning personal behaviour (Mann, Tarantola et al. 1992).

A critical review of the lessons learned from prevention of sexual transmission of HIV in sub-Saharan Africa pointed to the recent discovery of the "structural"[77] and "societal"[78] factors in the likelihood that transmission will occur, in comparison to the better known "individual"[79] and "infrastructure"[80] factors (Lamptey P. et al. 1997). This explains why most programs until now still intervene almost exclusively at the individual level, for example, identifying and acting upon individual risk factors using epidemiological methods. Consequently very few intervention programs address the "*long-term, complex, and difficult issues*" (op. cit. p. S65) related to structural and societal aspects, and the identification of vulnerable factors related to those. The consequence of this acknowledged gap is leading to the reassessment necessary to work out the perfect ingredients and mix of the "cough syrup." (ref. Fig. 1.1) The local responses has the ambition to reconcile all four levels and set "*comprehensive, integrated, and multisectoral programs,*" (op. cit. p. S63) as a necessary new approach identified to slow the HIV/Aids epidemic in Africa.

Due to the complexity of these different levels, the need to combine "epidemiological, cultural and economic studies… to illuminate a different part of level of the whole picture" (Carael, Buvé et al. 1997), and design appropriate interventions in specific context is recommended. It is the backbone of the Local Responses approach and explains the present case study design.

Taking into consideration these recent developments, the local responses launched by UNAIDS and WHO aims to provoke plans and responses more for a local- than for a national-driven responses,[81] given local levels were up to now insufficiently reached by national plans. The local responses at the District level attempts to link the national level to the reality and needs of the local level. It is

---

[77] factors related to laws, policies, and developmental issues
[78] factors related to societal norms that encourage high-risk sexual behavior
[79] factors that directly affect the individual and that the individual has some control of changing
[80] factors related to the health system that directly or indirectly facilitate the spread of HIV
[81] UNAIDS has published in 1998, three Guides to the strategic planning process for a national responses to HIV/ AIDS: situation analysis, responses analysis, strategic plan formulation

hoped that the cumulation of several local responses experiences in each country at the local levels will be instrumental to refine the national strategic plan in each country as well. This contrasts with the opposite top-down original approach in the late eighties and early nineties expecting trickling down effects at the local level and which proved to be a wrong assumption.

The present concern and priorities to work through local levels are also found in industrialised countries. Taking the example of the USA, one of the key approach to battle the HIV pandemic acknowledged recently is to "*achieve higher degrees of coordination across a broader scope of program activities, particularly at the local, implementation level*" (St. Louis M. et. al. 1997).

In 1996, an early UNAIDS' definition of an expanded responses was leading to some major orientations already which clarifies the approach used and gives evidence of the overlaps with the PHC approach:

> *"An expanded responses calls for social change, including the integration of HIV/AIDS into national development policy, creation of supporting environments, strengthening of community action, developing individual skills and reorienting services towards providing prevention rather than curative interventions.*
>
> *Most responses to the pandemic are primarily driven by risk reduction measures.*
>
> *In order to expand the responses we need to analyze individual and broad societal factors influencing the HIV pandemic. This analysis and its impact can be enhanced by broad participatory process of reviewing available information, sharing experiences and facilitating a common vision of responding to HIV/AIDS.*
>
> *The expanding responses recognizes that the social environment and individual risk behavior are closely concerted. It enhances the value of individual decision-making while relating behavior and behavioral changes to some of their underlying causes.*
>
> *Vulnerability reduction implies a long process of profound cultural, institutional and environmental change in most societies. The setting of short and long-term goals for action aimed at reducing*

vulnerability are required to create a manageable plan of action out of daunting, seemingly overwhelmingly challenges.

This expanding responses must be based on the prioritization of needs at the national and community level, and requires the mobilization of the appropriate human, material and financial resources. It also requires concerted action by individuals and communities, as well as governments and private agencies, both in the short term and over long periods" (UNAIDS 1996).

The present current understanding of the Local Responses and Health Sector Reform is summarised in a recent UNAIDS publication, "Expanding the global responses to HIV/AIDS through focused action" (UNAIDS 1998) discussed earlier (ref. Section 1.1).

In conclusion, based upon the literature review, and the practical field work and exchanges we had over the past two years, and to take a step further Lamboray's original question on "do health reforms pass the HIV test?" we may in turn ask: "Is the Local Responses and Health Sector Reform for HIV/Aids passing the Primary Health Care test?"

The present literature review supports what the local responses originally advocates, and that the approach is based on sound concepts. Those are laid in the combination of using the principles of Primary Health Care approach, with the search for the best mix of practical strategies and interventions, finally with striving for the improvement of the overall systems in which HIV/Aids function through the Health Sector Reform. On the other hand, due to the nature and weaknesses found in this combination, international and national institutions, policy-makers, technicians, and managers may still be skeptical to fully support the local responses now and in the years to come. They are the senior decision-makers who are the Primary Health Care (PHC) skeptics, and will not embrace any more what may be perceived as one of a U.N. agency latest fad. They are the managers who consciously or not may be inclined to the vertical approaches to responding to HIV/Aids. Finally, they are those who will only be converted once results are documented with hard data show and positive results.

We shall argue and document next how with relatively little inputs and scientific stimulus we were able to make an important step to respond locally to HIV/Aids through the present initiative along the PHC approach. This occurred with the technical and financial support of the country national and international partners, and of UNAIDS and GTZ in particular. It is a way to address the UNAIDS Executive Director's plea for the donor nations to invest more into Aids because of the single greatest threat it represents to global development today, instead of the present "minimal" contributions (Piot 1999).

1.2.3 HIV/Aids Strategies and Interventions and Local Responses

As pinpointed by P. Piot in the *Preface* of the most recent Report on the global HIV/AIDS epidemic: after 15 years of action against the epidemic, important insights into effective responses are many (UNAIDS 2000). Ironically. Effective responses need a „nationally driven agenda", a „single and powerful national AIDS plan involving a wide range of actors" (multisectoral response), „social openness increasing the visibility of the epidemic and countering stigma", „social policies that address core vulnerabilities", „the engagement of all sectors (not just health)", „a recognition of the synergy between prevention and care", „support to community participation and targeting interventions to those who are most vulnerable, including young people before they become sexually active", „forward-looking strategies" (op.cit. p 7). In addition, as pinpointed in the report, *„two decades of experience show that behavioural prevention can make a serious dent in the rate of new infections and change the course of the epidemic"* as reported with the review of existing tools and skills (op. cit. p. 55-77). Community-based responses, or the Local Responses, is one among the different ingredients to have effective national responses (op. cit. pp. 108-115).

What is missing up to now for effective responses are effective local responses, hence the nature of the approach and of the study in Gaoua communities and district described in the present research study.

"Expanding the Global Responses to HIV/Aids through Focused Action" requires a two pronged expansion of the global responses with political commitment:
"- First, there needs to be an improvement in the quality, scope and coverage of continuing prevention, support, care and impact alleviation.

- Second, there needs to be new action directed at the societal factors which enhance people's vulnerability to HIV and AIDS" (Piot 1998).

Piot further recommends that *"past efforts to reduce individual and person risk must now be combined with actions to reduce vulnerability through changes in law and policy, and through longer processes of cultural, structural and environmental change."*

A recent conceptual framework with four determinants (macro factors, socio-economic environment, sexual behaviour, and biomedical) could be used for an improved understanding of the various determinants of the HIV epidemic looking and assessing more systematically those. (Barnett and Whiteside 1999)

The Local Responses and Health Sector Reform being an approach, rather than a clear cut strategy or intervention, it relies in the end upon existing HIV/Aids strategies and interventions to be implemented in order to reach and document changes and successes.

Following the local responses situation analysis of mid-1997 in Gaoua District, Burkina Faso, the Consensus and Planning Workshop took place several months later in early 1998, and clarified the context of the local responses (Appendix 1A). The partners from the public and private sectors, established how ill-equipped and -prepared the technical planning and the management teams were to design clear cut strategies and interventions with the local district partners in responses to the problems identified in the situation analysis. At the local level, while prevention strategies are evolving rapidly, those for care and support are even more recent and still at the experimental stages (Gilks, Floyd et al. 1998). As a consequence, the planning and implementation of strategies by local managers working in high prevalence areas, who need to combine and tackle the epidemic from both the preventive and curative angles, become a daunting challenge. In addition, the care and support strategies for Aids largely depend of activities to be implemented outside the walls of the hospital just like the bulk of the preventive activities are for HIV.

What is, in the late nineties, or little over ten years of experience only, the status of development of strategies and interventions available to combat HIV/Aids? What is the state-of-the art of those? Are they as straightforward for HIV prevention or mitigating (care and support) Aids purposes as the following illustration of the "One bug. One drug. One shot" slogan (advertised to treat uncomplicated gonorrhoea) may at first suggest?

Fig. 1.2

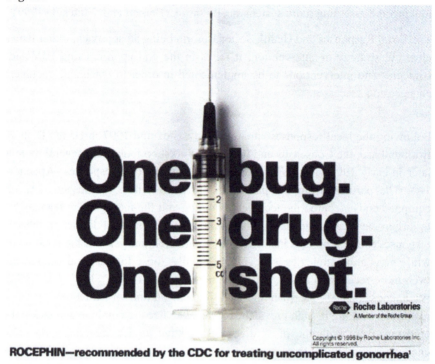

ROCEPHIN—recommended by the CDC for treating uncomplicated gonorrhea'

HIV/Aids Strategies and Interventions--
recommended international standards for preventing HIV and mitigating Aids?

Even if numerous strategies and interventions are available (next paragraph), the above question is still open, given the state-of-the art of development of HIV prevention and effectiveness to prevent sexually acquired HIV is only in the incipient stage of development in the public health field. For the patients who need special strategies, care and support because of Aids, the field is new too. We can draw a parallel with the present research to the development of a highly active anti-retroviral therapy, or of a safe and efficacious vaccine in the bio-medical field. We have the ambition to contribute with the present research to a so-called systemic (i.e. systems based) HIV prevention and mitigation vaccine development over the years to come (C. Pervilhac 1997). Yet, the slow and difficult status of development of HIV prevention is seldom recognised as such in the literature or in international conferences. To revisit the image of the best "coughing syrup" (1.1), the development of the local level responses is still being studied and the machinery needs to be simplified. In addition, in contrast to the bio-medical developments with "sensational reporting" (Piot 1998), public health advances and progresses are more often reported in the international news media as gloomy developments with limited impact on a growing epidemic.

Despite the promises shown in the development of the bio-medical field, prevention remains in the short and long term the most feasible global strategy for the control of HIV/Aids, justifying local responses-related research such as the present one.

Which strategies and interventions?

Based on WHO/GPA training manuals,[82] a "strategy" is *"a major means of achieving an objective which may include one or more interventions"* and an "intervention" is more specifically *"a set of activities through which a strategy is implemented"* (WHO 1995). At present, surprisingly, no documents or articles exist which give a comprehensive view of existing HIV/Aids strategies and interventions, a sign of a rapidly evolving field of research still.

To fill in this gap, based on information and materials gathered at the 12th World AIDS Conference, we reviewed and categorised the types of strategies and interventions into prevention, care and support, and additional ones. We sub-divided the strategies into a "typology of intervention programs" (Cohen and Trussell 1996) according to the foundation on which they are based (Table 1.1).

The known relative easy access of populations to the institution-based programs are attractive to the various partners, potentially cost-effective in comparison to other programs. In addition, being mainly health-institution based, or medically driven, they are often largely favoured by the powerful medical lobbying groups in comparison to the public health ones, and they are the ones that have had the most experience over time. The community-based programs with the community participation component necessitates time, special techniques, logistics support, are less cost-effective and have been well-studied in the PHC

literature, as well as in the context of Aids (UNAIDS 1997). The population-based programs are for the most part, relatively new programs and are still being experimented upon.

Such useful classifications are not used in planning exercises, and more complicated economic analysis appear to prevail in the current setting of priorities instead.

---

[82] The training manuals targeted to National AIDS Program Management" by WHO/ GPA have had limited distribution and applications due to the UNAIDS mid-nineties policy changes. These manuals were not known in Burkina-Faso in 1987 either at the national or local levels.

Table 1.1 Summary Table of HIV/Aids Strategies

1. Nine major HIV Prevention Strategies	2. Six major Aids Care and Support Strategies	3. Eight additional Complementary Strategies
Institution-based programs:		
1.1. Promoting and distributing condoms (WHO-GPA 1995; D'Cruz-Grote 1997)	2.1. Clinical Management (drugs for opportunistic infections and STD, and ARV therapies...) (WHO-GPA 1995; WHO-GPA 1995; Gilks, Floyd et al. 1998; Girma and Schietinger 1998)	3.1. Tuberculosis treatment, control, and prevention (Gilks, Floyd et al. 1998)
1.2. STI treatment, control, and, prevention (syndromic approach)(WHO-GPA 1995; Gilks, Floyd et al. 1998)	2.2. Nursing Care (Gilks, Floyd et al. 1998) (WHO-GPA 1995; Girma and Schietinger 1998)	3.2. Epidemiological and behavioural surveillance (WHO-GPA 1995; Gilks, Floyd et al. 1998)
1.3 Provision of safe blood for transfusion (WHO-GPA 1995; Gilks, Floyd et al. 1998)		3.3. Training of health care staff of volunteers in health and other sectors (Gilks, Floyd et al. 1998)
1.4. Prevention of perinatal transmission of HIV (WHO-GPA 1995; UNAIDS 1997)		3.4. Improving the systems for delivering care(WHO-GPA 1995)
Community-based programs:		
1.5. Promotion of safer sexual behaviour through education (Gilks, Floyd et al. 1998)	2.3. Voluntary testing and counselling (WHO-GPA 1995; Gilks, Floyd et al. 1998; Girma and Schietinger 1998)	
1.6. Reduction of the vulnerability of specific population groups (WHO-GPA 1995; WHO-GPA 1995; USAID 1998; Hunter and Williamson n.d.)	2.4. Home-Based Care (WHO-GPA 1995; Girma and Schietinger 1998)	
1.7. Prevention of unsafe drug use among injecting drug users (WHO-GPA 1995; Gilks, Floyd et al. 1998)	2.5. Social Support (WHO-GPA 1995; Gilks, Floyd et al. 1998; Girma and Schietinger 1998; Hunter and Williamson n.d.)	

Population-based programs:

1.8. Provision of condoms through social marketing (Gilks, Floyd et al. 1998)	2.6. Promotion of Human Rights issues related to HIV (WHO-GPA 1995)	3.5. Eliminating barriers to providing HIV-related services to youth and women, to vulnerable groups, and to people living with HIV (WHO-GPA 1995)
1.9. Promotion of safer sexual behaviour through mass media (WHO-GPA 1995; Gilks, Floyd et al. 1998)		3.6. Increasing the capacity of non-governmental, community-based, and private sector organisations to respond to HIV (WHO-GPA 1995)
		3.7. Community and District mobilisation and sensitisation (D'Cruz-Grote 1997)
		3.8.Policy Support (The World Bank 1997) (WHO-GPA 1995)

Source: C. Pervilhac, based on a literature of the references on the availability of strategies and interventions in HIV and Aids of relevant materials from 12th World AIDS Conference

The review is not exhaustive but merely aims to identify the numerous strategy options, over twenty, which are offered to district program managers to expand the responses. Taking as a conservative estimate an average of five interventions for each strategy, a huge spectrum of over one hundred options is available to managers. HIV/Aids planning, prioritising, and finding the best mix of the strategies (the "cough syrup" presented in the introduction) is complex and outcomes are difficult to measure. This contrasts with the straightforward vaccination preventable diseases, i.e. one vaccine and one shot with at the end a direct visible effect or positive and measurable outcomes. It goes far beyond the past clear cut "core set of prevention indicators" developed in the early nineties by the previous WHO/ GPA. Those were limited to the knowledge of prevention practices, the condom availability and use, the sexual behaviour change, the quality of STD case management and the HIV/ STD sero-prevalence (Mertens T. et al. 1993).

The above wide spectrum of complicated strategies contrasts with the much clearer set of policies and guidelines currently promoted for STD control (UNAIDS 1997) (UNAIDS 1997; UNAIDS 1998), or for Tuberculosis control (De Cock K. 1996; UNAIDS 1997). STD or TB program technicians or managers may consciously or not avoid to mingle into complicated "comprehensive" HIV/Aids programs, and find in turn more satisfaction in their own limited, nevertheless important, "selective" programs.

While the strategies mentioned above aim to expand the global responses by addressing the current acknowledged needs in prevention, support, and care, those addressing the "impact alleviation" and the "societal factors" which enhance people's vulnerability to HIV and Aids still remain to be clarified. As of 1995, WHO/ GPA had already developed training modules for prevention, support, and care only. But then, no modules had yet been developed about the strategies "to promote action to reduce social and economic consequences"(WHO-GPA 1995), giving evidence of the difficulties to identify clear strategies. This is still true at the end of the nineties. The status of the latest developments of "Efficient and Equitable Strategies for Preventing HIV/Aids" (The World Bank 1997) is disappointing in this sense. In the "Research Report" (op. cit. pp. 123-132), improving strategies to influence individual choices seems to be mainly a concern of containing costs which reflects in turn among some Agencies their present priorities and concern in running programs, e.g. social marketing of condoms. In relation to the "impact alleviation" and "societal factors," the current status seems to point more to problems than to spell out clear strategies or solutions, for example in the difficulties of:

170

- altering social norms, e.g. traditional polygyny, traditional custom of "levirat" (ref. findings of community level study, Section 4.1) marriage, marriage and childbearing, large families for a woman's social status and economic well-being,
- improving the status of women with low social and economic status who cannot insist upon male sexual fidelity and the negotiation of safe sex,
- reducing poverty and the impact of poverty on the decisions people make about risky behaviours.

At present HIV/Aids strategies are more often run under the form of a patchwork of different vertical and independent programs, based on the Agencies' interests and managers' expertise, instead of a harmonious prevention-care continuum. The epitome of such a strategy is the HIV prevention through the social marketing of condoms which is run as a strict vertical program. It is found across Africa run by Population Services International (PSI/USA) funded by the Kreditanstalt für Wiederaufbau (KfW), with current reviews emphasising more the economic program efficiency than the above considerations, as per our recent experience in Rwanda (Pervilhac and Kielmann 1999).

Where to focus interventions?

The correct choice of strategies and interventions at a local level is further complicated as experienced in the 1998 Planning and Consensus workshop (ref. Section 4.3.1) as well, by the problematic of prioritisation of approaches either for a general population and/ or targeting vulnerable groups. Prioritising vulnerable groups at the local level with the best program managers available in the country, and additional support of outside expertise, proved to be a difficult exercise with simple prioritisation methods still lacking. It is indeed a much more difficult choice to identify vulnerable groups to combat HIV/Aids than to prioritise for the Expanded Program of Immunisation for example for which for example there are clear cut age groups suggested as standard policies to vaccinate children for specific antigens.

Almost twenty years into the epidemic, a recent review of targeted and general population interventions for HIV prevention in the USA, recommended both approaches to *"match the needs of an evolving epidemic"* (Sumartojo, Carey et al. 1997). The question is not so much to choose one or the other, but *"to determine how best to use and combine these intervention approaches"* (op. cit. p. 1206), a premise applicable in general to all countries.

In sub-Saharan Africa, the heterosexual mode of transmission combined with the determination and identification in the late eighties, early nineties, of more vulnerable groups, and the avoidance of stigmatisation, have justified general population interventions. Yet the traditional health education of the late 1980s, or such diffused interventions, have not induced the widespread behaviour change expected. More specific programs need to be designed preferably by "targeting interventions to specific target audiences" (Cohen and Trussell 1996). Vulnerable groups in the late 1990s are now better known and can be better targeted.

Despite the fact the strategies and interventions are available, numerous barriers exist to reach vulnerable groups. Taking the example of border migrants in the case study of Burkina Faso, we identified (ref. Section 5.1.7) at least five major categories related to population, paradigmatic and epidemiological, program conception and design, organisational and institutional, and political and economic issues.

The technical difficulties of tailoring interventions for each vulnerable group at a local level combined with the financial cost to support such interventions can explain the lack of support to embark into such efforts as well. In addition to be more convincing to donors and agencies, cost effectiveness studies on HIV prevention targeting, such as the one carried out in the USA and giving evidence of substantial benefit (Kahn 1996), still lack in sub-Saharan Africa.

Let us take the above mentioned example of Social Marketing of Condoms (SMC) strategy in a recent review of HIV/STD Prevention in Rwanda (Pervilhac and Kielmann 1999). That strategy is by nature better equipped and has the mandate to reach vulnerable groups, and yet, the following gaps were noticed. Many important vulnerable groups (STD patients, Persons Living with HIV/Aids, returnees and refugees) had not yet been adequately addressed, even if several groups (several women's groups, urban youth, the military, and clients of non-traditional outlets) had already been reached by the program.

In conclusion, the review of HIV/Aids strategies and interventions documents a rapidly evolving field with a wealth of new experiences, combined with the danger of the emerging curative strategies and interventions taking much attention, energies and resources from the preventive aspects. Strategies and interventions targeted to vulnerable groups have not yet had the attention they merit in sub-Saharan Africa. Yet the knowledge gained over the recent years, and the future needs to respond to the changing epidemic, will hopefully bring those in the forefront soon. Much remains to be done to simplify for local use the offer and correct choices of mix of strategies and interventions, of the development of clear country specific guidelines, and to develop prioritising schemes to select the vulnerable groups at a local level.

1.3 Systems Approach of the Research

To identify the social and behavioural sciences research priorities to prevent and mitigate Aids in Sub-Saharan Africa, a panel of experts in the mid-nineties confirmed the necessity to direct more research to "contextual interventions" or indirect interventions as a weapon against HIV. Efforts have been biased up to the mid-nineties towards "proximal interventions" that attempt to interrupt HIV transmission directly targeting individual perceptions and behaviours, and overlooking often the large context within which those perceptions and behaviours are shaped. The new approach attempts to change the environment in which the HIV/Aids epidemic and many other communicable and non-communicable diseases are deeply rooted (Cohen and Trussell 1996).

Recently, through consultative workshops which took place in different parts of the world between 1997 and 1999, leading researchers and practitioners from different parts of the world examined the global use of communications for HIV/AIDS prevention, care, and support, reported in „Communications Framework for HIV/AIDS" (UNAIDS and PennState 1999). In the majority of non-western contexts, the family, group, and community play a greater role than individualism (as opposed to collectivism) in decision making. The group of experts identified five domains of context that are virtually universal factors in communication for HIV/AIDS preventive health behaviour: government policy, socio-economic status, culture, gender relations, and spirituality. Beyond the individual health behaviour approach driving up to now communications interventions in Western societies, these interrelated domains form the basis of a new framework suggested as a flexible guide to adapt in the developing world for HIV/AIDS communications interventions. The Local Responses is based on this emerging framework. It goes beyond the more traditional and well-know diffusion of innovation theory used to inform health promotion programs. The framework recognises that the individual is a product of the context, and for the HIV/AIDS Local Responses (beyond strict „communications" consideration) strategy to have a meaningful effect, intervention programs should begin with one or a combination of these domains. The framework specifies that „*effective approaches can only be developed and refined when the framework for each region, nation, and locality is locally derived*"(op. cit. p. 22). This explains the nature of present research based on the recommended „*community-based approach*" (op.cit. p. 52), introduced with the comprehensive situation analyses conducted at the community and district levels (Chapter 4).

At the same time, a comprehensive review of "Communications programming for HIV/Aids" (UNAIDS 1999) summarised the state-of-the art of publications on communications which cut across all programs. The review is encouraging in documenting how much has been done over the past ten years in adapting communications strategies to HIV and Aids.

The social, cultural, policy, economic factors are a combination of structural factors that influence individual and group behaviours and need to be taken into account by the contextual interventions. More than a decade of work has indicated that proximal and contextual interventions are necessary to reduce the spread of HIV, as well as to mitigate its impact (Mann J. et al. 1992).

The generic "District Responses Initiative Protocol for Field Assessments and District Case studies" (UNAIDS January 1997) which has been adapted for the present research is therefore largely based on contextual and country issues. The combination of developing and attempting to carry out a bi-dimensional research to understand, explain, and act upon both proximal and contextual interventions, is daunting but courageous from UNAIDS, and a much needed initiative. It also can explain some of the scepticism encountered in this early stage still of the development of Local Responses by Development Agencies, besides a few such as the German Technical Co-operation (GTZ), or the Co-operation for The Netherlands.

The same panel identified operations research as a high priority in order to improve the effectiveness, cost-effectiveness, and quality of institutional and community-based responses (op. cit. p. 196). The emphasis is not so much on individuals as the main units of analysis, but more on the understanding of contexts, e.g. communities, organisations, policies etc. This explains the choice of a problem-solving systems approach to the present research, along the method proposed in the original protocol. We adapted a phased approach to this action-research (Figure 1.3), drawing from experiences described in "Operations Research Methods," (Blumenfeld 1985) and clarified in the Methods section (Chapter 3).

Fig. 1.3

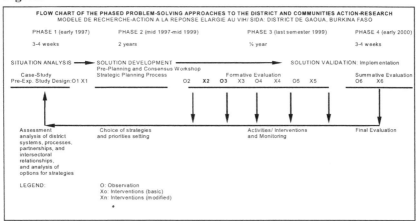

FLOW CHART OF THE PHASED PROBLEM-SOLVING APPROACHES TO THE DISTRICT AND COMMUNITIES ACTION-RESEARCH
MODELE DE RECHERCHE-ACTION A LA REPONSE ELARGIE AU VIH/ SIDA: DISTRICT DE GAOUA, BURKINA FASO

This Flow Chart (Fig. 1.3) illustrates Phase 1 of Problem Analysis, or the Situation Analysis at the Community level (4.1), complemented by the one at the District level (4.2), carried out in early 1997. A long process follows in Phase 2 of Solution Development (4.3), between mid 1997 to mid 1999. Finally, the outcomes of Phase 3 of Solution Validation or the implementation took place for the convenience of the study over a very limited time period of 6 months only (last semester 1999), and were complemented by Phase 4 of auditing the developments (early 2000). The results of these two Phases are documented jointly separately (4.4), as well as the national scaling-up and international dissemination (4.5).

The first phase focuses on an improved understanding of the communities and district systems, the second phase prioritises the interventions, the third phase implements and monitors interventions which will be multisectoral and community-based driven, and the fourth phase evaluates the whole study.

Systems analysis seeks to determine the components of the health and other systems interacting with health, how those interact with one another and with inputs into the systems. It also seeks to understand how the health system is influenced by the external environment (op. cit. p.7). In the context of the health sector reform, the health system has multi-dimensions which includes the vast spectrum of health policy, resources, organisational structure, management and support systems and service delivery. It becomes in turn the basis of the agenda for research in health policy and systems development (Cassels 1995; Janovsky 1996). This multi-dimensional aspect adapted from a systems model

(Blumenfeld 1985), illustrates the additional complexity and ambition of the present research (Figure 1.4).

Fig. 1.4

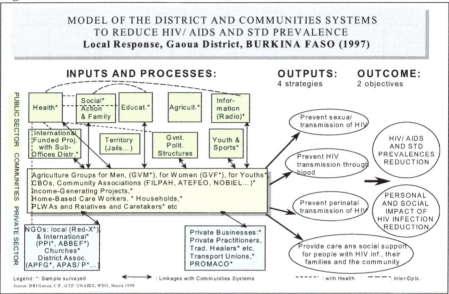

The present model is designed for the action-research to concentrate on the inputs and processes, and particularly the interaction between the communities at the core of the model, and the public and private (voluntary and private) sectors. This focus, over a certain period of time on the up-stream of the system, is too often overlooked in the hasty design of interventions, and yet is essential to develop sound effective strategies (outputs) which in turn lead to impact (outcome).

The present research cycle can be illustrated based on a recent community-oriented health systems planning research (Rohrer 1996). The planning and interaction between the communities and the service providers start with a community needs assessment, followed by an organisational performance assessment. Both processes in turn can improve the overall systems design that is finally evaluated as well (communities and providers' responses).

The evaluation approaches described previously are a contribution to improve the program evaluation aspect of HIV prevention practices with among others the determination of the most informative mix of formative, process, outcome and impact evaluation (Swiss AIDS Federation 1998). They go far beyond the original mere concerns of and emphasis on paying mainly attention to outcome by monitoring the epidemic through sentinel sites.

To implement the Local Responses, UNAIDS launched the process in early 1997. The present research is based on two personal country visits to Burkina Faso in mid-1997, and in the first semester of 1998. It is part of broader general process of the Local Responses with other concurrent events between 1997 and 1999 documented separately (Appendix 1A), and a continuous relationship with the development of the activities over a three years period.

Five case study countries in sub-Saharan Africa with three districts in each were selected to allow to field test the Local Responses generic instrument proposed. An agreement between UNAIDS and WHO, and the German Technical Co-operation (GTZ), identified GTZ to be responsible to carry out the studies in one district of Burkina-Faso, and of Uganda in which the German Co-operation has projects.

The present research is grounded on a combination of empirical research directly based on a field case study, with a three years documentation of the full process. We hope that it will contribute to the success of the Local Responses approach into the XXI Century.

1.4 Outline of the thesis

Section 1 sets the context of the research, its rationale and theoretical background, including a review of the Primary Health Care Approach, Health Sector Reforms and current HIV/Aids Strategies and interventions (Chapter 1), and they justify altogether the aim and objectives of the study (Chapter 2). Finally, the study site, the research methodology and data collection and analysis are described (Chapter 3).

Section 2 of the thesis (Chapter 4) presents the overall results of the study. It is related successively to the four different Phases of the research illustrated earlier (Fig. 1.3 Flow Chart of the Phased Problem-Solving Approaches to the District and Communities Action-Research). The findings of the two situation analyses (Phase 1) at the community level encompassing community determinants and factors of vulnerability (4.1), and at the district level the responses of the public and voluntary sectors and the policy environment (4.2). These analyses set the stage for the Local Responses. Different facets (4.3) are then presented, related to the development of the solution with a consensus-building and pre-planning exercise of the local partners, followed by the strategic planning (Phase 2). Finally, following a brief implementation of the approach in the last semester of 1999 on a small scale (Phase 3), the last sections present the early outcomes (Phase 4) (4.4), and the national and international dissemination (4.5).

Finally, section 3 of the thesis (Chapter 5) discusses the former results sequentially (5.1 to 5.5). It includes a discussion on the development of a new tool called the Rapid Organisational Review (5.6), and a review of applications and limitations of the Local Responses approach taking the example of the migrants, as a specific vulnerable group (5.7). The limitations of the study follow (5.8), and, finally, the overall results in light of the original hypotheses (5.9). The key methodological (5.2.1), policy (5.2.2) and research (5.2.3) recommendations arising from the study are highlighted for conclusions, followed by the bibliography (Chapter 6).

We turn next (Chapter 2) to the aim, objectives and research hypotheses of the study.

References

AIDSCAP, The Francois Xavier Bagnoud Center for Health and Human Rights of the Harvard School of Public Health, et al. (1996). The Status and Trends of the Global HIV/ AIDS Pandemic. XI International Conference on AIDS, Vancouver.

Baier, E. (1997). De l'impact du VIH/ SIDA sur les familles/ communautés rurales et de la nécessité de concevoir des stratégies multisectorielles en vue de prévenir la pandémie et d'en atténuer les effets dans les zones rurales (Orientation: Afrique). Rome, FAO.

Barker, C. and M. Turshen (1986). "Primary Health Care or Selective Health Strategies." A Review of African Political Economy 36: 78-85.

Barnett, T. and A. Whiteside (1999). "HIV/AIDS and Development: Case Studies and a Conceptual Framework." The European Journal of Development Research 11(2): 200-234.

Bererr, M. and S. Ray (1993). Women and HIV/ AIDS. London, Pandora Press.

Blumenfeld, S. (1985). Operations Research Methods: A General Approach in Primary Health Care. Chevy Chase, Maryland, Center for Human Services.

Caraël, M., A. Buvé, et al. (1997). "The making of HIV epidemics: what are the driving forces?" AIDS 11(suppl B): S23-31.

Caraël, M. and B. Schwartländer (1998). "Demographic Impact of AIDS." AIDS 1998(12 (Supplement 1)).

Cassels, A. (1995). "Health sector reform: key issues in less developed countries." Journal of International Health Development 7(3): 329-349.

Cassels A. et al. (1998). "Better Health in Developing Countries: Are Sector-Wide Approaches the Way of the Future?" The Lancet 352: 1777-1779.

Chabot, J. (1984). "Primary Health Care will fail if we do not change our approach." The Lancet(August 11 1984): 340-1.

Ching-Bunge, P. (1995). Report of the Questionnaire Survey on the Use of Combined Messages and the Integration of AIDS/ STD Information into Family Planning Programs in Developing Countries. Eschborn, GTZ.

Cohen, B. and J. Trussell, Eds. (1996). Preventing and Mitigating AIDS in Sub-Saharan Africa. Washington D.C., National Academy Press.

D'Cruz-Grote, D. (1997). Prevention of sexual transmission of HIV/ STD in developing countries. Experiences and concepts. Eschborn, GTZ.

De Cock K. (1996). "Editiorial: Tuberculosis Control in Resource-Poor Settings with High Rates of HIV Infection." AJPH **86**(8): 1071-73.

FAO (1997). Impact du VIH/SIDA sur les systèmes d'exploitations agricoles en Afrique de l'Ouest. Roma, FAO.

FAO (1997). Les populations rurales d'Afrique face au SIDA: un défi au développement (Synthèse des travaux de la FAO sur le SIDA). Rome, FAO.

Foltz A.-M. et al. (1996). Decentralization and Health Systems Change: Burkina Faso Case Study. Geneva, WHO.

Frenk, J. (1994). "Dimensions of Health System Reform." Health Policy **27**: 119-134.

Gilks, C., K. Floyd, et al. (1998). Sexual Health and Health Care: Care and Support for People with HIV/ AIDS in Resource-Poor Settings. Liverpool, Department for International Development.

Girma, M. and H. Schietinger (1998). Discussion Papers on HIV/ AIDS Care and Support. Integrating HIV/ AIDS Prevention, Care, and Support: A Rationale. Arlington, USAID, Health Technical Services Project.

Grodos, D. and Xavier de Bethune (1988). "Les interventions sanitaires sélectives: un piège pour les politiques de santé du tiers monde." Social Science and Medicine **26**(9): 879-889.

Hemrich G. et al. (1997). HIV/ AIDS as a cross-sectoral issue for Technical Cooperation. Eschborn, GTZ.

Hunter, S. and J. Williamson (n.d.). Children on the Brink. Strategies to Support Children Isolated by HIV/ AIDS. Arlington, USAID.

Janovsky, K., Ed. (1996). Health policy and systems development An agenda for research. Geneva, World Health Organization.

Kahn, J. (1996). "The Cost-Effectiveness of HIV Prevention Targeting: How Much More Bang for the Buck?" American Journal of Public Health **86**(12): 1709-1712.

Lamptey P. et al. (1997). "Prevention of sexual transmission of HIV in sub-Saharan Africa: lessons learned." AIDS **11**(suppl B): S63-S77.

Mann, J., D. Tarantola, et al., Eds. (1992). AIDS in the World: The Global AIDS Policy Coalition. Cambridge, MA, Harvard University Press.

Mann, J. and D Tarantola (1998). "AIDS - die globale Bilanz." Spektrum der Wissenschaft: 34-35.

Mann J. et al., Ed. (1992). Assessing vulnerability to HIV infection and AIDS. AIDS in the World. Cambridge, Harvard University Press.

MAP (Monitoring the AIDS Pandemic Network) (2000). The Status and Trends of The HIV/AIDS Epidemics In the World. XIII International AIDS Conference, Durban, South Africa, UNAIDS.

Mayhew, S. (1996). "Integrating MCH/ FP and STD/ HIV services: current debates and future directions." Health Policy and Planning 11(4): 339-353.

Mertens T. et al. (1993). "Evaluating National AIDS Programmes: New Core Indicators." AIDS Health Promotion Exchange 4: 13-16.

Mhalu, F. (2000). The Disaster of the HIV Infection/AIDS Epidemic in sub-Saharan Africa: Who will be accountable for the many lost opportunities for prevention and control brought about by silence and denial? Stockholm, International AIDS Society (AIDS).

Mills, A. (1994). "Decentralization and accountability in the health sector from an international perspective: what are the choices?" Public Administration and Development 14: 281-292.

Moore, M. (1996). Public Sector Reform: Downsizing, Restructuring, Improving Performance. Geneva, WHO.

Murray, C. and A. Lopez, Eds. (1996). The Global Burden of Disease A comprehensive assessment of mortality and disability from diseases, injuries, and risk factors in 1990 and projected to 2020. Boston, Harvard University Press.

Mutangadura, G., H. Jackson, et al. (1999). AIDS and African Smallholder Agriculture. Harare, Southern Africa AIDS Information Dissemination Service (SAfAIDS).

Newell, K. (1988). "Selective Primary Health Care: The Counter Revolution." Social Science and Medicine 26(9): 903-906.

Oulai D. et al. (1993). The Impact of HIV/ AIDS on Education. Paris, UNESCO.

PANOS Dossier (1988). AIDS and the Third World. London, The Panos Institute.

Pervilhac, C. (1998). "The Role and Approaches of the European Schools of Public Health in Improving Public Health Managerial Skills of the Human Resources from Developing Countries: Challenges into the Years 2000." Zeitschrift fur Gesundheitswissenschaften Journal of Public Health 6(Heft 3): 283-288.

Pervilhac, C. and K. Kielmann (1999). Mid-Term Review HIV/ STD Prevention (Social Marketing) Ministry of Health Republic of Rwanda KfW. Heidelberg, University Hospital Ruprechts-Karls-Universität of Heidelberg Department of Tropical Hygiene and Public Health.

Pervilhac, C. and W. Seidel (1995). Training for better District Health Management. First European Conference on Tropical Medicine, Hamburg, Public Health Promotion Centre DSE Berlin.

Piot, P. (1997). "Executive Director of UNAIDS outlines challenges ahead and some of achievements so far". Press Release. Nairobi: 2.

Piot, P. (1998). Current Sate of HIV Prevention -Advances and Challenges. 2nd International Symposium on HIV Prevention, Geneva, the Swiss AIDS Federation.

Piot, P. (1999). UNAIDS Appeals for more Funds in International AIDS Fight. Geneva, UNAIDS.

Piot P. et al. (1990). "The global epidemiology of HIV infection: Continuity, heterogeneity, and change." Journal of Acquired Immune Deficiency Syndrome 3(4): 403-412.

Rifkin, S. and G. Walt (1988). "The Debate on Selective or Comprehensive Primary Health Care." Social Science and Medicine 26(9): 877-977.

Rohrer, J. (1996). Planning for Community-Oriented Health Systems. Baltimore, United Book Press, Inc.

Sayagues, M. (1999). "AIDS Hits Uganda's Villages." Africa Recovery in Development and Cooperation(5): 18.

Silva Saavedra M (1996). AIDS and the Developing World. HIV-Ausbreitung und Prävention. A. Krämer and C. Stock. Weinheim und München, Juventa Verlag: 147-160.

St. Louis M. et. al. (1997). "Editorial: Janus Considers the HIV Pandemic - Harnessing Recent Advances to Enhance AIDS Prevention." American Journal of Public Health **87**(1): 10-12.

Stein, Z. (1996). "Editorial: Family Planning, Sexually Transmitted Diseases, and the Prevention of AIDS-Divided We Fail?" AJPH **6**: 783-4.

Sumartojo, E., J. Carey, et al. (1997). "Targeted and general population interventions for HIV prevention: towards a comprehensive approach." AIDS **11**: 1201-1209.

Swiss AIDS Federation (1998). HIV Prevention Symposium Report. 2nd International Symposium on HIV Prevention, Geneva, Swiss AIDS Federation.

Tanbanjong, A., Piyanat, et al. (1998). HIV and Health Care Reform in Phayao From Crisis to Opportunity. Bangkok, UNAIDS and PAAC.

Taylor, C. (1987). "Ten Years after Alma-Ata: Health Progress, Problems and Future Priorities." International Health News(September).

The World Bank (1993). World Development Report 1993: Investing in Health. Washington D.C., World Bank.

The World Bank (1997). Confronting AIDS Public Priorities in a Global Epidemic. Washington D.C., Oxford University Press.

Topouzis, D. and J. d. Guerny (1999). Sustainable Agricultural/Rural Development and Vulnerability to the AIDS Epidemic. Geneva, FAO and UNAIDS.

UNAIDS (1996). Expanding the Response. Geneva, UNAIDS.

UNAIDS (1997). Children with AIDS: a Crisis Mature. Geneva, UNAIDS.

UNAIDS (1997). Community Mobilization and AIDS. Geneva, UNAIDS.

UNAIDS (1997). Mother-to-child transmission of HIV. Geneva, UNICEF UNDP UNFPA UNESCO WHO World Bank.

UNAIDS (1997). The Orphans of AIDS: Breaking the Vicious Circle Children Living in a World with AIDS. Geneva, UNAIDS.

UNAIDS (1997). Report on the Global HIV/ AIDS Epidemic. Geneva, UNAIDS-WHO.

UNAIDS (1997). Sexually transmitted diseases: policies and principles for prevention and care. Geneva, UNAIDS.

UNAIDS (1997). Tuberculosis and AIDS. Geneva, UNAIDS.

UNAIDS (1998). Expanding the global response to HIV/ AIDS through focused action. Reducing risk and vulnerability: definitions, rationale and pathways. Geneva, UNAIDS.

UNAIDS (1998). The public health approach to STD control. Geneva, UNAIDS.

UNAIDS (1998). Relationships of HIV and STD declines in Thailand to behavioural change A synthesis of existing studies. Geneva, UNAIDS.

UNAIDS (1999). Communications programming for HIV/ AIDS: An annotated bibliography. Geneva, UNAIDS.

UNAIDS (2000). HIV and health-care reform in Phayao *From crisis to opportunity*. Geneva, UNAIDS.

UNAIDS (2000). Report on the global HIV/AIDS epidemic June 2000. Geneva, UNAIDS.

UNAIDS and PennState (1999). Communications Framework for HIV/AIDS A New Direction. Geneva, UNAIDS and PennState.

UNDP (1997). Human Development Report 1997. New York, Oxford University Press.

Unger, J.-P. and J. R. Killingsworth (1986). "Selective Primary Health Care: A Critical Review of Methods and Results." Social Science and Medicine **22**(10): 1001-1013.

USAID (1998). USAID Responds to HIV/ AIDS A Strategy for the Future. To increase use of improved effective and sustainable responses to reduce HIV transmission and to mitigate the impact of the HIV/ AIDS pandemic. Washington D.C., USAID.

Vaughan, P. and R. H. Morrow, Eds. (1989). Manual of Epidemiology for District Health Management. Geneva, World Health Organization.

Walsh, J. (1988). "Selectivity within Primary Health Care." Social Science and Medicine **26**(9): 899-902.

Walsh, J. A. and K. S. Warren (1979). "Selective Primary Health Care: an Interim Strategy for Disease Control in Developing Countries." New England Journal of Medicine **301**(18): 967-974.

Walt, G. (1994). Health policy: an introduction to process and power. People, governments and international agencies -who drives policy and how it is made. London, Zed Books.

Walt, G. and P. Vaughan (1981). An Introduction to Primary Health Care Approach in Developing Countries. London, Ross Publication.

Warren, K. (1988). "The evolution of selective primary health care." Social Science and Medicine **26**(9): 891-898.

WHO (1978). Declaration of Alma Ata. International Conference on Primary Health Care, Alma Ata, World Health Organization.

WHO (1980). Discussion Paper Selected Primary Health Care Interventions (Field Test Version). Geneva, WHO.

WHO (1995). Achieving evidence-based health sector reforms in Sub-Saharan Africa. Background paper for an inter-country meeting, Arusha, WHO.

WHO (1995). Decentralisation and Health Systems Change: A Framework for Analysis. Geneva, WHO.

WHO (1995). Interventions and Policies. National AIDS Programme Management. A Training Course. Geneva, WHO. Global Programme on AIDS.

WHO (1996). Integration of Health Care Delivery Report of a WHO Study Group. Geneva, WHO.

WHO-GPA (1995). HIV/ AIDS Care and Social Support. Geneva, WHO.

WHO-GPA (1995). HIV/ AIDS Problem, Control Activities and Target Populations for Prevention. Geneva, WHO.

WHO-GPA (1995). Interventions and Policies. A Training Course. Geneva, WHO.

Wisner, B. (1988). "GOBI vs PHC? Some dangers of selective primary health care." Social Science and Medicine **26**(9): 963-969.

CHAPTER TWO:
AIM AND OBJECTIVES

In light of the background and introduction to the present research (chap. 1), this chapter formulates the research study aims and objectives (2.1), and the study hypotheses of this operations research (2.2).

2.1 Aim and Objectives

The study described in this thesis aims: first, to improve the knowledge and gaps (under the form of research conclusions) of how to plan and implement HIV/Aids strategies in rural settings in Africa by testing an approach called the Local Responses; second, to document critically a three years process in Gaoua District, Burkina Faso, including some early results.

This research study had the following four objectives (C. Pervilhac Expanded Study Protocol for District and Communities Social and Health Systems, WHO/UNAIDS/GTZ, Apr. 1997, p. 3):

1. to develop a rapid appraisal method which can be a resource to assist district and communities in determining their options for approaches to meeting social and development challenges of the HIV/Aids epidemics at the District level
2. to carry out situation analysis with respect to:
      2.1 the community needs and priorities (vulnerability factors),
      2.2 the links and determinants of the public and private sector institutions in the district systems;
3. to apply the findings to improve the planning and management at the District level (identification of the key factors and priority interventions which can improve the responses);
4. to broaden the lessons learnt from the present research to international implications and applications (if outcomes are not yet possible to measure over the next three years time period of the present research, processes may be used as proxy indicators).

In the present study, we defined the "public sector" as the various Ministries, and the "private sector", as the non-profit and for one, i.e. Non-Governmental

Organisations (NGOs), Churches, voluntary sector, community-based organisations and businesses.

2.2 Study Hypotheses
The Operations Research can be, in turn, broken down into **three hypotheses** that will be tested through different Phases (ref. chap. 1, Fig. 1.3 Flow Chart of the Phased Problem-Solving Approaches to the District and Communities Action-Research):

- **First (phase 1), the feasibility of using a systems approach to analyse the situation at a local level (district and communities),**

- **Second (phase 2), the possibility, based on the findings of the situation analysis, to design and stimulate well tailored priority interventions,**

- **Third (phases 3 and 4), to give as a consequence evidence that a number of activities can be implemented successfully over a short period of time by taking stock of the existing and potential partners' inputs.**

We turn next to the methods (chap. 3) used for the study.

CHAPTER THREE:
METHODS

Burkina-Faso was the first of the five countries selected to carry out the Local Responses, and to pioneer the generic instrument in a district case study (May 1997). It was soon to be followed by Ghana, Uganda, and Zambia in the second half of 1997, and finally, Tanzania in early 1998. The Burkina-Faso case study methodological set-up presented next was discussed briefly in Geneva and in Accra before the country visit, and the study was followed by a number of technical and follow-up meetings related to the Local Responses between 1997 and 2000 (Appendix 1A).

The local responses case study is innovative in that it attempts to tackle some of the uncomfortable situation of systems research methodologies, joining Peter Piot's opening remarks at the Symposium on HIV Prevention in Geneva (1998). Evidence of prevention success needs to be documented not just using "*experimental studies, randomized controlled trials for example*" but "*may come from comparative studies of intervention effectiveness,*" as well as "*other valuable evidence derived from efforts to evaluate complex programs of intervention in the pursuit of predetermined objectives. While this approach may be methodologically 'messier,' it may be a more realistic way of proceeding since we know that complex and multi-levelled programs of intervention - not social 'magic bullets' - are most likely to work...*" and not just the "*promise of technology.*" The society for success is based on "*both individual persuasion and societal enablement*" necessary to develop successful programs and interventions (Swiss AIDS Federation 1998).

This joins the Ottawa Charter for Health Promotion as one of the first internationally endorsed documents to recognise the importance of supportive environments for health. The local responses is further rooted on earlier claims formulated in an agenda for research of "Health policy and systems development":

> "... The challenge (lies in developing) methods for understanding context and process, and the need to take a holistic approach to analysis in contrast to the reductionist research tradition of the bio-medical sciences. There is a need to legitimate analytic research approaches that feature broad-based, often qualitative assessments, identify a range of policy options, indicate what specific conditions are associated with success (or

failure) and under what circumstances, and provide some guidance on how to identify opportunities and implementing change" (Janovsky 1996).

We first present next the study site and the rationale for the district selection (3.1). We then review successively in the research methodology (3.2) the following points, and when necessary bring up some of their current developments or limitations which explains the depth of this chapter: the methodology selected grounded on the original generic protocol; the action-based operations research type on which the present case study is based; the systems model, the "pre-experimental design" before and after prospective intervention study concentrating more on the structural and systems factors; the qualitative methods; the sampling units based on systems and groups; the assessment of existing tools. Finally, we present the data collection used (3.3), followed by the data analysis (3.4).

3.1 Study site

The political and economic background of Burkina Faso explains the context in which the decentralisation (4.2.3) takes place (Foltz A.-M. et al. 1996). The country became independent in 1960 and had been accustomed to a highly centralised quasi-military rule. Traditional rulers who were allowed to maintain some influence in exercising customary law with an authoritarian slant. During the next twenty years the country experienced three republics with policies influenced by Marxist-Leninist regimes, and interspersed with coups and military regimes. Meanwhile, the economy, based mainly on agriculture, had severe setbacks during the Sahelian droughts of the 1970 and 1980s. The present President Blaise Compaoré took power in 1987 in a bloody coup, and a new Constitution was approved in 1991. In that period, and pursued until the mid-nineties, the Government began its structural adjustment program (curbing external current account deficit, reforming taxation and customs, combined with funds channelled into primary education, health, and financial administration) negotiated with the World Bank and the International Monetary Fund. By 1995, Burkina Faso had weathered the devaluation better than most countries in the Franc Zone; nevertheless, it had also experienced only a disappointing growth in GDP (1%), and its budget deficit stood at 9.5% of the GDP, the worst showing in the Franc Zone. The political stability makes Burkina Faso one of the countries benefiting from large external assistance, and is often taken as a model for the Sahelian region. Despite this, the Regime, even though recently democratically re-elected (Nov. 1998), and run through a National Assembly with almost no opposition, suffers from serious internal growing dissatisfaction becoming increasingly visible (Jaffre 1999).

Gaoua District, located in the south-west Poni region of Burkina Faso, shares more than a third of its borders with Côte d'Ivoire and Ghana. It is hilly, and benefits from some of the best rain falls in the country (tropical vegetation) which profits in turn the agro-pastoral activities such as farming corn, and millet, and in animal husbandry. The population of over 250,000 in 500 to 600 communities is largely rural; Gaoua District capital with 17,000 inhabitants is growing rapidly (10% annual growth rate). Among the seven different ethnic groups, the four main ones (Lobi, Dagara, Mossi, and Birifors) speak identical languages as the bordering communities of the Upper West Region of Ghana and of Côte d'Ivoire. Within the District, however, the cultural diversity and distinct traditional values of each ethnic group create important barriers in social communication between communities or villages. Gaoua is a well-known reservoir of migrant workers for the coastal plantations in Côte d'Ivoire and the gold fields in the Ashanti region of Ghana. The rural District is remote and relatively isolated from the capital Ouagadougou. Until recently, it has received relatively less attention than other Districts in the allocation of Government and international development resources. In Gaoua town, the HIV prevalence among pregnant women was reported at 12.5 percent in 1992, and 5.7% in 1994, in the routine HIV surveillance District/ Regional hospital-based. Although it is one of the best sources of information for estimating HIV prevalence, it underestimates the magnitude of HIV infections (Burton A. et al. 1998). The study revealed and confirmed that AIDS is experienced and recognised as a major health problem by the population of the District.

It is one of the four health Districts of the Regional Province of Gaoua (or Poni Region). The decentralization process started over two years ago is not yet fully operational. It benefits from one Regional Hospital (150 beds), and twenty health centres.

We selected Gaoua District out of ten Districts in which GTZ works with the Ministry of Health in Burkina Faso based on the following criteria classified by order of importance:

- First, the district suffers from a high prevalence of infection based on the most recent available HIV sero-prevalence surveillance data (5.7% in 1994) among pregnant women at the District/ Regional Hospital of Gaoua. As such it is one among the ten Provinces considered as high risk zones in the World Bank Project (1995).

- Second, the district is weak in terms of systems: HIV/Aids programs and projects are young and not yet either well planned or implemented in the health and other sectors[83], and the district has been relatively neglected in the allocation of scarce resources (lack of personnel, drug shortages etc.).

- Third, the district is located in a border region with Côte d'Ivoire and Ghana, with highly mobile populations who are also known to be attached to their traditional values and difficult to access.

- Fourth, the District capital, Gaoua, is also the headquarters of the new Poni Regional Direction of Health, an important entity in the Health Sector Reform, and a good base to ground the work, gain political support, and extend later to other Regions and Districts.

- Fifth, due to some of the above constraining factors, the District does not benefit from any research-action projects like other Districts supported by GTZ, but does benefit from a GTZ supported Agriculture Project in thirteen villages close to Gaoua.

Ironically during our first visit, the national media was paying more attention to a new more visible epidemic related to the strange disappearance of male genitals, in comparison to the silent pandemic of HIV devastating communities across several Provinces of the country, such as the Poni region. The sex disappearance epidemic had just hit Ouagadougou, as illustrated (Fig. 3.1) in the headlines of the national newspaper "*Le Journal*" (Some 1997). It was raging across the capitals of West Africa, and had already made some victims in different countries among witch crafters originating from other countries.

---

[83] Scepticism expressed at the national level in selecting this District was often expressed as "Why go to Gaoua? -Nothing is going on there."

sexes à Ouagadougou

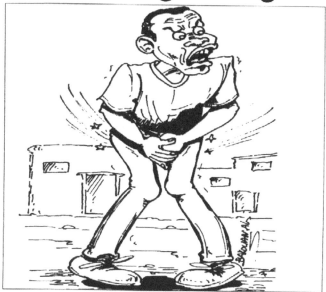

Fig. 3.1
Source: Lierme Some, "Disparition de sexes à Ouagadougou Des victimes témoignent...",
Quotidien ouest-africain d'information Le Journal du soir,
16 mai 1997, p. 1

3.2 Research Methodology

The UNAIDS/WHO District Initiative Project First Working Draft Protocol for Field Assessments and District Case Studies (UNAIDS/WHO 1997) proposed a "multi-stage approach" for the development of the Initiative. The development of the Local Responses in Burkina Faso followed the similar stages with a few modifications (indicated in the footnotes):

1. the development of the district responses concepts,
2. the development of protocols and tools for country visits and case studies,
3. country assessment visits by WHO/ UNAIDS joint missions working with national institutions and UN Theme Groups on HIV/Aids,[84]
4. a consultation in Geneva to review the protocols and tools[85] in line with countries' systems and experiences from field visits,
5. national case studies in 3 districts of each country,[86]
6. review and analysis of the country case studies for agenda for action,
7. national consultative meetings[87] on the development of the local responses.

For the purpose of the local responses in Burkina Faso, we adapted an "expanded study protocol" described based on a review of the UNAIDS/ WHO generic "Protocol for field assessments and district case studies" (UNAIDS/ WHO January 1997).

Type of Research

Operations research is known as a powerful analytical and decision-making tool to resolve a problem-solving process and find practical solutions. It can be used to test new interventions and improve the cost-effectiveness of service delivery. The operations research methods used for the present health systems research design are based on operations research methods developed for Primary Health Care (Blumenfeld 1985). They have been tested and applied successfully in many projects world wide. Measuring the outcome of community-based preventive intervention programmes have been documented the need for more problem-orientated, inter-disciplinary and multi-sectoral approaches (the findings of the review of cardiovascular studies would certainly apply to those of HIV/Aids too) (Brannstrom and al. 1994).

Measuring intervention at community level has been the recent challenges borderline with epidemiological methods (Susser 1995; Fishbein and al. 1996; Lawson and al. 1996). Community forces that influence change need to be better understood because of the "complexity of community dynamics", and a balance

---

[84] Both in Burkina Faso and Uganda the local responses case studies combined this stage with stage 5

[85] A more detailed inventory and analysis of tools which could support the local responses was accomplished in early 1999 (ref. Section 5.1.5)

[86] In agreement with UNAIDS/ WHO, both in Burkina Faso and Uganda, the case studies supported by GTZ took place in one district only

[87] National consultative meetings were held in each country through the UN Theme Group, and two international meetings took place in Dar-es-Salaam (May 1998), and Geneva (June 1998)

needs to be found for "risk targeting" between "public health (community) intervention model," and the "medical (individual) intervention model" (Feinleib 1996).

The three years **action-based operations research** consists of four Phases which can be distinguished under the form of a Flow Chart of the Problem-Solving Approaches of the Action/ Operations Research for Districts and Communities (Fig. 1.3 Chap. 1):

- 1st Phase: 2 months (1 week preparatory period, 3 ½ weeks visit, 3 weeks data analysis). Supported by a consultation visit.

This phase forms the core part of the present thesis (next Chapter 4). It consists of a descriptive or information-building systems situation analysis to describe the roles of partners and links within and between systems and to determine the correct mix of strategies and interventions. Based on the Model of the District and Communities System (Chap. 1 Fig. 1.4), the situation analyses focuses on the Inputs and Processes of the various systems. In particular, they analyse the Communities Organisation System as the heart of the model, and its internal functioning and linkages with other systems, and the District Health System as well. The rapid assessment of problems of district systems, processes, partnerships, and interrelationships prepares for in the next Phase the consensus on objectives, and options of priorities for strategies and interventions.

How each system in turn can and will contribute to improve the responses to HIV/Aids outputs, and finally outcomes are further planned for in Phase 2, implemented in Phase 3, and reviewed in Phase 4.

In addition to the above, Phase 1 allows:

- first, to identify the most appropriate questions to answer in order to facilitate the improved HIV/Aids responses,

- second, to identify and test the tools selected and their usefulness to collect the data, and whether they serve the purpose expected given the important questions to answer,

- finally, to set the correct stage for the next second Phase.

- 2nd Phase: 1 to 1 ½ year. Supported by two consultation visits: first, by the present researcher for a pre-planning and consensus workshop, second by the UNAIDS country "broker"[88] for a strategic planning workshop.

The solution development Phase 2 was much more complex and critical than the original one, originally planned as short and simple process driven by the local decision-makers and managers. It took place over a longer period of time (more than one year). This can be explained by the delays encountered in the feedback of the situation analysis (half a year), combined with the additional duration to analyse and act upon the data at the national and local level. In parallel to these unofficial solution developments at the national and local levels, "official" solution developments needed to take place. Two outside consultants supported this process: for the pre-planning and consensus workshop, and for the strategic planning process both described in this thesis (Sections 4.3.1 and 4.3.2 respectively).

The solution development, with the results of the situation analyses leading to a sound consensus and planning exercise locally, is therefore a critical long bridging period between the situation analysis and the solution validation. Whether the results of the situation analyses are shelved, like many studies end up to be, or acted upon, depend of the original involvement of local partners and understanding of the process, and of the dialogues at different levels. It also depends of the planning exercises which, as documented next (4.3), are more difficult to carry out than other classical planning program exercises.

- 3rd Phase: 2 years. Supported by periodical visits 3-4 times per year of the country broker.

This phase consists of the implementation of interventions (X1 to Xn as per Fig. 1.3 Chap. 1) by the local actors. The solution validation of the research is done under a number of on-going formative evaluations (O1 to On... as per Fig. 1.3 Chap. 1).

- 4th Phase: 3-4 weeks. Outside external review team.

The summative evaluation (Jan.-Feb. 2000) planned as a classical external mid-term review took place following the 3rd Phase. The present study documents the original outcomes (4.4), and the national and international dissemination of the

---

[88] the "country brokers'" concept to have a permanent 3-4 months per year consultant facilitate the process in each country was introduced as an appropriate way to support the local responses in each country and accepted as such in the Health Reform and HIV Workshop (Geneva, June 1998)

experience (4.5), and discusses the lessons learned (5.1), and the overall results of the evaluation (5.1.9).

The local responses intervention and its successes may, like the control tobacco and smoking studies, be based on "mass change... followed by multiple, multilevel interventions which, in turn were founded on causal inference from observational studies only" (Susser 1996). The success may therefore "emerge only after two decades of research and action" (op. cit. p. 1715). Pioneer health systems researchers working in HIV/Aids also need to develop their own "systems responses," over a longer period of time (10 to 20 years Phases 3 and 4). Hence, they can be compared to the virologists and immunologists who necessitate this time-period presently to discover a safe and effective HIV vaccine, or the pharmacologists to develop the anti-retroviral therapies.

Systems Design Research

Due to the nature of the research rooted in an improved understanding of systems, we designed a **systems model** illustrated in the "Model of the District and Communities Systems Aimed at Reducing HIV/Aids Prevalence and STD Prevalence" (Fig. 1.4 Chap 1).

The model has two entry points:
- from a research perspective, it illustrates the various systems operating at the district level, the institutions and individuals within those, and the main links between the "Communities Organisation System" and "District Health System" due to the importance of these two systems;
- from a managerial perspective, it illustrates the Inputs and Process originating from the various systems which lead in turn to improved Outputs, and finally will contribute to the ultimate Outcome of the intervention which is to reduce HIV/Aids prevalence and STD prevalence.

Partnerships are illustrated under the form of linkages first, with the Communities at the centre of the model, second between Public Sectors, and third between the voluntary for profit and non-profit, and public sectors.

Research Design

For the purpose of the present research, the study design is a "**pre-experimental design" before and after prospective intervention study** with a classical pretest-posttest design of the form:

O1   X   O2

where "X" represents the combination of the situation analysis (Phase 1) and the plans (Phase 2), and O1 the baseline at the time of the situation analysis, and O2 the first formative evaluation.

The various systems (inputs and process) are considered as independent and intervening variables that in turn will affect the dependent variables, or contribute to the outputs and outcome. Instead of "variables," the local responses research protocol (UNAIDS Apr. 1997) prefers to identify "factors" which can influence HIV transmission and are grouped into four levels, two of which are essential (indicated in bold) to the present research:
- super-structural factors: (extraneous variables) background or environmental factors which neither individuals nor governments can change in the short or medium term (ex. unstable politic system, economic inequities, rapid urbanisation, presence of refugees in border regions),
- structural factors: not controlled by individuals but can be addressed by Governments (ex. laws, customs),
- systems factors in Health, Communities, Agriculture, Education:[89] controlled by Ministries or influenced by the private sector (ex. quality and accessibility of services),
- individual factors: directly influenced by intervention programs (ex. behavioural changes).

The local responses case study in Burkina Faso (as well as the one in Uganda) focused on critical information related to poorly understood structural and systems factors of relevance to HIV/Aids which can be influenced.

Less emphasis was placed on data related to the larger super-structural factors which cannot be influenced but which nevertheless need to be identified and known, and on the individual factors which are better known because of the strong Information Education Communication (IEC)/ health promotion programs. Such key methodological choices influencing the Local Responses case studies would merit further discussion,[90] and yet were never revisited during the various technical meetings over the past two years.

---

[89] our definition is broader than the UNAIDS one restricted to "health services" alone and is "systems" based
[90] we differ here from the UNAIDS study protocol (Apr. 1997 draft) which recommended emphasis on super-structural and structural factors

The original classics of "Experimental and Quasi-Experimental Designs for Research" (Campbell and al 1963) analyses the pros and cons of different types of design. The present pre-experimental design cannot control for many confounded extraneous variables that can jeopardise the internal validity of the results. For example in the case of the Local Responses such factors as the "history" or changes in events over time, or the "maturation" or changes over time in biological processes of the communities may have affected the changes despite the Local Responses process.

The study design limited by time and budget constraints did not allow the use of a control, non-experimental site. If the Local Responses were to be truly experimented and validated it would need to compare the progress with another control, non-experimental neighbouring district. The ideal "true experimental design," under the form of a pretest-postest control group design, would then be:

District of the Local Responses: O   X   O2
                                      1
Other district: O   O4
                                      3

For the purpose of the Local Responses formative and on-going evaluation taking place, we recommend at least an improved "quasi-experimental design" such as the time series design of the form which necessitate periodic (for example twice yearly) careful review (using the same evaluation instrument):

O1   X   O2   X   O3   X   O4 etc.

The limitations of this study design are discussed in more details separately (5.1.8).

Research methods
The local responses first Phase consists of a rapid assessment situation analysis and inventory taking of the key partners from the communities, and public and voluntary for profit and not for profit sectors based on **qualitative methods**, as recommended in the original generic framework protocol (UNAIDS/ WHO 1997).

The Local Responses benefits therefore of the recent developments and recognition in the nineties of rapid assessment and qualitative methods as sound and much needed scientific methods, which have been neglected up to now in comparison to the quantitative methods. In the mid-eighties, social scientists pointed to the validity of and need for qualitative research methods (Borman and al. 1986; Krenz and al. 1986). It includes more recently the development of software for analysis (Tesch 1990), and methods described in a recent comprehensive masterpiece in the field of qualitative research (Denzin 1994). Developments of Rapid Rural Appraisal (RRA) methods originate from the field of agriculture with the early work of Chambers (Chambers 1981; Chambers 1992) and some RRA were reviewed comprehensively in "qualitative research methods" (Jefremovas 1995). The relevance of such applications in the field of health research and interventions has been recently acknowledged (Vlassof and al 1992). As a result, numerous manuals have been developed for public health purposes in the nineties to clarify either the methodologies of rapid appraisal (Rifkin and al 1991; WHO 1991; WHO 1991), or the specific qualitative methods (Maier and al. 1994; WHO 1994).

The present research is based in particular on the qualitative research methods[91] and definitions that were used in the field during a workshop (Kikwawila Study Group 1994), with the results, in turn, documented separately (Kikwawila Study Group 1995).

The community level study surveyed ten to twelve **key informants**[92] per community which encompassed a balanced mix of males, females and youth, based on the pre-selection of the best types out of a list of thirty potential ones the experienced surveyors identified (Appendix 3A).

In addition, two **focus groups** of youth males and females, between 16 and 25 years, were completed.

In parallel, the district level study surveyed a dozen of **key informants** or **group discussions** of representatives from the public and private institutions. In addition, this was accompanied by a **review of documents**, if available.

---

[91] the researcher attended this workshop, and facilitated a module on qualitative methods introduced for the first time in the European Course in Tropical Epidemiology (13th Course, Barcelona, Sept. 1994)

[92] among the choices were the following: chief of village, administrative chief, responsible of associations, (1 male and 1 female) teacher, agriculture technical delegate, traditional healer, artistic traditional chief, (1 male and 1 female), responsible for cooperatives, (1 female and 1 youth) traditional birth attendants, president of the Parents Pupils' Association

Sampling Units

In order to step beyond the classical individual level of organisation used in the population sciences (e.g. individual behavioural studies), Susser's "eco-epidemiology" (Susser 1996) paradigm appears to be the most appropriate model for the systems design research needed. It emphasises how beyond the individual level analysis, complex contexts such as groupings, communities, cultures, and legal systems and their effects need to be understood. As recommended by Susser, groups can be used as units of study, as long as the different levels of organisation and "study units" are recognised. This is justified because "variables *special to groups* are present wherever groups are constituted and at all levels of the organisational hierarchy…" and "we are clearly dealing with dynamic systems rather than static situations" (op. cit., p. 1714).

The original District Responses Initiative Protocol for Field Assessments and District Case Studies (UNAIDS/ WHO January 1997) stated as general objectives that the local responses "working with countries, will undertake assessments of the responses situation within each selected country as well as specific district systems." We designed the "Model of the District and Communities Systems" (Fig. 1.4 Chap. 1) on which we drew the "Units of Analysis and Sample Checklist of Specific Problems related to District Systems" (Appendix 3B) to analyse these specific District systems. This was based on the above recommended new "study units" for "complex contexts." We further outlined the Types of Studies and Tools that could be used for the study (Appendix 3C).

The community level study concentrates on the heart of the model, or the communities organisation system who are the clients, but can also be the providers of services through their associations, or trained health workers. The district level study reviews the various other systems from the public and private sectors found at the district level (ref. next section 3.3).

For the community level study (Community Organisation Systems Sampling), four communities were selected by convenience sampling to represent the communities organisation system. They were surveyed within the time constraints of the study (two days per village): two rural (remote villages), and two semi-rural (one district capital neighbourhood and one small border town neighbourhood). All communities could be accessed within an hour drive from the District capital even under heavy rains. Each rural community represented the main ethnic groups found in the District.

For the District level study (Systems Sampling), we sampled all public institutions (N=14), and an approximate equivalent number of various private ones (N=15). The private ones included the largest international and national NGOs, then the most important Community-Based Organisations of different types already active. At least one representative or a group of representatives from each system (public and private) was sampled. Each system can be divided in turn into a number of sub-systems or units of analysis. For example, the health system which is studied in more details comprises the following sub-systems:

- infrastructures (district hospital, peripheral health units),
- managerial (different committees and district health management team),
- programmatic (various programs[93] and their support services[94]),
- community (local committees, local associations, groups, and primary health care workers, i.e. village health workers, traditional birth attendants, traditional healers...).

Assessment of existing tools

One of the hypotheses testing of this action-research is that first, a systems approach is feasible with existing tools, and second, local capacities can apply those.

In sub-Saharan Africa, like in the United States, the challenges lie in turning fragmented local delivery systems into co-ordinated primary care systems (Rohrer 1996). Older epidemiological, or population-based perspectives adapted from older health systems models (Donabedian 1973) may still be insufficient to reach this aim, or to develop the HIV/Aids improved responses at a district level. This explains the combination of different approaches and tools used.

Originally, we aimed among different hypotheses to test the feasibility and use of different but complementary approaches, using the lenses and applying various existing tools with a set of questions from the different following disciplines: epidemiology, anthropology, policy, sociology, and economics.

The study attempts in light of the aforementioned objectives to answer several general questions (Appendix 3C) based on a list of issues which needs to be addressed in each country for each unit of analysis in each system:

---

[93] example: HIV/ AIDS, immunization, diarrheal diseases, malaria control, respiratory infections
[94]example: training, health management information system, logistics, health promotion

- How well each system in the district performs?
- What are the different district systems leaders' roles through a self-analysis?
- What are the stakes of each organisation or individual?
- What are the types of organisations running each system?
- What is the community managed responses to HIV/Aids?

The approaches and purposes of each tool are the following, with additional references for those in the previous Chapter 1 (1.1 to 1.3):

1) *The epidemiology approach*: Assessment of the present performance of each system, using epidemiological existing indicators (WHO 1996).
Purpose: to assess each performance systems based on documents, available information, and external reviews of reports; monitoring behavioural changes and evaluation of existing services capacity.

2) *The anthropology approach*: assessment of the community managed responses. The approach is based on community participation assessment (Bjaras 1991; Schmidt D. et al. 1996), and qualitative methods of research to assess community participation (Kikwawila Study Group 1994; Nakamura Y. et al. 1996).
Purpose: to assess the communities' roles in responses to HIV/Aids and their perceptions of other systems' roles, support, including the estimation of the degree of the community participation.

3) *The policy approach*: Self-analysis of roles and other systems roles from different district systems' leaders (e.g. Position Map). It is based on political mapping approaches, and exists under the form of a software for political analysis and policy advocacy tool (Reich 1994), with a stakeholder analysis for an improved responses, policy networking map, and transition assessment.
Purpose of the Stakeholder Analysis: to describe the consequences, actors, resources, and networks involved in a particular decision, and explain how and why the decision process was taken (improve the communication process among organisations), and finally to assist decision-makers in choosing strategies to influence the politics of formulating or implementing a decision.

Purpose of the Policy Network Mapping: to understand how different organisations related to each other in practice (key decision-makers, access to influential individuals, direction of influence and degree of conflict among organisations, potential flow of interests and conflicts...), as opposed to the connections shown in official agreements or organisational charts.

Purpose of the Transitions in Progress: to understand the dynamic environment in which the public policy occur, particularly in light of the current sector reforms.

4) *The sociological approach*: categorisation of the type of organisations running each system. There exists no experience, and no specific succinct guidelines in the context of district level[95] to apply some analysis techniques of organisational theories (Mintzberg 1982). Those encompass power, environment, technical systems, age and size of organisations. An attempt is made to understand some of the more "innovative organisations" or "operating adhocracy" (projects) from the private sector vs. the "machine organisations" (centralized government bureaucracies) from the public sector, and their interactions (Mintzberg 1989).

Purpose: First, to improve in each system the understanding for each institution of its type of organisation, and forms of politics and games that can influence the strategies of HIV/Aids responses and improve the efficiency of their implementation. Second, to analyse the past, present, and future roles of each organisation or individual and their main enabling and constraining factors; to assess the organisation's position vis-à-vis the proposed decision or policy related to the improved HIV/Aids responses.

5) *The economic approach*: costing analysis assessment and capabilities (Creese and Parker 1994).

Purpose: to be able to select the most cost-effective combinations of interventions.

Our experience during the study did not support the original hypothesis that existing tools of different disciplines are already sufficiently developed to be applied to the local responses. As a consequence the state-of-the art of the development of the existing tools cannot be used easily with local capacities at the district level. Due to our own limited expertise, time and resources constraints, we confined our original large ambitions to concentrate instead to the testing of approaches and tools essentially to anthropological methods for the community level study, and epidemiological and sociological methods for the district level study. We pointed to the importance of understanding more the cost of interventions and activities at a district level in order to be better able to take this dimension into consideration in the final weighing of priorities.

---

[95] personal communication with H. Mintzberg, March 3 1997

In conclusion, based on the wide interpretation by each Local Responses study team for the five different country case studies of which tools to use and questions to ask, it was not possible in the follow-up Technical Workshop (Dar-es-Salaam, May 1998) to draw any conclusions about their strengths and weaknesses. Suffice it to say that different country team leaders concentrated on different approaches and tools with a fair amount of success to analyse the situation in the different districts. The aggregated amount of experiences cumulated, and a special exchange concentrating on each approach used, would allow to enrich substantially the state-of-the art of the local responses methods. The testing of the different approaches by a multi-disciplinary team as originally planned is pending some of the financial and design constraints mentioned previously (*Research Design*).

Following the Local Responses study, a detailed inventory of tools accomplished in early 1999 which could be used and adapted for the local responses shows the gap which still lies ahead to disseminate and promote the local responses approach (Section 5.1.5). A package for the local responses such as the rapid assessment of district health system (Nordberg 1995) still remains to be fully tested and validated.

3.3 Data Collection

For the situation analysis (Phase 1), a couple of days were necessary at the national level, before and after the study for technical briefing and debriefing visits to various authorities. Two different teams collected the data in parallel over a two weeks period, with an additional three to four days necessary before data collection in order to pre-test and finalise the protocols:

- The community level study: headed by a country national sociologist, with applied knowledge of use of qualitative methods, with two teams of two or three people (depending if a local translator was needed or not);

- The district level study: headed by the international principal investigator (present researcher) as public health specialist with a sociology background, accompanied by a country national specialised in Information-Education-Communication (IEC) in HIV/Aids. When necessary, the support of a local district health staff was sought to co-ordinate the visits, and to facilitate the access to the communities.

The two team leaders of each study team were responsible for the adaptation of the questions, testing, implementation of the study and data collection quality, and preliminary analysis of findings.

The original local responses generic framework (UNAIDS 1997) recommended the studied be carried by "multi-disciplinary HIV/Aids local (or country) team." The qualifications sought reflect well the diversity and complexity of the nature of the present study. Unfortunately, they are almost impossible to find all at once: "broad social sciences and health systems research and analysis experience and capacity... multi-disciplinary... previous links with institutions from national and district levels... sustained presence in the country...involvement in health and health sector reform... acceptance by UN Theme Group and Ministry of Health."

In country, we could not gather that ideal "multi-disciplinary HIV/Aids team" (of 10 to 12 members) coming from different systems to develop, test, and carry out the different types of studies, because of the non-availability of the expertise on a short notice. We were additionally limited by funds to hire a large team. We overcame the difficulty by concentrating on using at least the local expertise (a local Non-Governmental Organisation) to carry out the community level part of the study.

The participatory nature of the exercise, and its ownership at the local level, were stronger in Phase 2, the solution development, and Phase 3, the solution validation or implementation, than Phase 1, the situation analyses. The GTZ project staff and UNAIDS and WHO were encouraged to play more the roles of co-ordinator and facilitator, and to be only another mere stakeholder in this initiative rather than to be the main engine or driving forces.

3.4 Data Analysis

Preliminary data analysis for Phase 1 was done daily on the spot for the two studies.

A rough outline of impressions of the findings of the studies was done immediately following the full field work. Two levels were involved: the District level to the District Health Management Team, and the national level with the Directorate General of the Ministry of Health, and the U.N. Theme Group.

After the survey, two weeks of data analysis for each study by each team were necessary.

Finally, all the data were then reviewed and compiled by the principal investigator in a country case study report for GTZ, and UNAIDS/WHO.
The present research was supported under a grant from the Federal Ministry for Economic Co-operation and Development ("Bundesministerium für wirtschaftliche Zusammenarbeit und Entwicklung"/ BMZ). The Aids Control and Prevention in Developing Countries, Health Population and Nutrition Division of the German Technical Cooperation (GTZ or "Deutsche Gesellschaft für Technische Zusammenarbeit") was the implementing Agency. Unfortunately, GTZ suffered budget constraints at the end of 1997 which did not allow a smooth follow-up of local of activities by the country and district offices as planned originally. The major national and international donors are moving in the direction of supporting large-scale public funds for the HIV vaccine development, (European Commission 1999) instead of public health prevention strategies such as the present local responses. Fortunately, however, UNAIDS has continued the implementation of the research findings through its national Office located in Ouagadougou, Burkina-Faso, and the UNAIDS country broker's nomination.[96]

Despite these constraints, the GTZ Head Office, Eschborn, has kept a strong interest in the Initiative and been able to keep the networking going, particularly through its Regional Aids Support (RAP) office located in Accra, Ghana. In addition, a number of international and national meetings and conferences (Appendix 1A), took place in 1998, and have allowed to gain local and international recognition and to facilitate the exchange of experiences.

In conclusion, we structured the local responses under the form of an action systems research. It is based on the best methodological set-up presently possible under several constraints: first, the limited state-of-the-art of developments of community-level interventions and of tools development; second, limited financial resources to monitor the case study development closely. The next chapter documents the findings of the situation analysis at the

---

[96] the present researcher is not UNAIDS "country broker" allowing the present analysis of process, outcome and outputs to be analyzed even more objectively as an independent researcher

community level (4.1), and at the District level (4.2), with the original planning stages (4.3).

We advocate here for the development of the Local Responses approach on a large scale, to apply more rigorous quasi-experimental design and systems approach identified in this section. This in turn will allow to document and to validate scientifically the processes and outcomes over time

References

Bjaras, G. (1991). "A new approach to community participation assessment." Health Promotion International **6**(3): 199-206.

Blumenfeld, S. (1985). Operations Research Methods: A General Approach in Primary Health Care. Chevy Chase, Maryland, Center for Human Services.
Borman, K. et. al. (1986). "Ethnographic and Qualitative Research Design and Why It Doesn't Work." American Behavioral Scientist **30**(1): 42-57.

Brannstrom, et. al. (1994). "Towards a framework for outcome assessment of health intervention Conceptual and methodological considerations." European Journal of Public Health **4**: 125-130.

Burton A. et al. (1998). "Provisional country estimates of prevalent adult human immunodeficiency virus infections as of end 1994: a description of the methods." International Journal of Epidemiology **27**: 101-107.

Campbell, D. et. al (1963). Experimental and Quasi-Experimental Designs for Research. Chicago, Rand McNally College Publishing Company.

Chambers, R. (1981). Rapid Rural Appraisal: Rationale and Repertoire. Sussex, University of Sussex.

Chambers, R. (1992). Rural Appraisal: Rapid, Relaxed, and Participatory. Brighton, University of Sussex Institute of Development Studies.

Creese, A. and D. Parker, Eds. (1994). Cost analysis in primary health care A training manual for programme managers. Geneva, World Health Organization.

Denzin, N., Ed. (1994). Handbook of Qualitative Research. London, Sage Publications.

Donabedian, A. (1973). Aspects of Medical Care Administration. Cambridge, Mass., Harvard University Press.

European Commission (1999). Development -HIV/ AIDS action in developing countries. Brussels, European Community.

Feinleib, M. (1996). "Editorial: New Directions for Community Intervention Studies." AJPH **86**(12): 1696-1698.

Fishbein, M. et. al. (1996). "Editorial: Great Expectations, or Do We Ask Too Much from Community-Level Interventions?" AJPH **86**(8): 1075-76.

Foltz A.-M. et al. (1996). Decentralization and Health Systems Change: Burkina Faso Case Study. Geneva, WHO.

Jaffre, B. (1999). "Un journaliste face au pouvoir Le Burkina Faso ébranlé par l'Affaire Zongo". Le Monde Diplomatique. Paris: 21.

Janovsky, K., Ed. (1996). Health policy and systems development An agenda for research. Geneva, World Health Organization.

Jefremovas, V. (1995). Qualitative Research Methods An Annotated Bibliography, IDRC.

Kikwawila Study Group (1994). Qualitative Research Methods: Teaching Materials from a TDR Workshop. Geneva, UNDP/ World Bank/ WHO TDR.

Kikwawila Study Group (1995). WHO/TDR Workshop on Qualitative Research Methods Report on the Field Work. Geneva, WHO.

Krenz, C. et. al. (1986). "What Quantitative Research Is and Why It Doesn't Work." American Behavioral Scientist 30(1): 58-69.

Lawson, J. et. al. (1996). "The Future of Epidemiology: A Humanist Response." AJPH 86(7): 1029.

Maier, B. et. al., Eds. (1994). Assessment of the District Health System Using Qualitative Methods. London, The Macmillan Press Ltd.

Mintzberg, H. (1982). Structure et dynamique des organisations. Paris, Les éditions d' organisation.

Mintzberg, H. (1989). Mintzberg on Management Inside our Strange World of Organizations. New York, the Free Press.

Nakamura Y. et al. (1996). "Qualitative assessment of community participation in health promotion activities." World Health Forum 17: 415-417.

Nordberg, E. (1995). Health care planning under severe constraints Development of methods applicable at district level in sub-Saharan Africa. Department of International Health and Social Medicine. Stockholm, Kongl Carolinska Medico Chirurgiska Institutet: 58.

Reich, M. (1994). Political Mapping of Health Policy A Guide for Managing the Political Dimensions of Health Policy, Harvard School of Public Health.

Rifkin, S. et. al, Eds. (1991). Using Rapid Appraisal for Data Collection in Poor Urban Areas. Primary Health Care. Bombay, Tata Institute of Social Sciences.

Rohrer, J. (1996). Planning for Community-Oriented Health Systems. Baltimore, United Book Press, Inc.

Schmidt D. et al. (1996). "Measuring Participation: its Use as a Managerial Tool for District Health Planners Based on a Case-Study in Tanzania." International Journal of Health Planning and Management **11**: 345-358.

Some, L. (1997). Disparition de sexes à Ouagadougou Des victimes témoignent. Quotidien Ouest Africain d'information Le Journal. Ouagadougou: 1-3.

Susser, M. (1995). "The tribulations of trials-intervention in communities." AJPH **95**: 156-158.

Susser, M. (1996). "Some Principles in Study Design for Preventing HIV Transmission: Rigor or Reality." American Journal of Public Health **86**(12): 1713-16.

Swiss AIDS Federation (1998). HIV Prevention Symposium Report. 2nd International Symposium on HIV Prevention, Geneva, Swiss AIDS Federation.

Tesch, R. (1990). Qualitative Research: Analysis Types and Software Tools. New York, The Falmer Press.

Vlassof, C. et. al (1992). "The relevance of rapid assessment to health research and interventions." Health Policy Planning **7**: 1-9.

WHO (1991). Epidemiological and Statistical Methods for Rapid Health Assessment. Geneva, WHO.

WHO (1991). Report on a Meeting on the Application of Rapid Assessment Methods to Tropical Diseases. Rapid Assessment Methods, Baroda, India, WHO.

WHO (1994). Qualitative Research for Health Programmes. Geneva, Division of Mental Health.

WHO (1996). Catalogue on Health Indicators A selection of important health indicators recommended by WHO Programmes. Geneva, WHO.

CHAPTER FOUR:
RESULTS

This chapter is the core of the study presenting the results of the work carried out in Gaoua District, Burkina Faso. The results represent the different Phases described in the Flow Chart (Fig. 1.3).

The findings of the situation analyses (Phase 1) have been compiled in details in the original Report submitted to the German Technical Co-operation (GTZ) (Pervilhac, Kipp et al. 1997), and in a summary of the findings presented at the Pre-Planning and Consensus Workshop (Pervilhac C. et al. 1998). An overall review of the study was presented at two poster sessions at the 12th World AIDS Conference (Salla, Sebgo, Pervilhac et al. 1998), and the 13th World AIDS Conference (M'Pele, Pervilhac et al. 2000).

We present first the situation analysis at the community level: first, the findings of the six community participation determinants (4.1.1) to measure the present and potential responses of the communities with key strategic priorities for each; second, the findings of the three main categories of factors of vulnerability (4.1.2) to measure risk reduction potentials among the "window of hope," the youth, are discussed, with the strategic consequences as well.

We then present the situation analysis at the district level with the Responses of the Public (4.2.1) and Private[97] (4.2.2) Sectors and illustrate this under the form of an institutional landscape. Then we present the policy environment in which the present study takes place in light of the Health Sector Reforms (4.2.3).

Following the situation analyses, the planning stage (Phase 2) is described with an early phase of consensus-building and pre-planning (4.3.1), followed by a strategic planning exercise (4.3.2).

The outcomes (4.4), representing the early efforts of implementation (Phases 3 and 4) are reported next, and the consequences on the national scaling-up and international dissemination (4.5).

---

[97] we call here "private" any non-public sector, i.e. voluntary for or not for profit, Churches, and the communities

4.1 Situation Analysis at the Community Level

The findings related to the community system presented in this section were collected mostly through the community level study, and partly through the district level study.

The present analysis takes one step further the former findings of the original situation analysis approach, by using next a more direct, concise, and applied analytical framework. It is hoped therefore that this framework can be used in future local responses baseline analyses and can maximise for planning purposes the profit combining at the same time the analysis with data presentation oriented for an improved applications of the findings.

4.1.1 The Essential Community Determinants

The assessment aimed to gain knowledge of the social milieu of communities, an essential component of public health prevention programs (Keeley 1999) in order to understand and improve the responses towards HIV/Aids at the community level. First the social characteristics, more difficult to change, but important to understand and consider in the process of community participation are reviewed, followed by five essential determinants of community participation: perceived community needs, health sector, perception of Aids, community organisations, and external partnerships (Table 4.1). The selection of the five essential determinants (determinants 2 to 6) which can strongly influence the community participation process is based on the adaptation of existing community participation assessment frameworks to the particular case of HIV prevention (Bjaras 1991) (Schmidt D. et al. 1996). The detailed questionnaire to the Key Informants at the Community Level is attached separately (Appendix 4A).

Table 4.1 Community characteristics (1) and critical determinants (2 to 6) with related questions to measure community participation for the Gaoua Local Responses Initiative

1. Characteristics
a. What are the formal and informal community structures?
b. What are the essential characteristics of these structures?
c. Are there more immediately visible vulnerable groups to HIV?

2. Perception of Aids
a. Is Aids a serious problem?
b. What is the impact?
c. On whom?

3. Perceived Needs
a. What are the most important health problems?
b. What are the most important needs?
c. How does HIV prevention rank among those?

4. Health Sector
a. What is the status of the old Primary Health Care network?
b. Are there communication agents from the village and functional?
c. What role does the closest Health Centre play in relation to HIV/Aids activities?

5. Organization against Aids
a. Are there structures organized to respond to some of the health problems?
b. For the problem of HIV and Aids is there any structure(s)?
c. Leadership and influential peoples' roles in relation to the above structures, and management?

6. External Partnerships
a. Who are the external partners?
b. What is their role(s), and in relation to health, and to HIV/Aids in particular?
c. Is the partnership an outside intervention or a true partnership?

The following summarised key findings of the situation analysis is based on information collected through various key informants (Research Methodology, chap. 3, 3.2) at the community level. They are recapitulated in a comprehensive table summarising the obstacles, opportunities, and based on those, the strategic priorities are suggested as well (Table 4.2). The data are aggregated for all four communities. For the purpose of specific interventions, e.g. rural vs. urban, or for specific ethnic groups etc., it would also be possible to analyse the data with the original transcripts separately to tailor specific strategies as well.

1) Community Characteristics
The characteristics of the urban communities are dominated by more formal (registered) and structured Associations, whereas the ones from the rural areas are more informal and less structured grassroots community organisations. The community characteristics are complex to understand due to the large diversity of ethnic populations who live in the villages or in town. Each community has its own characteristics and mix of populations, confirming the non-homogenous communities' composition. A core autochthonous group constitutes often the majority of a village (in Banlo, for example the Lobi), with the minorities from different origins (in Banlo, the Mossi and Peulhs). In general, each ethnic group has its own grouping, or associations by occupational activities, and leaders under the traditional village chief. The more visible and easiest groupings and associations found are the ones for males, but women have theirs as well, and the youth much less formal and visible ones (tea, sports…).

Some communities have large migrant populations, particularly among youth, and constitute therefore an important vulnerable group to concentrate upon, although targeting migrants call for many barriers of various nature to be overcome (ref. section 5.1.7).

In both rural and urban areas, influential people, or gatekeepers, (land chiefs, religious leaders, teachers, administrative delegates, health workers, traditional birth attendants, traditional healers…) are essentially male-dominated. They play different roles (social, cultural, economic…) on different population segments. Decisions are taken in group meetings which these influential people call. In addition, they have their own agents of diffusion of information in the communities. Such networks should be favoured over the more visible and favourite "project" entry points of administrative structures. The latter are too often more coercive, hence less participatory, or picking up individuals for training in isolation from their community organisations of support. Multiple

214

segments of the communities possess different types of social networks each with their own popular opinion leaders. An improved partnership with these various support community networks should allow to tailor and deliver improved and more sustained community-level HIV prevention interventions to those at greater risk, overcoming the challenges of community-level interventions described elsewhere (Keeley 1999).

Based on these findings the key strategic priorities identified are:
- to use Rapid Rural Appraisal (RRA)[98] to identify by ethnic background the important groups and associations to work with and their leaders,
- to reinforce and work through the hidden or less visible but existent women and youth community organisations instead of individuals,
- to stimulate the responses to HIV/Aids through the dozen of different groups/ associations in each village (feasibility and sustainability to be tested), and/ or through the gatekeepers, with particular attention to those directed towards women and youth,
- to identify communities with migrant populations and tailor special strategies in town through the Associations (more formal), and in villages the groupings (more traditional).

2) Perception of Aids at the Community Level

Aids is perceived as a serious problem in both rural and urban communities because it cannot be cured. It has already caused a dramatic increase in the populations of widows and orphans, and has had serious socio-economic consequences, including "contaminating mostly the youth, the engine of development" (ref. section 4.1.2). Voluntary support networks exist to support Aids patients through the direct relatives, friends, or religious groups, for example by bringing financial support or food. Care and support activities related to Aids patients are perceived to be more urgently needed than HIV preventive activities, as can be expected from an area experiencing a micro-epidemic of HIV over the past few years, and the fact that strategy has been largely neglected by existing programs.

---

[98] Local Responses recommend particularly the use of Participatory Rural Appraisal (PRA) methods, such as mapping techniques, to stimulate the ownership of the process from the beginning (ref. UNAIDS Technical Note no. 3, in press)

Some of the youth groups are able to identify themselves as the most vulnerable groups among their communities based on their approximate estimation of the number of men and women who have already died from Aids.

Based on these findings the key strategic priorities identified are:

- to develop the care and support[99] of Aids patients among the communities requesting those,
- to focus efforts among youth groups who perceive themselves as the most HIV vulnerable groups.

3) Perceived Community Needs

In addition to the perception of Aids mentioned above, other serious health problems identified by the communities are Meningitis, Measles, Malaria, Yellow Fever, and Tetanus.

Despite this, perceived community needs and priorities are often different than public health ones, and concur to the ones found in earlier Primary Health Care (PHC) needs assessment of the seventies and eighties. Priorities ranking indicates needs for infrastructures (health posts, mills for cereals, water pump or well, schools, teachers' residences, agricultural materials...) or systems development (small commerce, pharmaceutical depot...), in comparison to less immediately tangible public health preventive strategies, such as HIV prevention.

Based on these findings the key strategic priorities identified are:

- to respond to one of the community perceived needs through micro-development income-generating projects first, or in parallel, to HIV prevention,
- to introduce feasible and cost-effective immediate complementary public health measures (e.g. Measles and Tetanus Toxoïd vaccinations, or Malaria prophylaxis with impregnated mosquito bed nets and early presumptive treatments...).

---

[99] Care and support, or in French, "la prise en charge," is the common terminology used in Burkina Faso despite the fact the term is rather ambiguous and entails the additional financial support discouraging the local NGOs and Associations to commit themselves fully to this strategy

4) Health Sector at the Community Level

Most of the old village primary health care (PHC) workers are not functional any more. In addition, either the few still functional PHC workers or special communication agents, too often in isolation from their communities, have been trained by the national NGO (ABBEF) to sensitise the population and do demonstrations on the use of condoms to prevent HIV. In some of the communities where these workers are functional and where they are answerable and accountable to a larger community organisation they belong to, they can be tapped to for HIV/Aids strategies. The youth favoured the health personnel from the closest Health Centre to receive information related to HIV prevention, instead of the local less anonymous resource. As a consequence easy accessibility to information is a problem. Youth were identified as more open, receptive, capable of interpretation, eager to forward information and use those, and appeared therefore to be an ideal group to support their own volunteer peer advocators who are for the time being not tapped to.

Based on these findings the key strategic priorities identified are:

- at the community level, to benefit from the existing functional or ABBEF trained agents as dissemination agents of HIV preventive activities with the support of their community organisations, while avoiding at the same time revamping a full scale PHC workers' network,
- in the health centres, introduce an adolescents' reproductive health program,
- to introduce other less informal communication channels with the community, e.g. from the gatekeepers, and local Groups and Associations such as youth groups and their own peer educators (ref. section 1 above).

5) Community Organisation against Aids

Essential to the process of stimulating community participation is the assessment of the present and future potential of community organisations to Aids activities, and the improved understanding of their constitutions, decision-making, concrete contributions and spheres of influence.

In general, both rural and semi-rural[100] communities do not have any special structures organised to respond to Aids because they expect solutions (e.g.

---

[100] we prefer the use of "semi-rural", instead of "semi-urban" for the urban communities, either District capital, or Chefs Lieux d'Arrondissements, due to the original nature of the rural communities still largely dependent of agriculture for income

"magic bullet" such as a vaccine for example),[101] or support (e.g. information from NGOs) from the outside. For example in Kampti town, the youth mentioned four types of sources of information (market stands, theatre, informants from Ouagadougou, and national Aids Day), and deplored the majority of those (besides national Aids Day) did not take place anymore.

Influential people who are gatekeepers over different segments of communities or groups (religious, ethnic divisions, different types of crops, youth, administrative delegates, chiefs of land, tailors, traditional healers etc.) do not play any major role presently in the responses to Aids. Such popular-opinion leaders, yet, have been capable in each community to mobilise those and the resources necessary to participate in activities beneficial for the whole villages or neighbourhoods. Examples are numerous: purchase of a mill, training women for a small income-generating soap factory, building a school, installing water pumps, drilling for water, planting trees, building a health post, lodging facilities for teachers, working in collective fields, fabricating butter, building a market, improving the hygiene.

A number of activities in each community exists which are collective income-generating initiatives benefiting to different segments of population (e.g. women), to the benefits of specific community groups (shared incomes), or individuals (salaries), or both, such as collective fields, fabricating butter or oil or palm-wine. Large local active support networks of families, relatives, clans, religious groups, take place in case of serious problems (diseases, deaths…) to assist persons or families under various forms (food, physical, presents or materials, financial…). Several groups from different Churches have a support network for People Living With Aids (PLWAs) (hospital, home-visits in Gaoua). The potential of empowering those into self-help groups of people with HIV/Aids can be pursued. The creation of new Associations are sweeping west Africa, particularly among women and the youths due to the emergence of the civil society to face the shortages of their Governments (Hoth-Guechot 1996). Working with these Associations may be the new societies of hope for energetic responses originating from the local population, and still remain to be fully exploited.

Resource people (informants, youth groups) in each community are capable to identify and prioritise some of the needs and potential responses (prevention messages promoted through well respected channels such as youth groups, agricultural agent, church leaders, teachers…) to Aids at the community level. In

---

[101] the false expectations of overcoming the epidemic of HIV at the community level with the present vaccine development originated from radio sources in isolated communities

addition, influential people can be instrumental in stimulating and operationalising those. The willingness to contribute to the local responses to Aids by being Aids prevention advocates exists.

Based on these findings the key strategic priorities identified are:

- to inform the numerous existing structures and organisations at the community level that their contributions are essential, and that no ("magic") solutions can be expected from the outside in the near future,
- to stimulate sustainable or on-going community prevention activities through the existing local groups and Associations, e.g. youth-driven peer education, instead of outside interventions with ad-hoc information,
- to involve the influential people or gatekeepers of each community and develop preventive education materials tailored to their specific segments of populations or sphere of influence, and offer them a range of activities which can address the care and support activities,
- to investigate how part of local existing income-generating resources can benefit in turn some of the needs to stimulate local HIV responses,
- to stimulate and support local active support networks (e.g. Church groups) to assist People Living With Aids, and their families,
- to use resource people to identify and prioritise needs and potentials responses, and influential people to have communities act upon those.

6) External Partnerships of Communities

Numerous external partners build up fruitful collaboration with the communities through different sectoral activities others than health (agriculture, education, social affairs…), and are willing to contribute to HIV/Aids activities. Communities perceive themselves as recipients of an intervention of external partners, instead of being themselves partners in the interventions' deliveries.

External partners are little involved in HIV/Aids activities in general with the exception of one international NGO (Plan International Burkinabé). The latter operates in a few communities where other interventions are already taking place. In addition, GTZ provides some ad-hoc information activities (video films, market…) in the towns of Gaoua and Kampti, and the Ministry of Social Affairs has a few schools education activities in Gaoua town as well.

HIV prevention activities are limited geographically to very few among the most accessible communities (estimated 10%). They are ad-hoc, implemented and driven directly from the outside without the participation of influential individuals. They are largely general population interventions, ignoring more vulnerable groups (e.g. youth, migrants…).

Based on these findings the key strategic priorities identified are:

- the involvement of new external multi-sectoral partnerships in HIV prevention and Aids care and support activities,
- the development of HIV prevention and Aids care and support activities in larger geographical areas, covering less accessible communities, more sustainable, using local support organisations, and targeting some of the more vulnerable populations,
- the change of interventions and approach from externally-driven partners with their own of communities being passive recipients to communities as partners in interventions' deliveries.

The following Table (4.2) summarises the key findings of the situation analysis related to the determinants of community participation. The latter needs to be brought to the attention of program managers of the public and private sectors, and is necessary to build up community-oriented and participatory responses to HIV and Aids.

Table 4.2 Key summary findings of the situation analysis at the community level

Determinants	Obstacles	Opportunities	Strategic Priorities
1) Characteristics	Complexity (need special studies) based on ethnic origins, age groups, and sex	Numerous occupational (farming, palm wine…) groupings/ associations exist by sex and for youth	- Use of RRA methods to identify by ethnic background the important groups and associations to work with and leaders - Reinforce and work through the hidden but existent women and youth groups
	More visible male dominated assoc., but existing women assoc., informal youth groups	Possibilities to stimulate women and youth groups	- The responses to HIV/Aids can be stimulated through the dozen of different groups/ associations in each village (feasibility and sustainability to be tested), and/ or through the gatekeepers (key informants)
	Large migrant populations, different characteristics between urban and rural settings	To focus on a vulnerable group (migrant populations), and to use different entry points for urban and rural settings	- Identify communities with migrant populations and tailor special strategies - Use in town, the Associations (more formal), and in villages the Groupings (more traditional)
2) Perception of Aids	Cannot be cured	Perceived as serious problem	- to develop the care and support of Aids patients among the communities requesting those
	Negative socio-economic impact	Dynamic youth population	- to focus among the youth groups where those perceive themselves as the most HIV vulnerable groups
	Preventive not a priority	Care and support activities are a priority, and existing voluntary support networks	
3) Perceived Needs	In infrastructures and systems development	For small scale micro-projects development	- to develop micro-development income-generating projects - to develop the care and support of Aids patients in communities requesting
	Aids one among other public health problems	Aids is recognised as a serious problem	- to introduce other cost-efficient public health measures

	Prevention of HIV: low priority in comparison to care and support of Aids	Need to introduce care and support, and further introduction with justification of preventive activities	(vaccination…) - to introduce HIV preventive activities with a strong rational or information component justifying those
4) Health Sector	Functional PHC network minimal	Some communities have benefited from PHC support	- to benefit from the existing functional or ABBEF trained agents for agent of dissemination of HIV preventive activities
	ABBEF agents not motivated anymore but trained	National NGOs have been active for HIV prevention with some agents	- in the health centres, to introduce an adolescents' reproductive health program
	Health centres are not so accessible by all communities	Health centres well appreciated by youth	- to introduce other community health sector less informal communication channels, e.g. ref. 1 gatekeepers or local Groups and Associations
			- Target communities where youth do not recognise condom use as an important protection measure

5) Community Organisation	- Miracle solutions expected, and coming from the outside - No involvement of gatekeepers or leaders - No use of present local income-generating activities to respond to HIV/Aids	- Recognise importance and interested in preventive activities - Gatekeepers and leaders willing to contribute and important capacity to mobilise - Solidarity networks function for sick people and their families, as well as income-generating activities	- to stimulate sustainable or on-going prevention activities through existing local groups or Associations - to tap to local existing income-generating resources activities - to involve the local influential people or gatekeepers and develop materials tailored to their needs - to assist PLWAs and families with local active support networks - to use resource and influential people to prioritise and act
6) External Partnerships	- Minimal involvement of external partners in HIV/Aids activities - HIV prevention activities are geographically very limited, punctual, driven from the outside, not targeted to the more vulnerable groups (e.g. youth, communities with migrants) - Existing intersectoral partners untapped	- Some fruitful external partnerships exist in some domains - Some HIV prevention activities take place through external partners (NGO, GTZ, Social Affairs) - Intersectoral partners willing to participate (Agriculture, Development, Youth…)	- to involve new external multi-sectoral partnerships - to develop activities extending the geographical coverage, the less accessible communities, the sustainability, the use of existing local organisations, the targeting of more vulnerable populations (youth, migrants) - to have external partners promote communities' participation as partners instead of recipients

In summary, the findings point to the feasibility and value of identifying the characteristics of each community to build up a sensible partnership. Due to the advanced stage of the epidemics, communities are eager to enter into care and support activities, but they need to be guided through their own already existing community networks. Some more visible public health interventions, (vaccinations, malaria control) or micro-projects, may need to be introduced first to some communities to respond to their priorities before any HIV/Aids activities are accepted. This is an additional argument justifying the integration of HIV/Aids activities with other PHC and broader development activities. It also justifies the use of participatory methods for communities to recognise and act upon the disease. Aids prevention advocates need to be carefully selected among supportive groups and linked to the closest health centres, in addition to the district teams. Health Centres should offer in turn the broader Reproductive Health activities and support the community advocates. Existing active community organisations and their leaders should be the cornerstones of HIV prevention efforts and be active and supportive gatekeepers as their catalysts.

In turn, community participation was ranked based on six indicators (Table 4.3). A hectogram (spider web or spoke configuration) documents visually next (Fig. 4.1) the present situation of community participation using the above mentioned aggregated data based on the adoption of recent community participation assessment tools (Bjaras 1991) (Schmidt D. et al. 1996). It may be further exploited to observe the expected changes over the two or three year period during which the intervention takes place.

Table 4.3 Ranking scale for process indicators of community participation

Degree of participation

Indicators	Narrow	Medium	Wide
1. Community Characteristics	*Not considered or unknown*	Considered and known but not used correctly	Networks fully exploited
2. Perception of Aids	*Helplessness*	In between	A disease which can be overcome by the community
3. Perceived Community Needs	Others than health	*Development and Health related*	HIV prevention as a central need
4. Health Sector	Passive local health network	*In between*	Functional local health networks
5. Community Organisation	Not involved in public health activities	*Involved in public health but not in HIV/ Aids*	Involvement in HIV and Aids activities
6. External Partnerships	*None or almost none in health and externally-driven*	Some external involvement in health but still externally driven	Communities true partners in HIV/Aids activities

Legend: present estimates indicated *"in italic"*

Fig. 4.1 Hectogram Visualization of Community Participation to the DRI Gaoua District: 1997 and Planned Changes by Year 2000

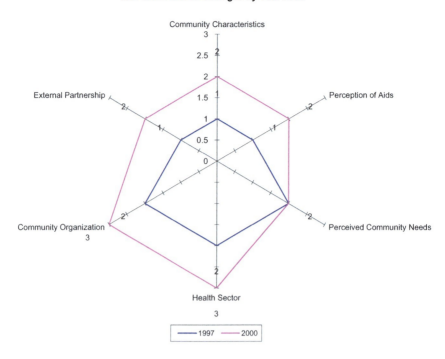

Based on the data collected as a baseline and their visualisation, besides a different forms of organised responses observed through the Health Sector and the Community Organisation, other components rate low still in the participatory process. By the year 2000, the local responses intervention should intensify and build-up on these two essential components of Health Sector, and Community Organisation[102]. At least three others should be instrumental in making good head-ways into the local responses as well: taking into consideration the various Community Characteristics when working with the communities, changing the Perception of Aids, and building up on the External Partnership. Finally, little changes may be expected in the short run for the Perceived Community Needs.

---

[102] unfortunately, the qualitative method used in early 2000 in Gaoua does not allow to compare the development of community participation with the baseline (other questions and communities)

4.1.2. The Factors of Vulnerability

In parallel to the analysis of community determinants, we collected and organised data into three broad categories (Table 4.4). They may allow to focus efforts to reduce the vulnerability of individuals and communities to HIV and Aids based on the known interaction of key factors: (i) personal factors, (ii) factors pertaining to the quality and coverage of services and programs aimed at prevention, care, social support, and (iii) socio-economic factors, such as norms, laws, social forces and impact alleviation (UNAIDS 1998). The literature and experiences abound in interventions related to the first two categories of factors, whereas the last one is less known. Influencing the environment to support personal behaviour change efforts, with additional elements such as social norms, relationships, environment and public health policies, is essential to complement the individual traditional approaches with risk reduction strategies (Keeley 1999).

The Focus Group Questionnaire for the Youth at the Community Level are attached separately (Appendix 4B).

Table 4.4 Critical factors and related questions to measure vulnerability and vulnerability reduction for the Gaoua Local Responses

1. Personal

a. Is Aids a problem among the youth?

b. What can be done to avoid Aids? Problems or difficulties with the use of condoms?

c. Changes in behaviours since Aids are known? More a problem of men or women? Due more to men or women (to identify any gender bias)?

2. Services and Programs

a. Are condoms available? Problems encountered to have access or buy condoms?

b. Availability of HIV testing and counselling services?
c. Availability of information about Aids, STD, Family Planning?

3. Socio-Economic

a. What is the impact of Aids among the youth? Among the community?

b. Is Aids feared among the youth? Why?

c. What can be done to avoid Aids among the youth? Among the community?

The following summarised key findings of the vulnerability factors are based on information collected through two focus group discussions in each community among 16 to 25 years old youth, males and females separately (Research methods, chap. 3). The full tables (Appendix 4C Vulnerability Factors: Original Findings) compiled in the original report (Pervilhac, Kipp et al. 1997) are recapitulated here under the form of a comprehensive table summarising the obstacles and opportunities. Based on those, the strategic programmatic priorities are suggested as well (Table 4.5). The data are aggregated next for all four communities. As per previous analysis of determinants, to tailor specific strategies for interventions, e.g. rural vs. urban or by gender, it is possible to analyse the data with the original transcripts separately.

Our findings concur with some of the earlier studies (Cros 1994; Cros 1995; Cros, Msellati et al. 1997) from ORSTOM accomplished in the region to document some of the local perceptions and descriptions of Aids which unfortunately did not have any applied programmatic consequences in the District.[103]

1) Personal Factors

In general youth possess a good knowledge of the main means of prevention (fidelity, condoms use, abstinence…), with evidence of individuals that are personally convinced and could in turn be convincing elements as part of a volunteer peer educators' network. In each group there is always a minority who does not know the exact causes of means of transmission. This leads in turn to false believes (e.g. sharing food with PLWAs, or stepping over their urine, or eating pork who ate the faeces of PLWAs, being close to PLWAs, etc.) which perpetuates stigmatisation. These findings were confirmed in the above mentioned ORSTOM studies. In addition, correct use may be a problem among a minority as well. Strategic priorities point to the need:

- to combat stigmatisation by overcoming local negative believes and behaviours on the transmission of HIV,
- to take stock of some of the youth males' and females' reservoirs of peer advocators,
- to carry out visual and practical demonstrations of the correct use of condoms (the "wooden penis" demonstration), and discuss problems (solidity, permeability, storage of condoms…) and negative believes ("condoms originating from America and disseminating Aids …").

---

[103] recent policies of the French government in 1998 and 1999 are attempting to have their research institutes (CNRS, ORSTOM) move into more applied research for the national authorities' benefits

The youth assert that some positive changes of behaviours (more abstinence, wearing condoms) are already occurring in their communities, but confirm some passivity to seek information and education about HIV prevention which are often too late, or do not care.

Strategic priority points to:

- to the need to promote group discussion for peer education to discuss delicate subjects and convince groups as a useful technique to approach the youth, and make information and education more accessible and timely (primary prevention), and convincing.

If a few males and females identify equal responsibilities of infections among both sexes, an important proportion of males blame females for being more responsible for the propagation of the disease. Strategic priority points to:

- the need to address gender issues by targeting male youth groups.

Several females gave evidence that successful negotiation with males for wearing condoms. Strategic priority identifies:

- the need to understand better the factors and means for the females successful negotiations of condoms among males.

In conclusion, we have documented in the analysis of personal vulnerability factors evidence of education and information that have been able to reach part of the youth already successfully. Several strategies and methods can catalyse further some of the present specific needs of the youth needs among both males and females.

2) Services and Programs Factors
Youth complained about the barriers to easy condom access, or to quality issues, more often in relation to the Social Marketing of Condoms (SMC) program. The public services played a minor role in the distribution of condoms. Strategic priorities address the need to:

- improve accessibility and quality of condoms distribution both through the SMC and public health services,
- train women sales force at the community level,
- increase accessibility of condoms for the youth through more anonymous distributors (e.g. peers) than the present ones (village shopkeepers who are relatives or lack discretion),

- study the feasibility of selling condoms by the unit instead of the present packaging of four condoms, in order to increase its financial accessibility for the youth.

Sources of information on HIV prevention need to be known and if possible, if not available within the communities, need at least to reach those. Existing media materials need to be distributed again or used in communities. Strategic priorities are to:

- let the youth, women, men know where they can find the closest information about HIV prevention,
- use, and disseminate existing materials to the groups (if too costly, at least to some of the gatekeepers and Aids prevention advocates).

Youth feel better informed about HIV than other areas of concerns as well, such as STD...). This finding is also congruent to the earlier ones from the ORSTOM studies mentioned earlier.[104] The strategic priority is:

- Health Centres need to offer the full Reproductive Health Services package (e.g. STDs, reference to testing and counselling...).

Care and support are perceived as a service to be received from the health infrastructures, and often not affordable. Strategic priority:

- address the accessibility issue of health services, and develop the care and support at the community level.

One young male commented on the importance of condoms and even suggested that a female condom would even be better. Female condom is "currently... the only safe, effective, female-controlled barrier method choice for preventing pregnancy and STDs, including HIV/Aids" (Gilbert 1999). It is currently available in seven countries in Africa, but not in Burkina Faso. This slow development of female condom experimentation contrasts wit the better known and larger efforts invested in the multi-drug therapies trials. Strategic priority:

- study the feasibility of female condoms distribution in more vulnerable groups.

---

[104] this finding appears to be a worldwide pattern based on similar findings of the 1998 Durex Global Sex Survey in 14 different countries with a sample of over 10,000 respondents and where the youth said they knew less about Sexually Transmitted Infections (e.g. 32% had never heard of Chlamydia) others than HIV (ref. C. Weilandt and C. Pervilhac et al., HIV Prevention Policy in Europe, WIAD/SPI, March 2000)

3) Socio-Economic Factors

The known impact of Aids among some communities and much feared disease may activate the collaboration of the hardest hit communities with more mobile populations to participate to HIV prevention activities (ref. section 5.1). Strategic priority:

- identify with rapid assessment methods the communities hardest hit by the epidemic and/ or with a more mobile, mostly young, population without stigmatising those.

Despite their remoteness, communities are aware of the existence or developments of multi-treatment drug therapies or vaccine that may negatively influence their support for HIV prevention activities. Strategic priority:

- inform on the importance and feasibility of introducing HIV preventive activities to protect the communities.

Condoms have a negative and shameful image. Strategic priority:

- Make condoms use a common and sensible feature of protection[105]

Deeply ingrained barriers involving cultural norms and values that may be contributing negative factors to the spread of HIV. e.g. ritual cleansing involving sexual intercourse after a woman is widowed, "levirat".[106]

Strategic priority:

- Overcome some of the negative cultural habits with feasible and acceptable alternatives

Negative impact on households with the young dying having as a consequence the loss of resources to cultivate field and to develop the village. Strategic priority:

- Extend existing small holder farming techniques (existence of a GTZ Agriculture project in the same area) tapping to the village Agricultural Co-

---

[105] "banaliser l'utilisation des condoms"

[106] tradition recommending or obligating the widow to marry one of her husbands' relatives

operatives (males and females), and to the employees of the Ministry of Agriculture equipped with motor-bike to cover their communities.

The following Table (4.5) summarises the key findings related to the factors of vulnerability to allow program managers to tailor more effective strategies and interventions for the HIV and Aids program

Table 4.5 Key summary findings of the vulnerability factors at the community level

Vulnerability Factors	Obstacles	Opportunities	Strategic Priorities
1. Personal	Exact causes of means of transmission still unknown with false believes inducing stigmatisation of PLWAs	Good knowledge of the main means of prevention (fidelity, condoms use, abstinence…)	- Combat stigmatisation by overcoming local negative believes and behaviours on the means of transmission of HIV
	Information and education seeking are passive	Some positive changes of behaviours (more abstinence, wearing of condoms) acknowledged in some communities	- Use group discussion for peer education (more difficult among females) to discuss delicate subjects
	Some males blame females of importing, or transmitting, or being negligent (prostitutes, not serious…)	In general an agreement that both sexes are responsible due to bad behaviours and being negligent	- Promote the use of condoms by addressing the bad experiences made by some youth, and reinforcing other positive experiences
		Some females are capable of negotiating successfully their partner(s) to wear condoms	- Address the males' blame on females in the youth education
	Many false rumours and believes still impinge upon the use of condoms among the youth	Condoms recognised and accepted as a good mean of prevention in almost all communities	- Exploit the successful negotiations of some females with their partners and study further the techniques involved
	Youth making bad experiences have no chances to discuss their problems with condoms and find alternatives	Openness to discuss difficulties and interests	

233

Vulnerability Factors	Obstacles	Opportunities	Strategic Priorities
2. Services and Programs	Logistics: poor storage, stock breakdowns, Health Centres play negligible role in condoms distribution	Improve quality logistics and bridge the gap between the social marketing condom (SMC) program and the public services and determine responsibilities	- Social marketing program needs to investigate and reassure Health Ctrs. Need to be active promoters of condoms
	Information on HIV prevention unavailable (except printed "STOP-AIDS" brochure in Kampti) or the sources of information unknown for youth or for women at the village level	Target HIV prevention to youth and women and clarify sources of information and disseminate some of the appreciated written existing brochures or former appreciated communication methods (videos, theatres....)	- Use youth or women groups from the villages or neighbourhoods to pass information. Specify sources of information, and use existing appreciated written materials. In Kampti the health centre needs to fulfil this role as well like in Gaoua - Need to promote availability and accessibility by and for women groups - Further investigate the pricing issue and sales strategy
	Less information on STD than on HIV in the Health Centres	Offer STD and Reproductive Health Services in Health Centres. Health personnel often well considered and appreciated for their expertise	- Improve STD and Reproductive Health Services in Health Centres - Offering quality testing and counselling services - Develop the care and support aspects in communities as well - Focus SMC in remote villages, and train women sales force at the village level. Study options for condoms sold by the unit at the village level.
	Lack of accessibility to testing and danger believes in mandatory testing for all travellers	Improve testing and counselling services and informing on best policy	- Explore feasibility of female condoms among more vulnerable groups.

234

Poverty does not allow to receive care in health services	Develop much neglected care and support component of Aids
Condoms seem less accessible for females than males (uncomfortable with the local known salesmen). Prices can be an issue for some individuals, males or females. Female condoms as perceived need.	Improve accessibility of condoms through improved SMC in remote communities and promoting female sales force. Reconsider sales by unit locally. Promotion of female condoms.

235

Vulnerability Factors	Obstacles	Opportunities	Strategic Priorities
3. Socio-economic	Aids cases cannot be detected and reported precisely at the community level	Known impact of Aids among the youth in the communities (approx. Aids cases known by youth), and psychological impact of surrounding deaths	- Benefit from the youth groups' capacities to identify the communities most struck by Aids with a rapid assessment of the approximate numbers of Aids
	Difficulty to assess exactly the financial impact of Aids	Known financial impact of Aids deaths among the youth and their communities (costs attached to care and support, or to lack of work force, or lack of future labour because the youth die and cannot have children)	- Reinforce the importance of preventing new infections with community-level interventions instead of hoping for treatments and vaccine in the near future
	Some community members knew and thought that multi-treatment drug therapies may be available soon, as well as a vaccine	Aids is a disease much feared by the youth due because it is a source of pains, cannot be detected easily, cannot be cured	- Target more mobile communities and groups within those without stigmatising
	Aids as a disease coming from another country	Prevent HIV infection in the communities by targeting communities with more mobile populations	
	Shame of the users of condoms	Condoms accepted among most of the youth	- Make condom use a common and sensible feature of protection
	Stigmatisation of Aids patients	Aids spread among the population at large	- Use local NGOs and Associations to combat negative cultural believes
	Negative cultural habits	Changing believes among the youth	

Negative impact on the village development and household income	Introduce small-holder agriculture farming techniques that require less labour, such as zero tillage, and less expensive inputs, including natural pest control.	- Tap to males and females co-operative groupings, and 32 employees Min. of Agriculture

237

A closer look at the various categories of vulnerability factors allows program managers to go beyond the first reaction commonly heard among national program managers of "déjà vu". As documented in the above Table, obstacles factors particular to the local situation to overcome can be identified, and in particular more opportunity factors as well. Those in turn lead to different strategic priorities which can be instrumental for the managers who can make, in consequence, an informed choice originating from the bottom-up to select the most appropriate strategy among the wide spectrum available (ref. chapter 1, Table 1.1).

In conclusion, the Community level study has brought a new community-oriented dimension to the planning and interventions approaches which was still missing up to now despite ten years of technical co-operation in this District of Burkina Faso. In addition to an improved understanding of the key vulnerability factors, some essential components of community participation to HIV/Aids are clarified. The present data can be used as baseline data for community interventions and progresses monitored over the next decade.

4.2. Situation Analysis at the District Level

The findings related to the district system presented in this section were collected mostly through the district level study, and partly confirmed with data from the community level study. The present data were analysed and documented in more details already elsewhere (Pervilhac, Kipp et al. 1997), similarly to the previous Situation Analysis at the Community level.

Program managers need to understand and master their environments at the District as much as at the Community levels. Current reviews addressing the present weakness of the HIV/Aids prevention programs point to the recent focus of efforts shifting from models aimed at changes in individual risk behaviour to models aimed at community mobilisation, with information-based campaigns displaced by intervention programs aiming at enabling and empowerment (Luger 1998). As a consequence, the local responses, in addition to the previous community level study (chap. 4), encompasses by nature an improved understanding of the intra-collaboration (e.g. within the Ministry of Health), and of the inter-sectoral collaborations (e.g. between different Ministries and between the Ministries and the partners from the private sector including the communities). This explains in turn the need to understand thoroughly who is doing what presently, who is not active among the potential partners and why, what is a common vision and the needs for the communities in the District, and how to improve policies and co-ordination in the District. Such an analysis aims to comprehend better the existing structures to support people instead of jumping directly and prematurely into implementing strategies, particularly in light of Health Sector Reforms (ref. section 1.2.2) which stimulated a District level responses. The failure of taking such a step leads, in turn, to responses to HIV/Aids that are limited, fragmented, inefficient, non-sustainable, not community-oriented, with insufficient resources, and often driven by the Ministry of Health without the support of other partners.

In light of this, the present analysis reviews first, the responses of the public sector, and, second, the one from the private sector. We have summarised and visualised the findings of the public and private sectors following these sections in an Institutional Landscape. Third, it takes the original findings of the situation analysis one step further in adding the review of the policy environment which were not covered during the study (ref. chap. 3 Methods), including aspects related to the intra- and inter-sectoral issues. Finally, we review the methodology and analytical framework we have used for the replication of the Local Responses.

The present analytical framework matches closely the "Managing AIDS project", a WHO Collaborative Study and the European Council of Aids Service Organisations between 1992 and 1995 (Kenis and Marin 1997). In the context of Africa, we do not know as of today of any other research approach than the present study. The degree of the organisational responses (being the dependent variable in the study) is defined as the degree to which an organisation or group of organisations responds to HIV/Aids. The responses correspond to the development of specific activities to deal with the problems of HIV transmissions and/or to reduce the negative personal and social consequences of HIV/Aids. Any organisation having at least one activity in the area of HIV/Aids in the study is considered as having organisational responses.

Three essential dimensions are assessed for each organisation:
- first, the types of activities (strategies, interventions, activities often summarised in objectives),
- second, the types of organisations (public or private, types of Non-Governmental Organisations such as Community-Based Organisations (CBOs), civil society organisations etc.),
- third, the distribution of the organisational across social groups (communities, vulnerable groups) and geographical areas (urban vs. rural,

border areas vs. others more accessible). The degree of the responses can be analysed on different levels (region, district, communities, households).

Our findings contrasted with the various original national experts' views that little or nothing was happening, i.e. little involvement of any institutions in the District of Gaoua, and that the situation was desperate with the consequence that other more active Districts than Gaoua should be approached for Local Responses. We observed among over half a dozen institutions surveyed in each of the public and private sector, that several partners in both sectors were already involved in some HIV/Aids activities. The profile is low and responses weak as we shall see next, with an institutional landscape not as crowded as Districts of higher profile and prevalence, for example in a similar Local Responses study carried out in Kabarole District, Uganda (Pervilhac, Kipp et al. 1997). The potential partners are numerous, and those could be involved at little additional costs in the Local Responses. Developing a common vision to the Responses and an improved share of roles and tasks between partners, under the leadership of one partner should be possible as well.

We developed an analytical framework (Table 4.6) to assess the degree of the organisational responses in the district and structured the detailed questionnaire (Appendix 4D) around these key areas. The framework has been adapted to be user friendly for program managers at the district level by categorising the questions and variables into the current categories of indicators (inputs, process, and outputs) they are familiar with. Those are currently used in public health development programs either by bi-lateral organisations such as GTZ (GTZ and ITHOG 1989), or WHO (WHO 1996), or more recently specific HIV prevention and Aids care programs (Ng'weshemi, Boerma et al. 1997).

The three categories fall into:

- Inputs or structural fix or independent variables, those which cannot be changed,
- Process or structural changeable variables, in turn those which can be either modified or influenced in the planning or implementation stages,
- Output or structural dependent variable, the result, or improving the degree of responses of each organisation from no, to at least one activity for the potential partners, and from weak or low to medium responses, or from medium to strong responses.

By including the degree of responses as an output indicator, the present model has the advantage to stimulate program managers to pay attention and enable the various organisations to play more efficient roles than they presently do, and monitor the changes over time as an organisational surveillance tool. After all, if individual behaviours can be influenced and change over times, organisational behaviours in relation to their responses and contribution to HIV/Aids can and should be influenced, and improve over time as well. To make an inventory from the beginning of the strength and weaknesses of these partners (inputs), and to analyse the factors which can or need to change over time (process) makes it a more powerful analytical and managerial framework in order to reach more effective responses.

Table 4.6 Analytical framework of the Organisational Responses with related questions to measure the degree of the organisational responses for the Gaoua Local Responses

1. Inputs (structural fix variables)

a. Is the organisation a public or a private one?

b. Is the organisation an active one or not in HIV/Aids? (at least one activity)

c. What is the experience of the organisation? (age, maturity…)

d. Is the organisation working on gender issues? (directed by women, targeting women and/ or women's issues…)

e. What is the organisation future development plan?

2. Process (structural changeable variables)

a. What strategies and types of programs is the organisation involved in, or plans?

b. What strategies and types of programs is the organisation planning to get involved in, or plans? (future role, willingness…)

c. In Reproductive Health, which activities other than HIV/Aids (e.g. STD, family planning,TB) is the organisation involved in, or plans?

d. Which geographical areas of intervention (semi-rural or rural), or plans?

e. Which vulnerable groups are the organisation involved with, or plans?

f. How much is the planning for the types of programs based on communities needs, or plans?

g. What are the human resource capabilities (volunteers, motivation, expertise…), present general expertise, and main constraints for the organisation contribution to a future expanded Responses

h. What are the stakeholders' relationships of the organisation with other partners from the public or private sectors (threat, competition, stimulation…)

i. Who should take the leadership role of an expanded Responses in the district and why?

The Institutional Landscape (next Fig. 4.2) illustrates some of the key indicators of the inventory taking at the district level. It identifies the organisations active (present partners) or not (potential partners), estimates the degree of responses of the active ones, visualises the co-ordinating and common vision development (reflected by the central arrow directed towards the centre with the identification of the co-ordinating body and Plan). It does not illustrate the strategies and types of programs that can be illustrated in another landscape (ref. 5.5).

Fig. 4.2

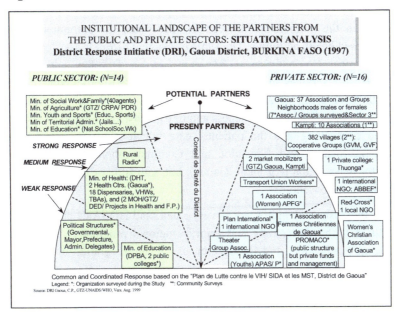

INSTITUTIONAL LANDSCAPE OF THE PARTNERS FROM
THE PUBLIC AND PRIVATE SECTORS: **SITUATION ANALYSIS**
District Response Initiative (DRI), Gaoua District, BURKINA FASO (1997)

PUBLIC SECTOR: (N=14)   *PRIVATE SECTOR: (N=16)*

POTENTIAL PARTNERS

Min. of Social Work&Family*(40agents)
Min. of Agriculture* (GTZ/ CRPA/ PDR)
Min. Youth and Sports* (Educ., Sports)
Min of Territorial Admin.* (Jails...)
Min. of Education* (Nat.SchoolSoc.Wk)

Gaoua: 37 Association and Groups
Neighborhoods males or females
(7*Assoc./ Groups surveyed&Sector 3**)

Kampti: 10 Associations (1**)

PRESENT PARTNERS

382 villages (2**):
Cooperative Groups (GVM, GVF)

STRONG RESPONSE

MEDIUM RESPONSE

Rural Radio*

2 market mobilizers
(GTZ) Gaoua, Kampti

1 Private college:
Thuonga*

WEAK RESPONSE

Min. of Health: (DHT,
2 Health Ctrs. (Gaoua*),
18 Dispensaries, VHWs,
TBAs), and (2 MOH/GTZ/
DED/ Projects in Health and F.P.)

Transport Union Workers*

1 international
NGO: ABBEF*

1 Association
(Women) APFG*

Red-Cross*
1 local NGO

Political Structures*
(Governmental,
Mayor,Prefecture,
Admin. Delegates)

Plan International*
1 international NGO

1 Association
Femmes Chrétiennes
de Gaoua*

Women's
Christian
Association
of Gaoua*

Theater
Group Assoc.

PROMACO*
(public structure
but private funds
and management)

Min. of Education
(DPBA, 2 public
colleges*)

1 Association
(Youths) APAS/ P*

Conseil de Santé du District

Common and Coordinated Response based on the "Plan de Lutte contre le VIH/ SIDA et les MST, District de Gaoua"
Legend: *: Organization surveyed during the Study   **: Community Surveys
Source: DRI Gaoua, C.P., GTZ-UNAIDS/WHO, Vers. Aug. 1999

The results of the situation analysis described next is a step to identify the actors, and their present competencies and limitations, which in turn can improve the share of responsibilities and tasks (ref. section 4.3.1).

4.2.1 The Responses of the Public Sector

1) The Ministry of Health

The study used different proxy outcome indicators of health services provision (e.g. immunisation coverage and contraceptive prevalence) to assess services provision. It confirmed the present state of disarray of public health services, in comparison to former achievements, e.g. the high vaccination coverage reached in the eighties.

The Ministry of Health (MoH) new annual District Health Plan encompassed HIV/Aids activities in which the District Health Team and various levels of the health care systems with the twenty health infrastructures and the hospital operating in the District already involved. The Plan covers training, supervision, improvement of services, delivering of equipment including sterilisation, and setting up community patients' care. It fails to clarify either the strategies to reach the objectives or to specify who are the partners involved others than

MOH or international bi-lateral agencies. Few Village Health Workers from the PHC days are still functional, and the large drop-outs may have exacerbated a lack of trust in the partnership between the MoH and the communities for community-based health activities. The MoH of Gaoua District is assisted by the German Technical Co-operation (GTZ) and German Development Service (DED) for Health Services in Rural Setting and Human Reproductive Health Project with three types of activities. First, the epidemiological surveillance which has problems of data completeness and of capacity for doing local testing. Second, the counselling and the patients' care which is quasi non-existent. Third, the Information and Education and Communication (IEC) which is functional for mass media (e.g. radio Gaoua), but with little or no activities for Communities and Households.

In addition, the District Health Team is very small, and HIV/Aids activities are in competition with other strong and priority national programs, such as the Guinea Worm Eradication, and Onchocerciasis.[107] The integration of activities has led to a one man show, or having a single program manager for all Communicable Diseases at the District level. Yet, for accountability and daily management purposes, it now becomes difficult to know "who is really in charge?" in contrast to earlier large vertical programs (e.g. EPI, CDD…) of the eighties.[108]

The communities and the organisations in the District perceived the MoH as the present leader in the public sector in the combat against HIV/Aids in the District. The MoH was identified as such because of its public health mandate, and its past and present activities. Based on the number of activities the MoH is presently involved in at the District level, even if insufficient in number and quality, we graded its present responses as "medium" in comparison to other public agencies. Hence, we used arbitrarily that structure as yardstick to assess the degrees of responses of the public structure.

2) Other Ministries
The rural radio ("Radio Gaoua") with the Director and managers have a long history of contribution, since 1996 at least, to information campaigns well adapted to and pre-tested among the local culture. Those have been financed by NGOs (Plan International and ABBEF), and by GTZ (Reproductive Health

---

[107] During our visit and study, experts from both programs were present and competing for the scarce time and resources of the District Health Team
[108] personal communication with Harry Godfrey, Consultant for the Guinea Worm Eradication, Carter Centre, Atlanta, USA (Gaoua, June 1997)

Project). The limitations of mass media campaigns to change behaviours are known to the technicians. The Radio was consequently rated medium on an equal footing to the MoH.

Two non-negligible but lower profile active structures were rated as weak responses: the Political Government Structures, and the Ministry of Education. The former, through the Mayor and the Préfet, and less so through the Administrative Delegates, are informing the public opinion about the danger of Aids and the importance of protection using condoms, even if not done systematically and efficiently enough. The latter, Ministry of Education, supervises all secondary schools in the Region and has recently in 1997 involved the teachers in a training program to educate school children; two public colleges are already active with sexual health and HIV/Aids education. We pointed to a few major constraints the school education program should overcome to have an impact on the youth. The program targets children between 13-15 years and may be more effective by targeting the 9-10 year children already to avoid early pregnancies, and to reach the young girls who drop out heavily from schools later. The teaching about Aids may be too academic and not practical enough (e.g. biomedical and lacking simple messages on de-stigmatising the disease a topic much in need of discussion in the whole district). Finally, didactic materials need updating (e.g. dissemination and use of the excellent flip charts of Plan International).

3) Potential Partners

The **potential partners of the public sector** are numerous and their contributions to improved responses important. By order of priority based on their present or future roles in relation to their capacities, coverage, and the present needs determined by the communities:

- The **Ministry of Social Work and Family**, with a small team of nine employees in Gaoua town and forty trained Agents could play the much needed role in the key strategy missing of home visits and psychological support through its "Service of Social Insertion." A recent restructure of the MoH which has left that Ministry on its own with little resources and a new role to be defined may have created hard feelings to collaborate together.
- The **Ministry of Agriculture**, in charge of the popularisation and efficiency of the agricultural sector in the whole Province has thirty-two employees

who are in permanent contact and speak the communities' vernacular languages. They also have the advantage of benefiting from their own transport (motor bikes). Some Agents are participating presently to the Guinea Worm Eradication program giving evidence of the feasibility of the inter-sectoral collaboration with the MoH. This could be an excellent entry point for training and supervising peer educators in the Agricultural Co-operatives Groupings.

- The **Ministry of Youth and Sports** (Education, Sports…) can reach several hundreds of youths through its Continuing Education program, and organises small well attended regional football events for the youth. An "Anti-Aids Cup" was an idea welcome and financially feasible, under the potential sponsorship of the Social Marketing of Condoms Project (PROMACO).

- The **National School of Social Work/ Ministry of Education** is responsible for the output of approximately thirty to forty social workers per year for the country. Despite twelve teachers trained for a month in 1996 on Aids/IEC, the social workers' curriculum and roles, particularly in relation to the care and support components, are still quite limited and cannot meet the new needs described above of the Ministry of Social Work and Family. A narrow partnership between the School interns and the Ministry operating in Gaoua could spearhead the efforts in that direction, and encourage the School staff to integrate such topics and applications in their curricula.

- The **Ministry of Territorial Administration** (jails…) welcomed the fact of introducing HIV/Aids prevention, at least information and education, among the prisoners of the jail located in town, particularly due to the high turnover of a large part of that population.

4.2.2 The Responses of the Private Sector

The programs from the private sector are largely community-based. Several actors in the private sector, particularly NGOs, could use other more cost-effective types of programs (institutional or media-based).

1) The Non-Governmental Organisations
We identified two key international NGOs active in the District, and by-and-large in the Poni region: Plan International, a branch from the United Kingdom, and the Social Marketing of Condoms Project (PROMACO)[109], a branch from Population Services International (PSI), USA.

Plan International covers 56 villages out of over 500 that the District encompasses with an "integrated development" project, but only 18 villages comprise an HIV/Aids prevention component under the form of community education and communication strategy. The villages have been selected by geographical priority: at least half a dozen around the high prevalence Kampti area, and half a dozen at busy road –crossings. In addition a second component of HIV/Aids prevention relates to school health programs.

The health education materials used (flip charts, T-shirts) and messages are well designed, of high priority (e.g. on de-stigmatisation) and culturally well adapted.

Potential remains in several domains: first, to improve the geographical coverage; second, to share and promote materials with other partners of the public and private sectors; third, to contribute with lessons learnt from the program to skills-building and diffusion of experiences to the other numerous present or potential district private and public sectors' partners; fourth, to play a pro-active role in leading the expanded responses in the District, instead of confining itself and be satisfied with limited direct interventions in a few villages.

In parallel to the above mentioned selection of the MoH as the yardstick for the public sector, the partners identified Plan International as the most visible and efficient private organisation working in HIV/Aids selected consequently as the yardstick for the private sector. With a large potential to improve performance still, it was rated as medium responses to HIV/Aids in the District.

---

[109] financed largely by KfW

The **social marketing** of the "Prudence" **condoms** by **PROMACO**[110] benefits from over 250 outlets in the District, with approximately 20 located in Gaoua and Kampti towns. Yet the qualitative studies, carried out at the community level, confirmed among the youth the lack of accessibility still to those, either geographic (particularly rural areas) or economic (high cost of packet vs. unit for youth), or social (among youth, fear of vendors' lack of confidentiality in small communities). In addition, storage breakdowns are frequent, and clients' complaints point to the deficiencies of the distribution systems either in the public (despite large stocks available permanently in the district capital) or in the private sectors. Besides the two direct and well appreciated "bals populaires Prudence" (Prudence dancing balls) sponsored in Gaoua town, PROMACO, through its local representative, is not participating as much as expected to local events and is oblivious of the public sector representatives and their activities and problems. The strategy used is not much different than any salesmen functioning in the area (Coca-Cola, Marlboro[111]...), whereas the "social" in the marketing should make a difference, instead of the mere sales of condoms, as cigarettes, for example. In conclusion, we rated PROMACO as weak responses in comparison to the large untapped potential of being a more active partner.

2) The Associations

Among large local formal community organisations (registered or well-structured), belonging to a type of civil society organisations, we identified one outstanding organisation, the "**Association of the Women of Gaoua**" (APFG). It focuses on women on socio-economic and cultural activities which can change women's conditions (family planning, circumcision, Aids and STD, hygiene and health, girls' schooling, persons and family rights such as women's violence or access to land). Local conferences are sponsored on such delicate topics. In a few villages around the district capital, the APFG carries out similar education and sensitisation about HIV/Aids transmission and prevention as Plan International. It also produces its own self-sustaining income generating projects (soap, plantation). It is the only organisation that can document an

active role, and shows concern, in the development of Community-Based Organisations (CBOs) or self-help groups capacities (training, demonstration, supervision...). As such the APFG was rated as having medium responses. It

---

[110] classified despite its attachment to the MOH as a private structure because of its private sources of financing and independent management structure from the MOH
[111] as we observed incidentally during our visit the PROMACO and Marloboro sales agents' presence and activities during our visit in the Gaoua town

was identified as being the main partner capable to lead the needed co-ordination of the private sector's responses in the district.

A smaller and more recent local Association created a few months before the visit, the "**Anti-Aids Promotion and Family Planning Association**" **(APAS/P)** was created specifically to respond to the problems attached to HIV and Aids. With its limited resources, it concentrated in Gaoua town on de-stigmatising the disease but lacks trained health promoters, and cannot really have their People Living With Aids (PLWAs) come out. They also visit Aids patients and their families and support them (washing, presents...). The few activities documented allowed to place already this organisation as an active partner with still weak responses.

Three smaller Associations have been capable to contribute to "medium" responses in the District given their relatively small capacities in comparison to other larger organisations. The **"Theater Group Association"** based on the findings of the community level study has been doing extensive and successful work in the promotion of HIV/Aids campaigns among communities in the District. Due to financial difficulties, this Association presently had a lower profile. The **"Transport Union Workers"**, a civil society organisation, benefited recently locally from one information session on HIV/Aids dangers and prevention methods by an outside team from Bobo-Dioulasso and had mobilised its workers to benefit from the information. It is well organised, with branches throughout the Region. A recent evaluation of the national Program with an increase of 65 to 79% in a two years intervention program on the use of condoms among truck workers documents quite a positive outcome; despite the authors' formulation of a different opinion, saying the condom use increased little (Testa J. et al. 1996). Two GTZ-financed individuals identified as the **"Market Mobilisers"**, a special project, have plaid similar roles of information as the two organisations just mentioned previously by holding regular sessions on market days.

One self-help group, the "**Christian Association of the Women in Gaoua**" with 130 women voluntary members functions in Gaoua town and the immediate surroundings. It plays already the role, informally and as a self-sufficient group, of supporting the PLWAs. Some members have been trained in management and family planning. The Association lacks financial means to extend their work (gasoline for mopeds...), and would like to become more involved and have more capacities towards the needed role of psycho-social care and support of PLWAs.

3) Potential Partners

In turn, the **potential partners of the private sector** are huge, and as such, their contributions to expanded responses remain to be tapped to. We have classified next by order of priorities (town first, less costs and a highly mobile population and probably more highly infected than rural) and feasibility of success these organisations:

- In Gaoua, 37 males or females **Associations and Groups by neighbourhoods and for the youth** as well, and in Kampti, 10 of those, are true self-help groups self-sustained or informal grassroots community organisations that could be at the heart of peers educators' support, local activities development.
- approximately **500 villages in the rural District with existing distinct males and females Co-operatives Groupings**, are Community-Based-Organisations (CBOs) similar to the ones mentioned for Gaoua above, but may need more nurturing, support and supervision than those.
- the **Red-Cross**, a local NGO, dynamic, with over 30 volunteers, one third females, with many qualified first aid workers. Would have much potential to support the psycho-social and care support component in urban areas (Gaoua, Kampti, and capitals of Departments, and jail), if they were provided minimum resources.
- one **private College** (Thuonga) in Gaoua, can add an HIV prevention information and education activity like among the public colleges mentioned previously.
- the **"Association for the Good Condition of the Family" (Association pour le Bien-Etre Familial/ ABBEF"),** international NGO, is dormant in Gaoua, but would have the potential to focus as well on the same component as the Red-Cross, but in rural areas.

In conclusion, we found the Associations to be a large untapped potential of existing resources of structures, people centred, to expand the Responses at the roots among the more vulnerable groups of women and youth.

Among civil society organisations, different Associations have different talents and a large potential to contribute to some of the needed strategies. To cite a few examples:

- the "Association of the education and training of orphan children" (ATEFEO);

- the "Association Souotaba" combining working professional and their talents from the health field (Medical Centre and Hospital) and Agriculture (CRPA, PDR/GTZ) which could instigate an intersectoral project with the Agriculture sector, or improve the quality of care in health infrastructures;
- the "Association of new ideas" (FILPAH) who has several community micro-projects particularly in literacy programs for school drop-outs;
- the "Association of the promotion of young girls and the prevention of Aids in urban area" for young girls from rural areas who need lodging in town to continue their education.

NGOs and Associations have increased by three folds over a three-year period from in the capital Ougadougou between 1994 and 1997 to reach almost one hundred (Desconnets and Taverne 1997). This rapid expansion translates the growing interest and willingness of the communities, and by and large the society, to organise itself to respond to HIV and Aids. Inventories have not been taken yet at the District level. It is encouraging though to find out in our study, in 1997, that the rural communities had organised themselves as well with a substantial number of formal and informal groups already committed or ready to contribute to the HIV/Aids activities.

4.2.3 Policy Environment for the Local Responses

This analysis is based on the situation analyses combined with a literature review of existing studies. It is not a focus of the present research and therefore will not be discussed any further (chap. 5).

The present micro-policy environment is little conducive or even counter-productive to expanded Responses towards efficient activities encouraged and shared between the present or potential public and private partners.

In the public sector, the Ministry of Health (MoH) is keeping its old prerogative of dominating and running the HIV/Aids activities in the District with a few privileged partners. Among those, activities with GTZ encompass the support of a few HIV/Aids activities related to the Market Mobilisers and IEC among the communities, the problematic HIV testing and counselling in the hospital, and the supervision of health personnel in the district. Neither the MoH, nor GTZ, are playing a leading force of empowering and delegating tasks within the presently active public institutions, nor are they encouraging some of the key public institutions to join forces in expanding the Responses. In addition, the

MoH is competing with some of the private institutions for some activities, for example school education activities, condom distribution, community sensitisation. Only the Rural Radio has been quite active as another public institution. Its mass media information in the Region, for example improving the knowledge of the danger of HIV and routes of transmission, has been successful. Still, its impact in de-stigmatising the disease among the communities has been quite insufficient, and therefore negligible. No policies or plans, up to this study, have addressed this major negative barrier which still urgently needs to be overcome.

In the private sector, the Plan International is dominating the activities but in isolation, within a limited geographical area, with little benefits for other private or pubic partners either to learn or strengthen their capacities. Private partners are competing, when not with the MoH, between one another for scarce resources. An atmosphere of conspiracy is even dominating between organisations with the fear of having its proposal "pirated."[112] Existing powerful and effective small Associations who could be the best multipliers either for sustainable community mobilisation, or for peer education, are overlooked.

No consensus exists among partners on priority areas, either by strategies or geographical or vulnerable groups, and the Responses are piecemeal with no overall orientation. All present partners in the institutional landscape looks in a dynamic environment as isolated actors functioning under centripetal or dispersing forces.

At a national level, co-ordination offices for NGOs, which should play a facilitating role between private partners and the public sector, are numerous and sponsored by international organisations. Those are, for example: the "Bureau de Suivi des

Organisations Non Gouvernementales" (BSONG), the "Secrétariat Permanent des Organisations Non Gouvernementales" (SPONG), the "Bureau de Liaison des ONG et Associations Nationales" (BLONGA). Their impact and usefulness to facilitate HIV/Aids activities at the District level appear to be negligible based on our observations.

The Local Responses approach attempts to remedy to the present weaknesses by creating a policy environment conducive to the expansion of more efficient responses. All actors work towards a common vision, as partners, of how the HIV/Aids responses should be organised in the District. Each partner contribute

---

[112] term commonly used by NGOs and Associations' representatives during the survey

to this common goal by taking into consideration the institutions' own strengths and limitations. The partners will function therefore under centrifugal or unifying forces co-ordinated by a District Health Committee (as illustrated by the arrow of the Institutional Landscape) in which the MoH becomes a leading and co-ordinating force. District Health Offices of the MoH have been requested recently to produce a five years "Development and Action Plan of the District Health" in the context of the Health Sector Reform. A common consensus exists that the public sector through the MoH should be more a steering and leading force in expanding the Responses, instead of carrying out activities itself, with roles focusing more on planning and evaluation of programs, and on training, i.e. steering more the boat instead of rowing.

A macro-policy review of the "Decentralisation and Health Systems Change: Burkina Faso Case Study" (Foltz A.-M. et al. 1996) gives evidence that the recent development of the Health Sector Reform creates an enabling context to the implementation of the Local Responses.

Foltz et al. documents that administratively it was only recently, after 1991, that decentralisation became a major explicit policy goal of the administration. Until the reforms, none of the administrative units of the country, whether Provinces, or Departments, or Communes, or villages, enjoyed actual functional autonomy of any sort in a country where political and administrative rule was conjoined in the one-party state. Budgets, personnel, and infrastructures were strictly controlled from the centre. This control extended to the Ministries themselves. The territorial decentralisation encompassed in the 1991 Constitution, and encoded in a series of laws passed in 1993, divided the country into decentralised collectivities in order to provide a framework for local democracy, and to assure local economic and social development.

The Health Sector in turn, under a condition to a World Bank Project financing in 1993, imposed the creation of the districts. The latter still had no juridical status as of 1995. This choice, not perceived as an indigenous policy preference and not accompanied by the necessary staff, funds, vehicles, equipment, infrastructures allocations, has led in turn to difficulties in making the District system a functional unit. In addition, confusion, when not conflicts, were rampant between the Provincial health directorates and the new District directors. Finally, to complete a process of a district health policy going nowhere, the health sector has in turn reached recently a consensus in 1995 to eliminate entirely the Provincial Departments of Health. The latter had no more autonomy than in 1983 when first established, and it was decided to move towards 11 Health Regions, each with its own hospital. As of 1995, none of the Regional hospitals was authorised to manage its own staff, finances, equipment or infrastructure, still making it an independent centrally run Unit from Ouagadougou, and downplaying its role as Districts and Regional referral centre. Hospitalisation for Aids, TB, Leprosy and Trypanosomiasis is free of charge for third to fifth categories of room in public hospitals by Presidential decree (May 1991). But the application of this decree is low because the hospitals suffer budgetary constraints, and the Aids patients are not identified correctly by lack of HIV test or mis-diagnosis.[113] The 53 Health Districts, created on paper by the Ministry, had no juridical status as of 1995, as well as no counterpart in the larger territorial administrative structure, and no resources allocated by the Ministry.

One of the main conclusions of the 1995 policy analysis is still very present in the positive, but still incomplete, present policy process developments that were taking place at the time of the local responses study:

> *"The multiplicity of levels involved, the multiplicity of institutions involved, and the contradictions among the different streams which arose from different objectives or from different advocates and supporters, created uncertainty about what decentralisation processes were actually underway. For example... autonomy of the provinces, as part of territorial decentralisation, could lead to provinces as the dominant decentralised unit in the health system."*
> (p. 16)

In 1997, we observed still the dominant role plaid by the Health Region in comparison to a power and resource-less District. The complexity to implement decentralisation --a mix of political, administrative, and technical choices-- is known for the health sector as a whole. The Health District and its District Health Team (DHT), as a consequence, will face difficulties to take a leadership role in the Local Responses to HIV/Aids in Gaoua District. Fortunately, the identical location of both the Region and the District authorities may confound and resolve the issue where the personalities' relationships and good will can overcome locally and temporarily, structural barriers. Still, this threatens the replicability of the Local Responses approach on a larger scale in other districts, even in the Poni Region.

---

[113] K. Ouedraogo, Key Correspondent (Burkina Faso), Fondation du Présent. "Services Under Strain –Burkina Faso, XI Pre-ICASA internet communication, 13.8.1999

A very big and real danger of "decentralisation" has been well described recently in the recent World Bank strategic planning document for Africa:

> *"Through health sector reform, HIV/Aids programs are being decentralised to districts without much-needed strong central guidance and sufficient resources."* (The World Bank 1999)

In 1999, an inter-country workshop on Health Reform and HIV (Reeler 1999) located in Gaoua District, with participants from the West Africa Region (Burkina Faso, Ghana, and Mali) and Thailand, identified the following main constraints related to the health system of the District:

- first, the insufficient accessibility to health care, either geographical or financial;
- second, the weaknesses in the performance of the health system due to the insufficient quality and quantity of health personnel and their high mobility, and specifically for HIV/Aids, the insufficiency of counselling for testing for HIV and lack of availability of testing facilities, and inadequate blood screening and safety;
- third, the underreporting of STD/Aids cases.

In conclusion, the Local Responses may facilitate the policy-making process to advance some of the key national policy areas and questions relating, to resolve, for example, the following issues raised through this study:

- How can the Regional Hospital still heavily linked to the central level of Ouagadougou play, at the tertiary level of care, a more active role at the District(s) level in the Poni Health Region (e.g. activities related to the HIV testing and surveillance, and counselling, to blood screening and safety)?
- How can the secondary level of care in the District (Health Centres) be functional as "community-managed health centres" through the introduction of the user fees? How can the Health Centres offer sufficient quality of care (drugs/ condom availability, and services for example in Reproductive Health, counselling in HIV/ Aids...) and improve the referral link between the communities and the hospital?
- How can the District Health Team, with reduced personnel and limited skills in HIV/ Aids, be empowered to play the role expected in the Local Responses with a supportive role from the Region Health Team?
- How can the political structure in the Region and in the Departments contribute to these different elements?

- How can the Co-ordination Offices for Non-Governmental Organisations located at the national level address the urgent problems of co-ordination at the District level, ironing out the competition between large international NGOs or between small Associations, while maximising their inputs to the Local Responses, and facilitating the financial mechanisms of the activities?

4.3. Planning

Following the Situation Analyses at the Community and the District levels (4.1 and 4.2), I initiated the Solution Development, or the planning process, through a "Consensus-Building and Pre-Planning" in country workshop. It had been originally planned at the beginning of the Action-Research, as a logical step following the "Situation Analysis" (chap. 1, Fig. 1.3). Observations follow to improve this step (4.3.1). The process was further catalysed and accelerated between mid-1998 to mid-1999 by the UNAIDS Country Broker into a full "Strategic Planning" process and document (4.3.2). These two steps show the long and critical period needed for "Solution Development" Phase, following the situation analyses to anchor ownership locally.

The different case-country studies and the new Local Responses approach were carried out in 1997 and 1998 with the first results collected already in 1999, such as the ones reported here for Burkina Faso (4.4). UNAIDS and some of the co-sponsoring Agencies, e.g. the World Bank or UNDP, needed to know what is the state-of-the art of the different tools which can be used to sustain and scale-up such an approach in other countries. After two years of the planning and first stage of implementation of the Local Responses process, the present researcher was mandated by UNAIDS to make an inventory and analysis of existing tools (5.1.5). The Local Responses will necessitate the adaptation of existing tools, or the development of new ones. We illustrated our experience in Burkina Faso limited to one facet of assessment: the "development of a new organisational tool", called the "Rapid Organisational Review" (ROR), based on the sociology of organisations (5.1.6). It aims to give insights into the public and voluntary structures functioning at the district level, and is illustrated under the form of institutional landscapes. If the solutions appear to be evident and easy on the paper, and despite the existence of some tools, we identified several barriers and constraints which need to be addressed in order to have more vulnerable groups participate and respond to HIV/Aids, taking the example of border migrants (5.1.7).

4.3.1 Consensus Building and Pre-Planning

The workshop aimed to plan and reach a consensus among the various partners on how to expand the responses in the District. To catalyse the transition from translating research case study findings into action, the workshop brought together all key partners from all Sectors, as well as the community representatives from the four communities where the study had taken place (chap. 1, Fig. 1.4). Consequently, representatives from each health system (communities, public, and voluntary for and not for profit) were invited in equal proportion (approximately 10 of each, or a total of 30).

The present researcher conceptualised and co-ordinated the Consensus-Building and Pre-Planning Workshop with the support of various international and local partners.[114]

The present findings were part of a formal Report addressed to GTZ (Pervilhac C. et al. 1998) with full detailed findings of the Workshop available in a separate Report (Nana and Sanogo 1998).

The workshop succeeded in accomplishing the following objectives:

- first, the institutional baseline data collected during the situation analyses were confirmed, or validated, during the workshop. All the partners outlined the various objectives and strategies in which they were presently engaged. The provision of care and social support for people, and socio-economic impact reduction were pointed as important strategies overlooked by all partners both from all sectors.

- second, several feasible Information Education and Communication (IEC) activities targeted to youth, women and migrants were identified by the four different communities (including resource and influential people, internal and external resources). Ten vulnerable groups were prioritised (youths, women of childbearing age, STD patients, international migrants, orphans as the first five of those) (para. 5.1.7 Migrants). A more detailed planning matrix, describing the youth and the women of childbearing age as vulnerable populations, was tested successfully by a group of technicians (Appendix 5A Matrix to Describe Vulnerable Populations). The matrix allows to assess for each vulnerable group dimensions related to: size of the population, risk behaviours, factors influencing infection, levels of possibilities of being infected or infecting others, relative

---

[114] GTZ Burkina Faso country team, the GTZ HQs Office, Eschborn, FRG., and GTZ RAP Office, Accra, Ghana, and national resource technicians (UNAIDS, WHO, National AIDS Control Program)

importance, present interventions, future interventions). Geographical areas of interventions could not be determined by lack of time.

- third, all the participants agreed as a common vision for 1998-2000/2002 to have the following five objectives to expand the Responses to HIV/Aids, accompanied by twenty one interventions (Appendix 5B Synthesis Table) identified to complete those:

1. The prevention of HIV/Aids infection to the target groups is secured
2. The multisectorial and community participation are secured
3. The care and counselling for Aids/STDs are secured by the health infrastructures and the communities
4. Aids is felt as a priority among target groups (importance, seriousness, risk behaviours)
5. The socio-economic impact of Aids and STDs is reduced in the district

- fourth, the key partners of the public and private Sectors in the District positioned themselves in relation to these interventions and clarified their inputs/ expertise, and limitations, in light of their experiences, human resources competencies, didactic materials, financial resources, existing interventions, population mobilisation. This represented a substantial improvement in comparison to the original (Ministry of Health) MoH 1997 HIV/ Aids Plan for Gaoua District found during the situation analyses. The MoH Plan was originally limited to six activities, MoH centered, had only a few other partners mentioned (GTZ and the NGO, Plan International Burkinabé), and the budget line items did not refer to the sources of financing.

- fifth, an informal co-ordination body for the private sector under the leadership of a local Non-Governmental Organisation (NGO), and an informal public sector co-ordination body with the existing District Health Team extended to a few other public sector partners, was identified to lead the Responses for each sector. The global co-ordination in the District falls as well under the mandate of an extended District Health Team structure encompassing representatives from all sectors. For the next six months following the Workshop, follow-up steps and dates were outlined with the institutions responsible and concerned.

In conclusion, the **2 main positive outcomes** of the Gaoua Workshop in the planning/ priorities setting process for the Local Responses were:

- the creation of an enabling positive micro policy environment with a consensus in planning and priority setting with an initiative based on the views of all three main partners of all sectors, and the communities' representatives together (in contrast with last year's MoH single and limited in scope planning exercise)
- the formulation of a five years common vision planning framework which fits well into the Five Years Plan of the Health Sector Reform, and which relates to five main objectives of HIV/Aids. Each main partner is positioned for specific intervention(s) in which the partner believes its institution large or small is most qualified and committed to.

4.3.2 Strategic Planning

Strategic Planning for the Local Responses Gaoua District
Mid-1999, or two years after the Case study took place, Gaoua District had elaborated with heavy inputs and guidance of UNAIDS a final comprehensive "Strategic Planning" document (Lamboray and M'Pele 1999).

We produced originally two documents of the Case study for Situation Analyses at the Community and at the District Levels (chap. 4), and for the Consensus-Building and Pre-Planning Workshop (4.3.1).

The mid-99 "Strategic Planning" document was based in addition on a series of the following eight other inputs and documents, produced over a one year period (between mid-1998 and mid-1999) by the country broker, with the last one on Health Sector Reform and HIV moderated by another consultant:

- "Analyse de la Situation et de la Réponse de la Prise en Charge du VIH/SIDA" (draft for the consensus workshop, third quarter of 1998): is a specific situation analysis of the much needed interventions in psycho-social support and care quasi-inexistent up to now.
- "Analyse de la Situation et de la Réponse de la Prise en Charge du VIH/SIDA" (Report of the workshop, end of 1998), and "Formulation du Plan Stratégique et Planification des Activités de Prise en Charge du VIH/SIDA" (Working document for the Planning Workshop, end of 1998): the situation analysis is finalized, and an original accompanying strategic planning document is drafted, addressing the psycho-social support and care only.

- "Guide d'Opération pour le Processus de Planification Stratégique dans le Domain Spécifique de la Prise en Charge du VIH/SIDA. Analyse de Situation et de la Réponse. Formulation d'un Plan Stratégique" (Jan. 1999), and "Etude de Cas Burkina Faso Processus de Planification Stratégique de la Réponse Nationale contre le VIH/SIDA dans le Domain Spécifique de la Prise en Charge des Personnes vivant avec le VIH/SIDA dans un District Sanitaire" (January 99): both documents addressing specifically as well the psycho-social support and care.
- "Plan de Lutte contre le VIH/SIDA et les MST dans le District Sanitaire de Gaoua" (Draft, January 99): is a the first comprehensive plan under the form of a draft, less than two years into the process of planning.
- "Health Reform and HIV Report of a workshop in Gaoua, Burkina Faso 15 to 19 March 1999": documents how the Local Responses into the health reform country process.

The Solution Development process (Phase 2) is presently cumbersome, time-consuming, costly, and hardly replicable if the tools and methods used are not more efficient, and simplified. This lengthy process gives evidence that the strategic planning approach recommended to implement the Local Responses is still in its initial testing stages, and merits further refinement. This is true despite the existence of the following modules, used throughout the process by the country broker: "Guides to the strategic planning process for a national responses to HIV/Aids" (Module 1, Situation analysis)(UNAIDS 1998), (Module 2, Responses analysis) (UNAIDS 1998), (Module 3, Strategic plan formulation) (UNAIDS 1998).

I pointed early on[115] to one of the major deficiency in the first (draft January 99) Planning document related to the huge number (27 strategies) which were to be executed by a limited District Health Team and their partners. Those were quite complex shared between Prevention (12 strategies), psycho-social and care (8), socio-economic support of PLWA (4), co-ordination and partnership (3).

Corrective action was taken through the elaboration of a quite well-balanced and feasible "Operational priority Plan 1999" in the final "Strategic Plan" limited to a few essential activities only:

- Health care/counselling: a large training component (traditional practitioners, social agents, association leaders, health care staff), provision of essential

[115] memo. of 18.3.1999 to UNAIDS Burkina Faso and Geneva of "Feedback on the Plan of Jan. 1999"

drugs and laboratory reagents, home visits and care in 8 sectors to support PLWHAs,

- Prevention: also a large training component of various essential collaborators (leaders from Associations, animators), social marketing of condoms, sensitisation
  and media coverage,

- Co-ordination: mechanisms set up, follow-up of implementation and supervision,
- Financing (one fourth of the 3 years budget for the 2nd semester plan).

4.4 Implementation and Outcomes

Three years after our original situation analyses (4.1 and 4.2) we present next some of the early outcomes of implementation of activities in Gaoua District.[116]

In the context of the present research, bounded by time limits, in the implementation phase (Phase 3), despite a very limited time span (second semester 1999), several outcomes were already visible, based on a recent formative evaluation (Phase 4).

The three-prone **prevention strategies** have allowed:

- First, the training of agents of changes (design of new training modules by the Technical Committee members with the NACP) to build up the skills and work with some of the vulnerable groups in the District:
  - 25 traditional practitioners of the District of Gaoua, 9 social workers, and 17 leaders (5 youth associations, 10 women associations, 2 military and police) participated in three different seminars to a five days sensitisation training with special training modules designed locally on the importance and means of prevention,
  - 28 animators or facilitators for HIV/Aids/STDs information and training activities of groups (5 radio Gaoua, 14 public services, 9 teachers of primary school, 1 each of agriculture, poultry, environment, primary inspection, militaries), and 9 Associations (Red-Cross, Catholic Women Association…), 14 public service employees (9 primary school teachers, 1 of each among livestock, agriculture, environment, primary inspection, military) to improve the

[116] The results presented here will be part of a UNAIDS *Best Practice* Collection, "UNAIDS Case study Gaoua District Local Responses: *The Burkina Faso approach" planned to be completed in August 2000 during a visit in Gaoua District (expected publication, late 2000)*

effectiveness of local communication adapted to the different audiences,

- and 5 communicators for radio information and education broadcasts.

- Second, for condom distribution, the social marketing of preservatives has launched additional community-based sales efforts. 10 condom sales males and females were trained, and equipped with bicycles, and supplies (cartons of condoms and promotion materials). They operate in a fifteen kilometre radius of Gaoua town (3520 condoms sold in December). In addition 14000 condoms were sold in new outlets. Over 10000 condoms were distributed freely through the public outlets in 1999.

- Third, a number of different health promotion, or Information and Education and Communication (IEC) activities using different channels have taken place:
  - the radio has developed messages in local languages with 180 broadcasts of sketches in French and Mooré, and have provided media coverage of activities for the promotion of HIV/Aids/STD coverage in the Region,
  - 9 local language stage performances by peers reached out-of-school youth in Gaoua town,
  - 5 inter-community contests on Aids control took place in 5 rural villages with 6 theatrical performances and 6 songs,
  - several sensitisation of communities took place among protestants and muslims, military men's spouses, associations of the disabled, teaching mothers; a local Association for women (APFG) have provided educational talks by peers on HIV/Aids/STDs in the local languages,
  - 2 educational talks by the Gaoua training centre (CRESA) reached approximately a total of 150 soldiers, and one educational talk a total of 150 prisoners in Gaoua jail,
  - finally, World AIDS Day in Gaoua carried out a number of substantial activities in Gaoua town (T-shirts on the theme related to youth), animation and theatrical performances and sketches and plays on Aids, football tournament, run, radio messages, evening show, drawing and poetry contest, training of traditional beer brewers, visit and provision of disinfectants to the Gaoua regional hospital patients, official ceremony by the High Commissioner, and over 4000 distributed free as promotion.

The newly launched **care and counselling strategies** started with massive training too:

- 42 health workers from the Gaoua regional Hospital and Kampti and Gaoua Medical Centres have been trained in care, pre and post tests counselling, screening, information, psycho-social support, and improved blood transfusion and safety measures,
- 7 additional health and social workers from the Gaoua hospital received complementary practical training for the medical care of People Living With HIV/Aids, and home visits in Bobo-Dioulasso at the regional hospital there, and at the voluntary screening centre (*Centre de Dépistage Volontaire*) and at the network of volunteers of PLWH+ (*Réseau des Volontaires+*).

In addition, it addresses also the following areas with a mix success due to their innovative aspects, but with encouraging signs that the population is becoming conscious of the availability of facilities and personnel equipped to support the communities:

- in the regional hospital:
    - 61 screening tests were done to volunteers in the hospital, 72 people were counselled, 6 People living with HIV/Aids were attended for care and counselling in the hospital, and 14 sick suffering from opportunistic infections were taken care of,
    - 7 health workers trained supported People Living With HIV/Aids on the spot but did not make any home visits, and social workers made 40 visits at the hospital,
- home visits and care (600 per semester) were planned in 8 sectors of Gaoua town with a minimum package of activities, but could not be implemented immediately. However, minimum home care is now feasible: the members of the Catholic Women Association supported 14 People living with HIV/Aids at home, with 728 home visits, and 10 visits by social workers,
- an Association of PLWH has been created but still has a low profile,
- drugs were ordered at the national level, as well as laboratory reagents for HIV/Aids, Syphilis, and Hepatitis B tests and delivered early 2000; they are planned for the Gaoua regional hospital and the urban Medical Centre of Gaoua town for patients, blood donors, pregnant women and those who volunteer for counselling.

The **socio-economic support** component could not yet take place by lack of funds, but the Catholic mission has completed an action plan for 2000.

Finally, several **co-ordination** activities allowed the smooth implementation of the above mentioned strategies:

- Functional and effective committees, with the meetings (10) held by the Technical Committee , and (2) by the Provincial Committee,
- The Technical Committee accomplished more than 30 supervisions, and received 1 visit from the NACP,
- The six-monthly plan was reviewed by UNAIDS, and the Committee members and progress reported in a semester "Assessment of 1999 activities", including an opinion survey of different partners, including community leaders and associations, of different dimensions of their perceptions of Aids,
- The design of an Action Plan for the year 2000.

Some of the early problems encountered in setting the Local Responses were:

- The mobility and insufficient number of health workers,
- The weak capacity in health and HIV/Aids of the various local partners, particularly non-health,
- Divergent, donor-driven disbursements and complex fund management procedures, accompanied by low coverage, reaching insufficiently the rural communities,
- Committees too large for effective management,
- The stigmatisation of the disease, and taboos surrounding it, still largely existing in the communities,
- VCT still under used,
- Strategies to reach PLWHAs and their families proven more difficult than expected.

4.5 National Scaling-up and international dissemination of the Gaoua Local Responses

Several indirect effects or results of the Local Responses in Gaoua District have spilled over at the national and international levels.

Burkina Faso National Response and International Contributions

Since 1987, the country has set up large-scale HIV prevention activities. The country is exploring, since 1998, different new approaches to become more effective in responding to HIV/Aids. Those are currently being formulated in the 2001-2003 National Strategic Plan which is in the process of being developed, and finalised by the year 2000. It involves the Health Sector and non-health public Sectors, as well as the voluntary and private for profit Sectors, who take the necessary time and attempt to define the best solutions to the problems and realities of the country, in contrast to quick fix solutions imposed from the outside. Several Ministries, in addition to the MoH, are presently directly involved in the planning of activities: Economy and Finances, Social Action and Family, Secondary Education, Higher Education and Scientific Research, and Communication and Culture.

The plan becomes a mean to articulate and agree upon a collective understanding of all key partners to respond to the epidemic. A United Nations (U.N.) Theme Group co-ordinates the national response and is comprised of the Government representatives with a dozen different representatives from key international U.N. and non-U.N. agencies (e.g. World Bank, FAO), expanded recently to involve other important stakeholders (bilateral agencies, the European Union, international NGOs, businesses), and representatives from the civil society (CBOs, social organisations). The national process and structures are strikingly similar to, and inspired by the ones described next for the Local Responses in Gaoua District.

Despite the fact the population is well informed and aware of the existence and modes of transmission of HIV, Aids is still considered to be a taboo. This taboo is recognised as a major barrier to prevention. This has direct operational implications on the need to tailor better Information Education and Communication messages, as well as other strategies (e.g. People Living With HIV/Aids organisations direct involvement), to overcome these barriers. Some vulnerable groups (youth, migrants, prisoners, soldiers) have not been sufficiently addressed, and some strategies (Voluntary Counselling and Testing or Care) are just nascent.

The civil society has been largely and increasingly involved in the responses to HIV/Aids based on the rapid increase in the numbers of registered NGOs and Associations. In 1997, approximately one hundred local NGOs and Associations were involved in HIV/Aids in the urban areas of Ouagadougou and Bobo-Dioulasso in an inventory accomplished then (Desconnets and Taverne 1997). Their numbers had tripled in three years. In Gaoua District, an institutional review, documents the same year dozens of them in a rural district, giving further evidence that the rural communities in the country are quite active as well. Still this essential reservoir of resources remains largely under-used, or untapped by programs. Yet, in 1997, it was felt that the social mobilisation is still weak in comparison to the severity of the Aids situation, perceived as largely the MoH's responsibility.

The President has declared recently Aids as a national disaster, rendering it a national priority. This political will to combat the epidemic has been translated into the creation of a National Solidarity Fund (January 99) for which funds still needed to be allocated by early 2000.

In 1999, the International Partnership against AIDS in Africa (IPAA) was launched bringing together a coalition of actors to work together to achieve a shared vision and common goals and objectives, based on a set of mutually agreed principles and key milestones to mount an *"extraordinary"* response. In this context, Burkina Faso was one of the six countries to conduct initial activities, with the agreement to develop a National Strategic Plan, and to mobilise resources, e.g. a special fund has been created for HIV/Aids.

Presently the intensification of the national response lies in four domains:

- institutional strengthening (still heavily centralised health system and limited managerial capacity of NACP),
- financial sustainability (increase the financial support for new strategies and the national and district levels, and finding mechanisms for effective transfer of funds to Districts),
- HIV drugs procurement policies and strategies and kits and materials for safe blood transmission,
- Necessary changes in law (for example in more effective channelling of funds).

In the international context, in May 2000, sixteen representatives from Ministries of Health members of the Organization for African Unity (OAU), met in Ouagadougou to prepare their health systems for both HIV prevention and care on an increased scale, and evaluating the Health Sector HIV/Aids control activities within the framework of the new International Partnership.

266

> *"... we need more information about the situation within the Burkina Faso itself, as well as coordinated efforts and a broad and transparent commitment to rolling back the epidemic."*
>
> (Christian Lemaire, UNDP, coordination of the UN system's response to HIV/AIDS in Burkina Faso)
>
> Source: OAU Meeting of Ministers of Health of the OAU, Ouagadougou, May 2000

National Scaling-up

Gaoua District has set up a model of decentralised HIV/Aids planning, with HIV/Aids activities that are integrated and multisectoral, and which reinforce the national policies of decentralisation. This model has been able to influence the making of national HIV/Aids and reforms policies through different means as outlined next.

Faced by the urgency to respond to the epidemic, the Government has not been satisfied with keeping Gaoua District as a *"pilot"* project but has been encouraging that the lessons learnt and the *"learning by doing"* approach used there are replicated as quickly as possible to other districts and regions. As early as 1998, following the original successful early steps of Local Responses in Gaoua, the Government involved local consultants to disseminate and be directly inspired by the experience of Gaoua District (Diébougou and Banfora), and others indirectly (Kaya, Fada N'gourma). As an example, the District Health Team of Diébougou Districtarticulated to the national level in late 1998 the need to offer individual and community counselling services, based on the experiences of Gaoua.

Some of the national legislation stimulated in turn local activities, for example, the new 1998 policy of the MoH to provide HIV-positive patients with free medication for the treatment of opportunistic infections, with drugs newly available in the District.

In 1999, two major national events triggered the advocacy of the local responses to HIV/Aids at the provincial and community levels with the sharing of the Gaoua experience on the implementation of an expanded response by the Gaoua Committees' members:

- the meeting of 45 High Commissioners of Burkina Faso (July 1999),
- the meeting of 44 Mayors of Burkina Faso (August 1999).

> "In 1999 we had a meeting of all the Burkina High Commissioners, and we presented our work in Gaoua; and we expect that all will follow our lead. And we did the same at a meeting of Mayors. These meetings went very well, and we hope that this year and in the years to come all the big towns will begin multisectorial plans like ours against AIDS. And in all the Provinces, they are going to create provincial committees like ours in Poni, tuned to their own particular problems, but working from the community."
>
> (President of the Comité Technique de la Lutte Contre le SIDA of Poni Province)
>
> Source: Robert Walgate, Open Solutions, Interviews in Gaoua District, February 2000

In addition, in that meeting, the High Commissioner of the Poni Region expressed the wish to expand the Response to encompass the three other Districts of the Poni Region as well. Following these meetings, several Districts expressed their interests and willingness to develop a similar approach.

The MoH decided to extend support to Local Responses to HIV/Aids in 11 Districts (one per Region) by the year 2000 in order to scale-up the national response. The different criteria to scale up the responses in Burkina Faso suggested are the following:

- Districts sufficiently large (i.e. approximately 250.000 inhabitants)
- A mix of urban and rural districts (rural areas are lagging behind in the responses)
- Evidence of effectiveness in Aids, and district participating to the Health Reforms

The steps suggested are to start the multisectoral and involvement of all partners on a small scale (one administative "Département", District and Regional capital) and if the experience is positive to scale-up to the whole District, then the Region, to identify the mechanisms to give the responsibility to the local political administrative authorities including the support structures, to empower the local district team to implement the response with the partners and identify the necessary technical, financial and logistics support.

A national Non-Governmental Organisation is foreseen to support the learning from Local Responses implementation throughout the country.

The planning framework and approaches used in Gaoua District have been adapted for the national strategic and multisectorial 2001-2003 plan of combat against HIV/AIDS/STI of Burkina Faso.

Finally, in year 2000, at the national level, in the public sector, many different Ministries, besides those mentioned in the planning process already, have been identified as potential stakeholders to HIV/Aids strategies and are presently carrying out their own strategic planning exercises. Those include: Water and Environment, Energy and Mines, Agriculture and Animal Resources, and the Army. Seven additional Ministry Departments, as well as large public and private enterprises plan a similar exercise. These developments give evidence that there exists a multi-sectorial involvement at the national level similar to the local level involvement of various stakeholders in Gaoua Region and District.

With a maximum of less than half a million $ U.S. for two years ($ 170.000 Gaoua District or $ 400.000 approximately for the Poni Region), the country can implement for approximately a mere 5 million $ U.S. Local Responses on a national scale in 11 Health Regions. It would in turn become a full-fledged national strategy like others that are presently foreseen (IEC, condom distribution…). This would represent a relatively small amount in comparison to the current budgets available in the country for population programs which range above 20 million $ U.S. for a five years period.

> *"The experience… of Gaoua is from that angle an example because it associates the higher administrative and political authorities with the various technical sectors and the Associations originating from the civil society and the private sector. This process needs an on-going and strong support from the central level and the necessary financial resources."*
>
> Source: Ministère de l'Economie et des Finances. Revue des dépenses publiques du secteur santé, Janvier 2000.

International dissemination

Catalysing the stakeholders' synergies to the benefits of HIV/Aids control activities is possible in any country, granted the understanding of their own cultural and socio-economic situations, and political will and commitment.

The "inter-country HIV and Reforms for Health workshop" (March 1999) with participants from national and district levels from Burkina Faso, Côte d'Ivoire, Ghana, and Thailand resulted in practical suggestions on how to make health system more effective in dealing with HIV/Aids, and to support communities to become "*AIDS competent*".

Technical meetings of the Local Responses network allowed to present some of the Gaoua findings (Tanzania 1998 and 2000, Zimbabwe 1999), and to compare those with the experiences collected from other countries, in relation to the different steps involved for implementation (Appendix B, Technical Note 1), and the measurement (Technical Note 3, to be issued in September 2000).

The Gaoua experience has stimulated a large debate internationally among major stakeholders from international agencies, including UNAIDS/PSR, and contributed directly to a global vision of how to stimulate locally "*AIDS competent societies*". The approach is gaining momentum and being disseminated in the West Africa Region rapidly (e.g. Ghana, Mali, Guinea). In addition, this experience has and is being shared and disseminated through a number of large international Conferences and Meetings over the past three years: the International AIDS Conference (Geneva, 1998 and Durban, 2000), International AIDS Conference for the Africa Region (Dakar, 1999), OAU Meeting of Ministers of Health from the Africa Region (Ouagadougou, 2000), American Public Health Association annual meeting (Boston, 2000).

Finally, in 2001, Burkina Faso will be hosting the International Conference on AIDS and STDs in Africa.

These different milestones indicate that Burkina Faso is deeply involved at the national level to overcome some of the major barriers to an effective national country program and to an acceleration of Local Responses. Burkina Faso is an important stakeholder in the Africa region and the different international discussions taking place on Local Responses.

Over a relatively short period of time between 1997 and 2000, the Local Responses of Gaoua District could plan using situation analyses and different planning methods, and implement HIV/Aids strategies in a rural setting. In addition, we could document the full process with visible outcomes of a few months of implementation only, and already national and international effects and benefits.

We hope the above framework (documented in this chapter) focusing on an organisational analysis for the Local Responses provides a useful analytical tool to the Local Responses. As a consequence we hope this process, with the development of the Rapid Organisational Review (5.1.6), contributes as well to the advancement of the sociology of organisations in the field of public health.

References

Bjaras, G. (1991). "A new approach to community participation assessment." Health Promotion International **6**(3): 199-206.

Cros, M. (1994). Araignée-sida et politique de santé en pays lobi burkinabè. Le Burkina entre la révolution et démocratie. R. Otayek, F. M. Sawadogo and J.-P. Guingane. Paris, Editions Karthala.

Cros, M. (1995). "Quête thérapeutique burkinabè en temps de SIDA De la capture du double à l'écoute du médicament." Champ Psychosomatique **2/3**: 89-101.

Cros, M., P. Msellati, et al. (1997). Faire dire, dessiner et narrer le sida Un vivier de sens en pays Lobi Burkinabè. Le sida en Afrique Recherches en sciences de l'homme et de la societé. Paris, ANRS ORSTOM.

Desconnets, S. and B. Taverne (1997). Annuaire des Associations et O.N.G. intervenant dans la lutte contre le sida au Burkina Faso, installées à Ouagadougou et Bobo-Dioulasso, 1996-1997. Ouagadougou, ORSTOM et CNLS.

Foltz A.-M. et al. (1996). Decentralization and Health Systems Change: Burkina Faso Case Study. Geneva, WHO.

Gilbert, L. K. (1999). "The female condoms in the US: Lessons Learned A Literature Review." AJPH **89**(6): 1-28.

GTZ and ITHÖG (1989). Indicators for District Health Systems. Eschborn, GTZ and IHTÖG.

Hoth-Guechot, M. (1996). "Mais laissons donc l'Afrique respirer." Croissance **396**: 12-13.

Keeley, J. (1999). "Community-Level Interventions Are Needed to Prevent New HIV Infections." AJPH **89**(3): 299-301.

Kenis, P. and B. Marin (1997). Managing AIDS. Organizational Responses in six European Countries. Aldershot, Ashgate Publishing Company.

Lamboray, J. L. and P. M'Pelé (1999). Planification stratégique et réformes pour une Réponse élargie face au VIH/SIDA dans un district sanitaire Gaoua-Burkina Faso Documentation des processus et des résultats Rapport Intermédiaire. Geneva, ONUSIDA/PSR/HRHIV.

Luger, L. (1998). HIV/AIDS prevention and 'class' and socio-economic related factors of risk of HIV infection. Berlin, WZB.

M'Pelé, P., C. Pervilhac, et al. (2000). The impact of a local response to HIV/AIDS in a rural district of Burkina Faso. 13th AIDS International Conference, Durban, South Africa.

Nana, L. M. and I. Sanogo (1998). Rapport de l'Atelier de Pré-Planification et de Consensus des Partenaires des Secteurs Public, Privé et Communautaire sur la Réponse Elargie au VIH/ SIDA au niveau du District de Gaoua, Burkina Faso. Ouagadougou, Ministère de la Santé, S.G., DGSP.

Ng'weshemi, J., T. Boerma, et al., Eds. (1997). HIV Prevention and AIDS Care in Africa. A district level approach. Amsterdam, Royal Tropical Institute.

Pervilhac, C., W. Kipp, et al. (1997). Report on the District Expanded Response Initiative (DRI) UNAIDS/WHO/GTZ Case-Study of Kabarole District the Republic of Uganda. Bonn and Alberta and Kampala, GTZ.

Pervilhac C. et al. (1998). Rapport de Synthèse de l'Atelier sur l'Initiative de la Réponse Elargie au VIH/ SIDA: District de Gaoua, Burkina Faso. Bonn, GTZ.

Reeler, A. (1999). Health Reform and HIV. Geneva, Health Access International.

Salla, R., P. Sebgo, C. Pervilhac et al. (1998). District Response Initiative (DRI): Fostering Partnership in HIV/ AIDS Control. Situation Analysis in Burkina Faso. 12 th World AIDS Conference, Geneva, Merck & Co., Inc.

Schmidt D. et al. (1996). "Measuring Participation: its Use as a Managerial Tool for District Health Planners Based on a Case-Study in Tanzania." International Journal of Health Planning and Management 11: 345-358.

Testa J. et al. (1996). "Evaluation d'une Action d'Information et d'Education sur le SIDA chez des Chauffeurs Routiers du Burkina Faso." Médecine d'Afrique Noire 43(1): 25-29.

The World Bank (1999). Intensifying Action Against HIV/AIDS in Africa: Responding to a Development Crisis. Washington D.C., The World Bank.

UNAIDS (1998). Expanding the global response to HIV/ AIDS through focused action. Reducing risk and vulnerability: definitions, rationale and pathways. Geneva, UNAIDS.

UNAIDS (1998). Guide to the strategic planning process for a national response to HIV/ AIDS Response Analysis (Vol. 2). Geneva, UNICEF UNDP UNFPA UNESCO WHO World Bank.

UNAIDS (1998). Guide to the strategic planning process for a national response to HIV/ AIDS. Situation Analysis. Geneva, UNAIDS.

UNAIDS (1998). Guide to the strategic planning process for a national response to HIV/ AIDS. Strategic plan formulation. Geneva, UNAIDS.

WHO (1996). Catalogue on Health Indicators A selection of important health indicators recommended by WHO Programmes. Geneva, WHO.

CHAPTER FIVE
DISCUSSION AND CONCLUSIONS

As illustrated in our present research work, the HIV/Aids is a complex issue (chap. 1 illustration, in fact with "several bugs, necessitating several drugs, and

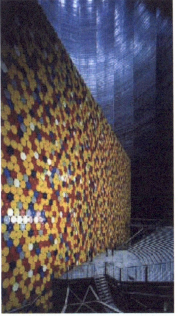 several shots") which as a consequence needs complex solutions, or responses. The constant search for the best patterns of responses in a country can be understood under the form of the following illustration. The managers and researchers are faced with a vast choice of strategies and interventions (illustrated here by the various coloured barrels) and are in constant search of the best mix of those, confronted with the various specific but also changing determinants of the epidemic. Yet, no definite pattern can emerge, as the responses are either community, or district, or country specific.

At best, the overall approach and its different steps through the Local Responses may be distinguished, improved, and adapted for replication.

Fig. 5.1 *The Wall, Installation in the Gasometer, 13.000 Oil Barrels, 1998-99, Christo and Jeanne-Claude, Oberhausen, Germany*

We first draw the main lessons (5.1) from the previous results (chap. 4). Then we discuss each specific result and step described previously (in chap. 4), to identify how the study methodology and the analytical framework for the diffusion of Local Responses can be improved: for the situation analysis at the community level (5.1.1), and at the district level (5.1.2), then for the consensus-building and pre-planning (5.1.3), and for the strategic planning (5.1.4) successively.

We then turn to three examples of the potentials but also limitations of what is known or can be discovered in relation to disseminating and applying Local Responses: with the current status of development of tools (5.1.5), the development of a new tool called the Rapid Organizational Review (5.1.6), and the applications and limitations of Local Responses looking at migrants as a specific vulnerable group (5.1.7).

Finally, we review the main limitations of the present study (5.1.8), and the overall results in light of the original study hypotheses (5.1.9).

In conclusions, based on this research study, we identify the methodological (5.2.1) and international policy (5.2.2) issues, and research priorities for the future (5.2.3).

5.1 Introduction to the Discussion: Lessons Learned

Although past programs have focused on interventions and strategies, or the *"magic bullet approach"*, the Local Responses approach places equal importance and emphasis on the environment in which those are implemented, hence the results for mobilising resources, structures and advocacy, and partnerships, presented next, before those for strategies.

Monitoring the Local Responses
It is too early to assess the impact (prevalence reduction) of the Local Responses in Gaoua District. Yet, the results, process and outputs data summarised next (M'Pele, Pervilhac et al. 2000), give strong evidence that the epidemic and its consequences are being addressed fully by the local actors with the potential to reverse the epidemic in the years to come. This situation contrasts to one described above and found in the earlier years, described in the 1997 baseline situation analyses (chap. 4).

The Local Responses uses a light combined system of bi-yearly monitoring and on-going evaluation. The monitoring matrix, or a progress report, is based on the review of activities planned, the period when those took place, the actors, the results and additional remarks which refer often to some of the main constraints encountered. The facilitator, with the Technical Committee members' support, reviews the activities together. The results are presented to and discussed with the members of the Technical and Provincial Committees. They are used for corrective or follow-up actions, and in addition, for the design of the new plan of year 2000.

⇨*Lessons learned: a light monitoring system with on-going review becomes a useful management tool for the local planning and implementing partners*

Mobilising resources
The situation analysis at the district level carried out in 1997 was unable to determine either the allocation of funds for the different activities, or the total

amount of funds allocated to HIV/Aids activities in the District with the exception of the Ministry of Health (MoH). At best the analysis identified that the MoH had earmarked $ 15,000 U.S. (5%) of its total 1997 health budget of $ 300,000 U.S. for HIV/Aids activities. Those were roughly shared for half to Information, Education and Communication (IEC) activities in the communities ("District Sanitaire de Gaoua, Plan d'Action 1997"), one fourth to care in the communities, and one fourth to health services. No funds were allocated to socio-economic, or coordination and advisory support.

In early 1999, the planning team established transparency by budgeting over a two years period (1999-2000): a total of $ 200,000 U.S. for all partners in the District for the whole District, or in comparison to the original 1997 MoH budget, five times more funds for a one year period. Although this budget seems to be large (half of the total 1997 MoH budget for the whole District), it represents a mere $ 1 U.S. per inhabitant.

In addition, the activities budgeted for by the different local actors reflected the new priorities in the District: over half were earmarked to both care and counselling (40%), approximately one third (35%) was earmarked to the former main and almost unique strategy of IEC for the prevention of HIV and STDs, socio-economic support (16%), and finally, a small but sufficient amount (9%) to co-ordination and advisory support.

Each partner in the District knew now the priorities (4.3.1). Consequently, international partners involved already locally (e.g. PBI, GTZ) could then mobilise their own resources to contribute to the Local Responses.

> *"Before this exercise, AIDS was the business of the health service alone. The new approach takes advantage of all local powers and potential - such as women's associations, youth associations, collaborations with other administrative sectors, the army, the truck drivers - all the different workers' groups. They came together to create a common plan, with common objectives, each one mobilising its own resources, and all with the support of Gaoua authorities. This gave us a much greater chance of success against the disease - and much greater credibility with outside donors...*
>
> (GTZ Gaoua technical advisor)
>
> Source: Robert Walgate, Open Solutions, Interviews in Gaoua District, February 2000

However, local resources were insufficient. Finally, knowing the budget and its allocation, the time was ripe to mobilise external resources for the District. A one-day meeting (June 1999) took place for that purpose in Ouagadougou with the various donors. In parallel, most importantly, the process was accompanied by the decentralisation of funds to the local Provincial Committee, giving it a special status along the current public reforms national policies.

"The funds are concentrated in Ouagadougou. It is essential to decentralise the resources, to liberate – completely - the Provincial Committee and the Comité Technique... After the preparation of a multisectoral plan of action, in collaboration with UNAIDS and the national programme, we held a meeting with international donors in Ouagadougou. They studied our plans, recognised its significance, and were convinced they should give them direct support at provincial level – that's to say their funds would and are coming directly to the provincial Comité Technique, in contrast to the usual method where funds go to the Ministry of Health before being distributed to provincial level. So that gave our work a completely original status."

(High Commissioner Poni Province)

Source: Robert Walgate, Open Solutions, Interviews in Gaoua District, February 2000

"The High Commissioner, having recognised the importance of the AIDS epidemic in his Province, emphasised the initiative taken by the Gaoua Health District to organise an extended and better structured response to the epidemic. He acknowledged the strong mobilisation of all the social strata on AIDS issue and reiterated the commitment of all the provincial leaders to untiringly work towards the success of the Provincial AIDS Control Plan. He announced a 5% contribution by Gaoua District to the cost plan and stated that henceforth a special budget line would be provided for HIV/AIDS control. He committed himself to implement the whole Plan together with the Poni population and welcomed the presence of international partners and the support that they would give to his Province under the AIDS Control Plan."

(from High Commissioner Poni Province' opening speech)

Source: HIV/AIDS and STD Control partners Meeting, Ouagadougou, 25th June 1999

As the groundwork had been completed over the past several months, several international partners found the Local Responses plan and suggestions credible and worth the investment, along the lines of their own policies, and consequently committed their institutions with different amounts (the World Bank 60%, UNAIDS 18%, UNFPA 8%, Plan International 6,25%, WHO 4,5%, and GTZ 3.25%), and the African Development Bank financing the working action plan for 2000. The total funding was shared between new international (75%), local former partners such as GTZ and PBI (25%), and the district and communities (5%).

Resources mobilisation gave confidence to the local partners about the credibility of their Plan and efforts. How the funds are disbursed successfully and used effectively among the
myriad of local partners remains to be fully assessed. Preliminary findings[117] though show that despite the structures in place, one of the main bottleneck caused by so many different sources of financing is the slow disbursement procedure from the external partners, and that the funds are reaching very partially the rural communities for the activities.

⇨*Lessons learned:* *expanding the resources means mobilising rapidly a minimal amount of external resources for the partners involved to start the process and building up the confidence of all local stakeholders, including the communities, but financial flow and disbursements locally with multiple sources are a major constraint to be overcome*

Structures and advocacy
The early steps of the Local Responses allowed the HIV/Aids program from being originally essentially a MoH's single vertical and unique concern to become a local program cross-cutting different sectors. It was concerned to establish partnerships not just by operational means (e.g. strategies, services) but to complement those with other means as well (e.g. institutional and structures, policies).

Early on, the Local Responses took stock of the local Government's deep concern and interests in tackling the epidemic locally.

One early visible and useful contribution was to implement in the Region a favourable policy climate, instead of waiting for national initiatives. For

---

[117] H. Binswanger, the World Bank, report of a visit to Gaoua District (June 2000) in "Scaling-up HIV/AIDS Programs to National Coverage" in the Local Responses satellite meeting on "Local Responses to HIV/AIDS: Going to Scale with Local Partnerships", 9th July 2000, Durban, XIII International AIDS Conference

example, in December 1998, the High Commissioner of the Poni Region passed an official legal decree (*"Arrêté"*) to create the Provincial Committee for the Control of HIV/AIDS and STD, and the Technical Committee, specifying their mandates. In addition, the High Commissioner signed an official declaration (*"Principes Directeurs de Lutte contre le VIH/SIDA et les MST dans la Province du Poni, District Sanitaire de Gaoua"*) which stipulated the six principles guiding the efforts and agreed upon by the different partners in an earlier workshop (ref. *"Determining the District objectives, activities, and priorities"*). Those became in turn an official and widely supported vision and ideals that the larger local society and local partners advocated and endorsed.

The committees and their different members are now active in sharing different tasks such as planning and supervising, making it a program locally owned and managed with powerful advocates of the Local Responses, in addition, supporting the fund raising for the Provincial Committee.

> *"We* (the Technical Committee) *coordinate and apply the programme of the Provincial Committee... For example, a youth association could decide on a certain activity according to the programme; they would work out their budget, supervised by the Comité Technique; and then the Provincial Committee would find the necessary resources from international partners."*
>
> (President of the Comité Technique, Gaoua, Army Officer)
>
> Source: Robert Walgate, Open Solutions, Interviews in Gaoua District, February 2000

As an example of technical inputs locally, in 1998 the local IEC regional team had planned a Campaign on Reproductive Health targeted to the youth, with the support of the National AIDS Control Program (NACP) technicians. The national level plays now an important role in supporting locally technical inputs, and at the same time is passing along and strengthening the technical know-how. In comparison to the situation described in 1997, the local team and partners have increased substantially their knowledge on the design of Local Responses, as well as the organisation and management of the Responses.

Health Sector Reforms are gaining impetus and facilitating the implementation of the Local Responses agenda in turn. In 1998, the Gaoua District Health Team was looking forward to the creation of the District Health Board as part of the nation-wide decentralisation of the Government. The decisions for district level activities is gradually moving to the local board, instead of going through previously via the central Ministry of Health in Ouagadougou.

The specific situation of HIV/Aids is now well known, as well as the priorities, as mentioned previously. The share of responsibilities between the different Sectors are well articulated by the main actors themselves, complementing and reinforcing the Health Sector.

"There are real difficulties at three levels: at the level of the person who is sick, there is no preparation so he or she can accept his or her seropositivity (HIV infection)... at the level of the family, they find it difficult to accept that a member of their family is affected by AIDS... What is going to happen to the sick person... to the family... misperceptions both of the disease and of the sick person... At the level of the health staff, are there any laws which can protect them when they announce the diagnosis? Can they be protected if they announce a person's seropositivity to another, without his or her agreement? I am talking about protection from aggression."

(Madame Kyéré, Directrice des Actions Sociales, District Gaoua)

Source: Robert Walgate, Open Solutions, Interviews in Gaoua District, February 2000

"Above all to improve the respect for AIDS victims in the community. If People Living With HIV/AIDS could be accepted in the society, that would already be a great victory. After that, there's a big programme: to intensify prevention measures; then to be able to provide medicines at the lowest possible cost for opportunistic infections to all those who are diagnosed HIV positive, to improve and hopefully prolong their lives. And then to work directly in the community. To support families affected. To support the sick person in the community. We are working on all these ways of taking care of those who are suffering from HIV and AIDS."

(President of the Comité Technique, Gaoua, Army Officer)

Source: Robert Walgate, Open Solutions, Interviews in Gaoua District, February 2000

The population is increasingly aware of the need for case-finding, i.e. to use the Voluntary and Counselling and Testing (VCT) services, but the persons who agree to be tested are still very few due to fear still. A situation which may change in the near future under the present strategies.

"... On... the community side, it's extremely important that people show to the AIDS patient that it is simply a disease, like any other, and that they don't abandon him or her. If a patient knows he won't be abandoned by his friends, by his work mates, then he could announce his state. But now, as soon as a person says he or she has HIV, everyone runs away."

(The doctor, at the hospital, Gaoua town)

Source: Robert Walgate, Open Solutions, Interviews in Gaoua District, February 2000

⇨*Lessons learned: The Technical Committee was not fully effective the first two years because of its large number of members, the poor distribution of tasks and lack of job descriptions, the poor dissemination of information among all local actors and partners, and the Committee's overall ill-defined role still. It wishes to become a body with more responsibility to co-ordinate and support the implementation. Remedial action has been taken locally in early 2000 to address these problems.*

Partnerships

A higher commitment and mobilisation of the different partners, public, voluntary and private, and communities, are visible based on their present involvement in HIV/Aids activities.

The local partners' guiding principle falls under the motto *"learning by doing"*. All partners learn from past errors, and take corrective actions to build upon those.

A new institutional landscape in year 2000 would indicate, based on the organisational markers (5.1.6), an increased number of active partners in comparison to 1997 (4.1 and 4.2), both in the public and voluntary sectors (NGOs, Associations and CBOs, Churches).

In 2000, 27 Associations, and 382 agriculture co-operatives were involved in HIV/Aids activities.

Activities covered mainly Gaoua town, and a few communities in the District, placing emphasis on the key social groups. Those were either some vulnerable groups (i.e. youth, women), or gatekeepers (religious leaders and communities, opinion leaders, and tradi-practitioners), and Community Associations. For the general population, the local Gaoua radio coverage in the District placed emphasis on messages in the local languages focusing on de-stigmatising the disease. Many Associations address some of the more vulnerable groups, e.g. women, youth, and promote effective strategies (Social Marketing of Condoms that are community-based, theatre) which was missing up to now.

"I think what's needed is education and information -so people can understand the disease...Yes (what is being done in Gaoua is effective) *with the associations that are mobilising people, the young are now aware of this disease. They think they now want to save their lives... I think in Gaoua* (town), *people now take care. But perhaps people who come here from outside do not. If the education continues, I think we will beat the disease."*

A young man with a baby at the Gaoua market

Source: Robert Walgate, Open Solutions, Interviews in Gaoua District, February 2000

"Well after training, we've covered eight small villages around Gaoua, and contacted 572 women, 140 men and 227 young people -nearly 1000 people so far- to make them aware of HIV and AIDS. We've used several methods, but the villages people seem to like our women's theatre best. Also young women in our associations are given bicycles and trained to explain and sell condoms -"social marketing" - in the village markets..."

(Association pour la Promotion Féminine Gaoua, President)

Source: Robert Walgate, Open Solutions, Interviews in Gaoua District, February 2000

The Voluntary Sector has been tapped to with different activities. For example, religious associations address groups who are more vulnerable, and pick up strategies such as care and counselling that were largely neglected up to now.

> *"We're working on two issues: first, the young men, who go to Côte d'Ivoire to make money, and come back with AIDS. And secondly, the young girls, who also leave for money to serve in bars in Ouagadougou and Bobo Dioulasso, they also often return ill, and die in their villages. And they leave behind orphans, and we try to take care in the Mission... We try to help women sick with AIDS, visiting them, alone and in the community. We try to support them at home, in the villages, with our prayer; and with some activities such as soap-making, and with information and education about HIV/AIDS..."*
>
> (President of the Association of Catholic Women)
>
> Source: Robert Walgate, Open Solutions, Interviews in Gaoua District, February 2000

NGOs are strengthening or creating new income-generating projects.

> *"The difficulties identified here are rural poverty; young people leaving the land, which is perhaps the greatest problem; and the proximity of Côte d'Ivoire and Ghana (where farming is easier): people migrate to improve their way of life. These are facts we work with. So we try to find ways of keeping people on land... (by) rural credit. For cattle rearing, for example. And anything that will bring them revenue."*
>
> (The Burkina Faso South-West Development Project Director)
>
> Source: Robert Walgate, Open Solutions, Interviews in Gaoua District, February 2000

In addition, the Defence and Security Ministry have joined in with information sessions among the prisoners, police force, soldiers, soldiers' wives. New recruits, e.g. the newly appointed military medical doctor, support these measures.

> *"...my role is as one of the doctors on this multisectoral group, for the expanded approach to AIDS. And as a soldier, I can say AIDS is a reality which affects us too. There's no real difference in the approach we must take to AIDS in the army from that in civil society. Our ages are from 20 to 50 years old; and most are unmarried. So all the STDs, including AIDS, are here... I intend to hold small meetings to explain how HIV can be contracted, and about the whole story of AIDS -and the other STDs. And to explain that for the moment our only means of attack on this disease is prevention, and convince them that AIDS is a reality in this region."*
>
> (New military Medical Doctor of the Gaoua regiment, Gaoua town)
>
> Source: Robert Walgate, Open Solutions, Interviews in Gaoua District, February 2000

New sectorial plans, designed with the World Bank support under recently strategies (The World Bank 1999), involve the Agriculture and Education Sectors (ref. Health Systems Reform workshop, Gaoua, March 1999). These Ministries fill up presently some of the gaps identified in the situation analyses to address better the youth, and the migrants, and develop poverty alleviation measures. These new plans encompass: strengthening HIV prevention among the youth, the workers and the agricultural communities; creating jobs and settling the young populations; initiating income generating activities; improving the standard of living in the migrant communities.

"...AIDS is not the property of the health system. You know that we local authorities, as well as having a role to advise in general matters of development, must also be promoters. The High Commissioner, the Prefects, the radio broadcasters, the journalists, the bar girls, the beer brewers, the religious leaders, the stall-holders in the market, the shop keepers, the clothes-makers – everyone is involved in the struggle against AIDS. The strategy must be "de-medicalized... It's not only for the men and women of the health sector, but for everyone who can be useful... Because if we confine the effort just to the health people, we will just look at them from afar and think we can let them get on with it. But it is we ourselves who must act."

(High Commissioner Poni Province)

Source: Robert Walgate, Open Solutions, Interviews in Gaoua District, February 2000

The Health Sector has changed its role from being a mere implementation agency of a few activities to become an important local and recognised stakeholder. It has now major inputs into having the public and voluntary sectors share a common vision, designing a plan based on local needs, and finally, stimulating the contribution of the various local partners.

In order to be effective in developing local responses, the situation analyses determined the need to accelerate and facilitate some of the health system reforms in particular "*to pass the HIV test*". This contrasts with the past situation of the majority of local actors being oblivious about policies and reforms. The four priorities identified fell into the need to strengthen the Health Information System, the Decentralisation, the STD and HIV/Aids care system (many service providers requesting more training and health education to play the information providers' role), and the partnerships in action.

> *"Reforms in different sectors must take place before any community can become 'AIDS competent...Health sector needs capacity building for health personnel in order to obtain better interaction with community members, to gain their trust and to know how their needs and how to respond to community needs."*
>
> (Abstract from conclusions, Gaoua District)
>
> Source: Summary of inter-country Workshop on HIV and Reforms for Health, April 1999

The Health Information System benefits now of a continuous and improved surveillance of HIV/Aids in the hospital (number of Aids patients, sero-prevalence among blood givers and among pregnant women), although behavioural surveillance is still lacking. Those data are reported under the epidemiological situation in the semester assessment of activities. Decentralisation has been stimulated by the Local Responses (e.g. local legislation, committees, planning, reviews). The 1999-2001 Work Plan emphasises purposely, early on, the training of health care providers to strengthen the STD and HIV/Aids care system, a process that started already in 1999. Finally, the local partners are stimulated to take stock of their competencies and desires as documented here. The Local Responses is not functioning in a vacuum but taking advantage and at the same time stimulating the reforms. This in turn makes it an enabling environment for the Local Responses to grow.

The communities are receiving well the messages and are active partners in the activities.

> *"Because what we can show in Gaoua is the real enthusiasm of the community, who have been committed from the very beginning of our plan. A real enthusiasm."*
>
> (President of the Comité Technique de la Lutte Contre le SIDA of Poni Province)
>
> Source: Robert Walgate, Open Solutions, Interviews in Gaoua District, February 2000

Finally, the needs to create an ethical, legal and social environment for taking care of the People living with HIV/Aids and affected by HIV/Aids, and ensure the greater involvement of People living with HIV/Aids was addressed as well. A project involving in Gaoua a national UNDP- United Nations Volunteers was drafted for this purpose.

> *"...I think to have associations prepare the family and the sick people is one thing; but the most appropriate would be to have an association of People living with HIV/AIDS ... an association of people who are seropositive, who are sick; this would be the right environment..."*
>
> (Association Pour les Femmes de Gaoua, President)
>
> Source: Robert Walgate, Open Solutions, Interviews in Gaoua District, February 2000

For the first time in Gaoua District, a branch of the national NGO, Initiative Privée Communautaire (IPC), Ouagadougou, for People Living With HIV/AIDS (*REVS+/IPC*), has opened in Gaoua town and participated to the technical meeting of the District (first trimester 2000).

⇨*Lessons learned:* Despite a positive partnership environment, setting up a local organisation of PLWHAs needs time to become accepted in the society and fully operational

Strategies

Although it may be too early in the process to measure any specific impact, the second semester 1999 activities (Phase 3 in Fig. 1.3) document a substantial number of activities and processes that are already addressing the issues identified in the earlier situation analyses.

The biennial Work Plan July 1999- June 2001 finalised in July 1999 (Phase 2 in Fig. 1.3), preceded since early 1997 by the steps described elsewhere (chap. 4), and setting the ground for implementation, is the milestone of the beginning of the implementation of Local Level responses.

By late 1999, the activities covered geographically the two larger towns of Gaoua and Kampti, and the small town of Broum-Broum, in addition to one hundred fifty villages[118] in other Departments Gaoua District.

The present HIV/Aids and STDs activities listed next are locally executed and owned by the local health structures and partners, and the communities. Along the present Health Sector and other Sector Reforms, the present strategies are decentralised and better integrated into the existing health services.

⇨*Lessons learned:* *The outcomes and impact of existing strategies still need to be assessed on the long term in the district, as well as their sustainability*

5.1.1 On the Situation Analysis at the Community Level

The main aim of this analysis (4.1) was to assess rapidly the situation at the local community level, the heart of the present systems analysis, in order to articulate a Local Responses responding to the local needs, with more effective strategies tailored to the existing communities. This study's particular methodological strength includes the use of existing participatory methods adapted successfully by a local national Non-Governmental Organisation (Population Santé Développement) to collect the data.

Applying participatory methods such as Rapid Rural Appraisals (RRA), even Participatory Rural Appraisals (PRA), are not the ultimate panacea of community participation and, although becoming fashionable in program design, have their own pitfalls (Kahrmann 1997). The author points to the difficulties in practising methods to design and implement projects in the Sahel taking the example of a farming project where the women are looking for pragmatic solutions for their own "daily battle of survival" and not so much for long-term solutions. Technocrats and local experts from the city are interested to resolve "how can the target group be made participatory?" from the above instead of getting involved with the problems of the rural population. We have faced a similar situation in the case of the RRA of Gaoua. The team was stronger at collecting the data, but weaker in presenting those in a useful and applicable way for program managers in a participatory fashion[119]. From the outset a difficulty lies in the RRA team's origins. Although Burkinabé, the team came from the capital city and had no direct obligations either over the consequences

---

[118] the exact number of rural communities (contrasting with the 30 reported recently by H. Binswanger during his recent visit) really active and on what basis needs to be verified

[119] the reader may refer in the future to the mapping techniques (biblio. Ref. Nyonyo V., D. Mayunga, C. Pervilhac, et al., TANESA, Tanzania), and Technical Note no. 3 (in press)

of the District findings or over the process of ownership by the communities. In addition, the problem was compounded by having no future local actors from the District Health team involved in the RRA. This was due to district personnel shortages at the time the study.[120] As a consequence, the above findings were in turn difficult to exploit for its original purpose of setting priorities in a planning situation at the District level (4.3.1). Finally, it remains still to be fully assessed how much participatory methods are stirring up more bottom-up participation during the intervention phase through the communities, committees, and private and public sectors supporting institutions.

We selected six dimensions or variables to measure the community participation's responses to HIV/Aids. The hectogram can be a useful and stimulating visualisation of a soft process such as community participation (4.1.1), and can encourage the monitoring of further progresses over time. Such methods were not yet known during the Primary Health Care (PHC) vogue of the seventies and eighties, and were only more widely publicised in the nineties. The method applied to community participation for the local responses merits refinement. Further studies may identify what are the most robust indicators (valid[121], specific[122], sensitive[123] and reliable[124]) and most useful to be acted upon, for example management, or leadership, as markers of the local responses progress, following the standards for selection of indicators in the field of Reproductive Health. In addition, the accuracy and standardisation of measurements (scale) of community participation to HIV/Aids need to be further developed. Finally, each community may have its own different baseline or web, and the aggregate of the four separate communities may be more representative of the communities in the District than the general aggregated estimates we have based our scores upon.

We used the essential categories of classifications proposed by UNAIDS, and found that those can be instrumental to complement the broad spectrum of risk reduction strategies which were wrongly in general limited more up to recently to individual risk factors. Further studies merit to address whether information collected by focus groups among men and women adults would be an added value or not to the identification of vulnerable factors, in comparison to the present study limited to the youth.

---

[120] we did not encounter this difficulty in late 1997 in the Kabarole local responses study, Uganda, with members of the District Health Team participating in the studies as observers
[121] valid: measures the factor it is supposed to measure
[122] specific: reflects only changes in the factor under consideration
[123] sensitive: reveals changes in the issue of interest
[124] reliable: gives the same value if its measurement is repeated in the same way on the same population and at almost the same time

The present study findings are based on aggregated data collected between key informants and focus groups. Further studies may also consider three additional types of analysis of the raw data for interventions purposes: by genders, by locations (rural vs semi-rural), and by ethnic groups. The major limitation of the study, due to time and financial constraints, was not to include the household responses. The importance of the latter was just thoroughly analysed recently on a literature review (UNAIDS 1999). An improved design of the present community level study encompassing household data could at the same time allow to make the link, expressed in a recent regional conference (UNAIDS 1998), between the HIV sero-surveillance, answering the "how much," and the behavioural surveillance, answering the "why."

Finally, the challenge of the community level study may lie more in the use and application of the findings than in the collection of data itself. Some vulnerability factors are much more complex and difficult to address than the mere identification of problems through a PRA or a RRA and can be the subject of controversies, or still pending solutions, for which no quick fix exists. For example, in relation to social norms and cultural barriers, a medical anthropologist from a well-known international research organisation has recently challenged the numerous organisations which combat the "levirat" as a traditional practice facilitating the spread of the epidemic, to reconsider their positions based on two observations (Taverne 1996). First, from an epidemiological angle, the "levirat" is containing the spread of the virus at least among family members only, whereas, if not, widows would have broader sexual networks among the general population. Although such statement would merit further documentation for example through more research in sexual networks (UNAIDS 1998), the argument is plausible. Second, from a social perspective, it represents presently the only efficacious social protection offered to widows. As an example of the cleansing involving sexual intercourse after a woman is widowed, it remains to be determined in Burkina Faso the extent of that practice still. No original local alternatives have yet been identified that we know of, in comparison to Zambia for example, such as the beaded ring around the waist of the widow (UNAIDS 1999). Identifying locally acceptable and positive cultural alternatives to reduce the risks of infection to HIV due to commonly and deeply rooted dangerous practices remain important under-developed more applied "projects" for anthropologists or ethnologists.

Under the Services and Programs, we could not investigate the closest formal supportive health structures, or Health Centres, to the communities. This was due to the nature of the team collecting data at the community level not qualified for such an assessment, and of the investigating team at the District level limited in number.[125] As a consequence, some technicians of international agencies (e.g. GTZ) may not have picked up so quickly on using some of the findings of the present study. Indeed intervention efforts prior to the study had been more invested and limited to that more formal level of care for the communities, and co-operation technicians were particularly interested to review these activities, and disappointed if not carefully assessed. Several observations of the formal Health System are nevertheless articulated in the District level findings (4.2).

The Community level study (4.1) has documented the feasibility of using RRA methods such as focus groups and key informants interviews, over a two weeks period, to comprehend the community participation at a District level, and their vulnerability factors. The RRA was not enough geared to participatory methods (i.e. using PRA). If the general impressions about the data are that the information is known already, a closer look to the above Tables (4.1 to 4.3 and 4.4 to 4.6) confirms their usefulness for local planning and interventions purposes, particularly identifying the local opportunities or strategic priorities. The challenge and success of community participation may not so much lie in mastering the tools of data collection than the use of the findings for prioritisation purposes in planning, and the design of programs. We would further recommend that such methods be not just limited to HIV/Aids program but more broadly based in the field of Reproductive Health encompassing at a minimum STDs, Tuberculosis, Family Planning. The local responses for HIV/Aids is now using planning tools which were still being tested or unheard of in the Primary Health Care (PHC) endeavour a few years ago.

The essentials to plan and design sound community-based programs in Gaoua District are now documented. This rapidly evolving field of research (UNAIDS 1999) is just starting to document current experiences with the top league models of African countries (Uganda,

Tanzania, Zimbabwe, Kenya, Zambia…), all English-speaking countries. Little or no documentation of the French-speaking countries exists (besides Sénégal), leaving out a large majority of the poverty struck Sahelian countries. The present case study can be further used to stimulate community planning in other Districts, and in turn be used for the national strategic planning exercises.

---

[125] in contrast we could carry out this analysis for the local responses case study in Kabarole, Uganda, late 1997

Although a young player in public health programs, HIV/Aids programs will benefit from such initiatives and approaches and become better equipped as a program to become part among other important old players to contribute actively to the comprehensive approach to Primary Health Care.

5.1.2 On the Situation Analysis at the District Level

The main aim of this analysis (4.2) was to assess rapidly at the district level the various systems, and their organisations as units of analysis. This in turn leads to an improved understanding of the organisations which have inputs into the community system, be it in the public or the private sectors (ref. chap. 1, Fig. 1.4), in order to expand the responses to HIV/Aids in the district.

The study design, similarly to an earlier WHO Collaborative Study and the European Council of Aids Service Organisations (Kenis and Marin 1997), focuses attention on the meso-level of organisations, here the district, by the nature of the Local Responses study. The district is the level at which organisations are located, instead of the more frequent traditional studies referring to the micro-level of individual behaviour, or the macro- (or national) level. The study extends to the community level as well to articulate further the bottom-up approach (4.1).

The institutional landscape, the dimensions contained and their measurements, has proven to be a more powerful management and surveillance tool of the Local Responses than the mere "inventory" of organisation suggested in the original UNAIDS/ WHO proposal (UNAIDS 1996).

The present limitation of the institutional landscape is that it does not illustrate the strategies or types of programs covered or not in the District. One of the original landscapes we developed contained the additional dimension of strategies[126], but was dropped after some technical feedback because the landscape became too complex to comprehend. A landscape for the strategies could be easily adapted though, by substituting to the measurement of the degree of responses that dimension (ref. section 5.1.6).

A further limitation is that people may not be used to visualise activities in a landscape form. In the presence of public health experts, often with a medical and/ or epidemiological background, data presentations are better understood in the form of numbers, rates, ratios and regular two by two, or other statistical

---

[126] strategies were classified into community-based, institutional-based, and media-based and social marketing

tables. We observed on a couple of occasions, difficulties for non-social scientists to comprehend the landscape. It needs therefore clarifications or some education first,[127] before overwhelming or losing the audience.

We assessed the degree of the responses of each organisation by reviewing its global activities based on the above inputs and process indicators for each organisation and given its present status and capacities. The method was criticised later for being too subjective.[128]

To improve the method, we used and validated a triangulation approach in the second Local Responses study carried out in Uganda at the end of 1997 (Pervilhac, Kipp et al. 1997). We developed a numeric scale to assess the depth of each organisational responses which based on scores fell into strong, medium, or weak responses. We were able to validate our observations and opinions by cross-checking the rating of the degree of each institution's responses based on our own observations and impressions, with the independent rating based on their own impressions only of each organisation between and by themselves. The second Case study in Uganda also demonstrates that methods can be improved and refined over time when repeating and replicating the tools in other national contexts.

Finally, the challenge of this tool lies also more in the use and application of the findings, like the community tools (4.1.1) than in the collection of data:
- Which institutions of which sector, within their limits, can improve their roles given the types of programs best tailored to respond to the communities' needs?
- What are the most cost-effective strategies to concentrate upon? Priority? Feasibility? Sustainability?
- How to bring in new partners into the picture (landscape), with the considerations just mentioned?

The Local Responses success is narrowly limited as well to an uncertain policy environment unveiled through the Health Sector Reform that we have just described. The latter can be an important confounding factor difficult to control for in the present methodological case study set up.

---

[127] we used a blank landscape first for people to comprehend its dimensions
[128] personal communications with a couple of UNAIDS-WHO experts following the presentation of the Burkina Faso findings at the UNAIDS Technical Meeting, Geneva, September 1997

We have moved purposely the measurement of the organisational responses as an output indicator so that programme managers do not overlook this essential component of the program in their plans and reviews. However, the ultimate aim or outcome of the Local Responses should not be lost of sight in the process, and that is to reduce the HIV/Aids and STD prevalence, and to reduce the personal and social impact of HIV infection (ref. chap. 1, Fig. 1.4).

5.1.3. On the Consensus Building and Pre-Planning

For the findings of the Consensus-Building and Pre-Planning (4.3.1), the three days workshop is a good method to catalyse the forces and reach a consensus quickly for all stakeholders/ partners together, and to move from a study into implementation in an organised and systematic fashion. The workshop contributed to have the partners share a common vision and their parameters (objectives, strategies) given their strengths and limitations. It answered the question on *"What"* can be accomplished for Expanded Responses? However, the workshop was not sufficient to answer the *"How"* can the Expanded Responses be accomplished, or what are the exact activities of each partner, what are the priorities, what is the Plan/ calendar? This next step was further addressed by the UNAIDS Country Broker nominated mid-1998 who carried out for this purpose a "Strategic Planning" workshop.

We concluded, to follow-up the workshop, that additional financing does not appear as a condition sine qua non to Expanded Responses. Based on a recent inter-country meeting which had just taken place in Dar-es-Salaam (May 1998), it was determined necessary to prioritise activities which can put the local actors (communities and various partners) into confidence, and which can have a rapid and visible success on the short term. The activities should be feasible with the limited existing resources. The workshop results were a step in this direction. We further recommended that interventions/ activities taking place on a quarterly basis be monitored carefully, and corrective actions be taken as on-going process over a one year period through a special technical support (identified mid-1998 as the "Country Broker"). The original thinking that existing resources to expand the Responses is sufficient was proven to be naïve but was based on the original thinking that a wealth of human and local resources exist already but are not tapped to. It overlooked the necessity to increase resources mobilised in support of HIV/Aids prevention and care activities.

This condition is stated in the original *Best Practice* on Expanding the Responses, as one among the six pre-conditions to fulfil equally (UNAIDS 1998) in order to increase the chances of succeeding in implementing a Local Responses.

In conclusion, the results were instrumental to consolidate and catalyse the various pathways to Expanded Responses with ambitious objectives fixed by the various local partners (Public and Private Sectors and Communities) in an original effort to increase the local ownership of the process.

The following main observations summarised in eight issues may allow to improve a future Phase 1 of Situation Analysis, and Phase 2 of Solution Development/ Priorities Setting, in other Districts of Burkina Faso, or other countries. Those may be instrumental to improve its in-country or other countries replication, should it be used to catalyse Responses. These issues show also that there is still much work to be done in improving the steps of Local Responses within the country.

1. Need to adapt the international terminology for interventions to the country national/ district one: the use of categories of objectives, strategies, and interventions based on the "Interventions and Policies" (National AIDS Program Management A Training Course, GPA/ WHO, 1995) to orient the workshop participants to a common vision was appropriate. The identification and language of "interventions" need to match the local realities and be more comprehensive particularly for care and counselling and social and economic impact reduction. The National AIDS Control Program (NACP) and the program managers at the local level would need in the future to design this framework of reference before such a workshop. It can in turn be used for the various Districts in the country.

2. Lack of benefits from the use of the Local Responses situation analysis findings for solution development: the study questions and approaches to encompass programmatic questions or aspects lacking for District and other program managers, targeted population interventions approach vs. the by and large "community approach".

3. Three key partners groups and the preparation and implementation of the workshop: community participants could not function well into a more academic room environment and needed more time and participatory methods as what they were offered in their own language. Group work exercises need to flow better into the general process for the various types of participants: either the exercises have

to be tailored foe each group of participants, from community representatives to public officials (different interests and aptitudes), or groups need to be involved in different workshops.

4. Consensus building was reached through plenary and pin-boards: the tight agenda and group works did not allow the original planned dialogue for exchanges of experiences, disagreements and controversies between the major stakeholders of different sectors. Group works which allow this fruitful and necessary exchanges, followed by debates in plenary would allow to overcome this problem, particularly on (re-) defining the major roles of some of the key actors (Ministries, NGOs, Associations).

5. Clarifications from external partners to District actors: local partners requested a number of clarifications from external participants (agencies, donors…). A better atmosphere can be created if all agencies can clarify their roles and potential inputs. As examples of issues raised are:
- directed to the MOH: the role and collaboration between the social private marketing actor, PROMACO[129] with 265 outlets selling condoms in the District, and the MOH with a limited impact of its 20 Government health facilities which have a restricted geographical coverage, suffer from condom supplies shortages, and distribute a very limited number of condoms per month.

- by local NGOs/ Associations: the role of the PNLS (World Bank credit) to stimulate local NGOs/ Associations via the new Plan International Burkinabé (PIB) acting as a local relay ("ONG relais") for those in the District,

- by some public Ministries and local Associations: the role of ABBEF in stimulating for example much needed interventions, e.g. care and counselling, and local fund raising (for ex. via PI) or including those in the new "Plan Stratégie 1998-2002" at the national level.[130]

6. Technical preparation of prioritisation of target groups, geographical areas before the workshop by technicians: a technical working group managed with great difficulty the prioritisation of target groups in the District, a concept that was non-existent in the previous plans and interventions. The adaptation from GPA/WHO 1995 Module 2 "Description of the Target Populations" and 4 of the "Determination of Priority Interventions" was well received by the technical group. However, also due to time constraints, the group could only describe a couple of priorities. The rationale for classification would merit further discussion

---

[129] the Social Marketing of Condoms project is a KfW funded effort but we noticed little communication and co-ordination between GTZ and KfW to implement this prevention strategy effectively at a local level
[130] Source: the national plan is budgeted for over 5.600.000.000 FCFA. ABBEF, IPPF "Su noog Zaka" no. 11 1er semester 1997, pp. 10-12

and attention by local planners and managers (ex. prostitutes classified last despite the fact that Burkina Faso rated 6th with 60% infection among 20 countries in terms of HIV prevalence infection in urban sex workers in Sub-Saharan Africa[131]). This low prioritisation may reflect the fear of embarking on difficult interventions, combined with the lack of understanding of potential entry points and local cultural unacceptability to consider prostitution issues. The important planning of priorities of geographical interventions with eight various locations to classify to provide guidance for the planning and interventions either for the public or the private Sectors was not carried out by lack of time. Mapping exercises as part of a situation analyses would resolve this difficulty.

7. Lack of planning of other program components related/ integrated to HIV/Aids: STDs, Family Planning, TB components were not discussed or considered. This should be addressed in the future to have HIV/Aids be part of the broader Reproductive Health package and agenda. The main reasons of this issue were:

- the situation analyses did not analyse these other components,
- the workshop was geared to a strict HIV/Aids expanded responses from the in-country users' (GTZ, MoH...) point of view,
- the workshop had to limit itself in its goals and objectives due to its experimental nature, and time constraints.

8. Monitoring and Evaluation Process: five categories of progress for Local Responses may be monitored over the next few months were discussed during the workshop:

- Documentation of the various stages defined in the workshop and their status completion, and solutions to constraints
- Detailed District Action Plan (yearly) by the MoH incorporating the findings of the Workshop and detailed Plans for each main Actor
- Documentation of activities (brief Quarterly Progress Reports with on-going internal evaluation) by each main actor , and comparing the new interventions 1 year later with the baseline of interventions collected in the Gaoua 1998 workshop
- Determination of the terms of partnerships between various actors (between public, but particularly between public and private) clarified for each intervention where the partnership is necessary
- Measurement: Inputs indicators encompassing institutional indicators. Process indicators encompassing personnel, activities, management, co-ordination,

---

[131] Source: A World Bank Policy Research Report, Confronting AIDS Public Priorities in a Global Epidemic, p. 89

logistics indicators, and HIV/Aids services (integration, quality of health services), and outputs indicators measuring the degree of responses.

5.1.4 On the Strategic Planning

The UNAIDS Strategic Planning
For the results of the Strategic Planning (4.3.2), as clarified in the recent UNAIDS Guides to the strategic planning (UNAIDS 1998; UNAIDS 1998), the traditional normative planning exercise is planned according to universal norms (e.g. a standardised treatment, vaccination, etc.). It applies to all beneficiaries, irrespective of their conditions or situations, and will produce its effects to the extent that it is reproduced accurately. Strategic planning contrasts with normative planning by adapting the norms to a given or changing situation, or taking into consideration a dynamic and flexible environment. It takes underlying determinants into account. Those vary according to the persons concerned (e.g. social class, religion, culture, gender specificity etc.) and according to situations that may alter rapidly over time.

Strategic Planning in the Private Sector
In the private sector, strategic planning has mesmerised many organisations since 1965. The massive use of strategic planning by the industry has been explained because "*as firms grew and became more complex... they needed a systematic approach to setting strategy. Strategic planning emerged as the answer*" (Porter 1987).

Recently, Mintzberg, a sociologist, world wide known expert in organisations (Mintzberg 1982), and management (Mintzberg 1989), argued in a milestone on the review of planning that "strategic planning" is far from being the ultimate panacea because of several fundamental fallacies (Mintzberg 1994). First, the difficulties of forecasting (particularly true in relation to the development of the HIV epidemic) are a major difficulty. Second, the detachment of planners and managers to strategy making is evident for different reasons. Among others: hard information are often limited in scope, not encompassing important ... non-quantitative factors (true in HIV/Aids with the lack of behavioural data), information are often too aggregated for effective use in strategy making, or arriving too late, and finally, there exists a surprising amount of unreliable hard information. Third, the failure to formalise gives evidence that innovation cannot be institutionalised.

In addition to the limitations of strategic planning, the author points to the real pitfalls of the original traditional planning too. Those are related to the lack of commitment of planning (with the exception of the "*Top*"), the inflexibility of plans, the biases of objectivity in light of the politics and policies, the obsession with control.

Finally, the author concludes:

> "We *have no evidence that any of the strategic planning systems - no matter how elaborate, or how famous-succeeded in capturing (let along improving on) the messy informal processes in which strategies really do get developed.*" (p. 296-7)

A closer look to Mintzberg's position in light of the application of strategic planning for the Local Responses, one would not recommend to HIV/Aids program managers to use strategic planning to come up with the best strategies and interventions in the District. The industrial sector has become more critical of strategic planning after thirty years of experience, and may be moving away from it in the nineties. Ironically, the health sector, late to catch up on the industry approaches, is attempting presently those with various degrees of success.

Strategic planning tools are used in development co-operation (e.g. logical framework) with well-trained experts, combined with additional outside expertise. We based our brief analysis on a recent review of the "logical framework"(Wiggins and Shields 1995). The logical framework usually consists of a four-by-four matrix which summarises the project, records the assumptions which underpin the strategy adopted, and outlines how the project may be monitored, all arrayed according to a hierarchy of objectives or an ends-means continuum. "(op. cit. p. 2) As a management tool, the framework emphasises objectives." Yet it is also acknowledged that "the logical framework is not by itself, however, a comprehensive tool for either planning or management" (op. cit. p. 4).

Germany's GTZ goal -orientated project planning and programming (ZOPP)[132], as a key part of its integrated project planning and management system, is perhaps one of the clearest and most detailed application of performance management to development programs. The authors point and refute some of the

---

[132] ZOPP (in German), or the GTZ "ZielOrientierte ProjektPlanung"

criticisms of the use of the logical framework such as a "rigid blueprint" which can lead to reduced flexible implementation and "learning process" (op. cit. p. 11). They counteract the criticism by documenting that the GTZ manual mention how the project matrix is expected to be revised at least four to five times during the project cycle (2-5 years), particularly as part of annual review and programming meetings.

We think that the criticisms are quite valid and are sufficient not to recommend the standard use of the logical framework to plan Local Responses (particularly out of "project context ", e.g. GTZ or USAID-financed). The Local Responses process we describe in this research must overcome the constraints of a limited "project cycle" and cannot afford the administrative time-consuming and technical dimensions bi-lateral funded projects entail.

It is still too early to know if the strategic planning approach is the best way to implement the Local Responses, and further replication, and research will answer this in five to ten years down the line. Our present review of the origins of strategic planning suggests that it is a planning tool better tailored to meet the needs of large businesses ran by well-trained north-American business managers. In the case of the various original UNAIDS Guides to the strategic planning process for a national[133] responses to HIV/Aids, those have been originally planned for the national level and better trained and supported program managers. In addition, even countries in Europe are moving away from Strategic Planning: "It is not envisaged that the forthcoming national HIV/Aids strategy will be in the form of a 'strategic plan.' It is likely that it will follow the format of 'An Evolving Strategy'"(U.K. Country Report 1999).[134] We remain sceptical whether its present form can meet the needs and capacities of planning for the Local Responses in the context of improving the local or district responses.

Despite the limitations of the present strategic planning process, the end product is satisfactory and much more powerful then what existed two years ago, thanks to the country broker's persistence, qualities, and flexibility. The process of taking the various partners through the various planning stages led early on to have a common vision on some of the priorities in the District and agreement on the tasks to be shared between numerous essential partners. As an alternative, the identification of an effective planning tool for HIV/Aids at the local (in contrast to the national) level merits further discussion and research.

---

[133] "bold" is our emphasis
[134] the researcher was involved in 1999 in a EU funded for the Review of HIV Prevention Policies in 28 countries in Europe

Strategic Planning and Health Sector Reform
One important aspect of the Strategic Planning process is the component related to the

Health Sector Reform due to the nature of the Local Responses. The HIV/Aids epidemic has put forward the weaknesses of the health systems in many countries which do not *"pass the HIV test"*, and can be better understood quoting the findings of the inter-countries (Burkina-Faso, Ghana, and Thailand representatives) Health Reform and HIV workshop which took place in Gaoua:

> *"Reforms, whether related to health or related to other public sectors, provide an opportunity to influence the way systems respond to their clients' needs. The HIV epidemic illustrates better than anything else the extent to which the responses is adequate or not."* (Reeler 1999)

The objectives of the reforms of the Health Sector in the new strategic plan of Gaoua District outlined the following:

1. an "individual/ client" (or community or district) centred action (vs. an original fix on combating the virus),
2. a common vision among all partners,
3. a consensus among all partners to prioritise and implement the program,
4. a capacity-building of communities, health systems and other sectors to respond to HIV/Aids,
5. bridging the gap between the politics and practice,
6. stimulating and supporting new partners,
7. setting up a Health System Reform of HIV/Aids.

To implement those, in relation to the Health Sector Reform, four priority areas were identified:

- Health Information System strengthening
- Decentralisation
- Strengthening of the Health System
- Partnerships in action.

Analysing the Health Sector Reform dimension is beyond the scope of this research, as mentioned earlier (4.2.3). Suffice it to say that for the program managers at the district level, the combination of tackling the above mentioned activities described in the Operational priority Plan 1999 with those of the Health Sector Reform can be daunting.

The combination of tackling the Health Sector Reform, combined with the strategic planning approach promoted presently, are part of the complicated and awkward tools and technologies illustrated in *The cough syrup transport system* (Fig. 1.1). Those will need improvements in the next few years to become a lighter system with a more feasible and replicable approach to the Local Responses.

Half a year into the implementation of the Local Responses, the process and outcomes were assessed through a Formative Evaluation described separately (4.4).

5.1.5 On the Development of Tools for the Local Responses

The World Bank's new strategic plan (The World Bank 1999) to combat the epidemic with African governments and partnership with UNAIDS stands on four pillars:

- "Advocacy to position HIV/Aids as a central development issue and to increase and sustain an intensified responses,
- Increased resources and technical support for African partners and Bank country teams to mainstream HIV/Aids activities in all sectors,
- Prevention efforts targeted to both general and specific audiences, and activities to enhance HIV/Aids treatment and care,
- Expanded knowledge to help countries design and manage prevention, care, and treatment programs based on epidemic trends, impact forecasts, and identified best practices."

The Plan is particularly useful in providing the basis of and rationale for the Local Responses approach described in the present research with the provision to "Build Local Capacity in National and Local Government, Civil Society, and the Private Sector to Lead and Implement Effective Programs" (p. 28). The Bank is setting up a special Unit called the "multisectoral AIDS Campaign Team for Africa" (ACTafrica), based in the Office of the Regional Vice Presidents which will, among other tasks, in collaboration with UNAIDS prepare tools for project development and evaluation.

To respond to this need, before the set up of ACTafrica, I was already requested by UNAIDS Department of Policy, Strategy and Research (PSR) Department, in early 1999:

- first, to develop a framework which summarised the various dimensions of each tool in a one to two pages "Explanatory Fact Sheet" (Appendix 5C)
- second, to make an inventory of the Tools used of the implementation of the Health Sector Reform and HIV Agenda in various national settings. The output of forty-five tools identified is attached in the "Summary Tables of Six Categories of Key Tools for the Implementation of the Health Reform and HIV Agenda in various National Settings" (Appendix 5D). Those are categorised into the logical key categories discussed next which are found in assessing and developing an expanded responses at the district level
- third, to review at least three or four of each using the Fact Sheet, the aim being of having some of the key ones reviewed as models. Twenty of those were reviewed in more details (Appendix 5E Sample of Seven Tools Reviewed). They are to be disseminated in late 2000 for countries on the recently available UNAIDS electronic "Local Response" network site.[135]

The World Bank Strategic Plan refers several times throughout its document to the fact Governments only need the tools, that those are being presently developed, and finally, that they need to be accessible to countries (p. 35) in order for them to respond more effectively to HIV prevention. This appears to be also the current thinking at UNAIDS. Our experience in the review of the tools, combined with the field level findings of the Local Responses case study of Burkina Faso, brings a caveat to this thinking though. We still have a long way to go to be able to offer simple and effective tools to country partners: the tools still need to be either further developed, or adapted and simplified, or tested, or a combination of those. We give an example next of a tool (section 5.1.6) we have newly developed to assess organisational aspects in relation to the Local Responses which is grounded on the sociology of organisations.

Specific limitations to each tool were reviewed and documented separately (Appendix 5E). We have found the following general limitations to some of the tools used as reviewed next for each category of tools. Those may in turn merit further research to develop standardised tools:

---

[135] "Local response to HIV/AIDS" available under "What's new" at www.unaids.org since July 2000

1) *For the Situation Analysis*: the existing UNAIDS Modules (Module 1 and 3) are more tailored to the national level, than to the district level, and the testing in Burkina Faso gave evidence that even with a country broker expertise the steps of the Guidelines were difficult to follow. A gap still exists between circumscribing the determinants of HIV and the specific factors of vulnerability and prioritising strategies and interventions.

Furthermore, the situation analysis does not allow yet to clearly prioritise vulnerable groups, and consequently the strategies and interventions used. The UNAIDS "Strategic Plan Formulation" (Module 3) does not address the last key step of the planning process, or how to develop targets and indicators and work plans.

2) *For the Institutions' and Sector's Capacity Assessment*: based on the angle and emphasis placed for this assessment, different tools need to be tailored and experimented upon still. For example, we developed the "Rapid Organisational Review" (ROR) tool based on the sociology of organisation theories and practice and tailored for the Local Responses (ref. next section 5.1.6). In Malawi, an emphasis on the problem of drug shortages led to an instrument tailored to the "Rapid Assessment of Access to Care and HIV/Aids-Related Drugs in Communities and the Health System" (Reeler 1999). In Tanzania, the struggle of various interests groups in the public sector led to an emphasis on "power relationships flows" with the "Mapping of Institutional Relationships and Decision-Making in Public Sector." That tool is based on an adaptation of M. Reich's "Policy Maker" and political mapping tool adapted for an institution and sector capacity assessment, and needs further testing too. It would also gain to be further developed for the mapping of power relationships at the District level. The UNAIDS "Responses Analysis" is limited to a few interventions only in comparison to the broad spectrum existing.

3) *For the Assessment of Existing Policies vs. needs and realities*: the original framework of analysis on "Decentralization and Health Systems Change" was developed and used by WHO was made for policy analysts. It still needs to be adapted and simplified (e.g. 27 "facets" of the framework) for lay people to be able to use for the Local Responses. The same for the "Health Financing Reform" tool. The numerous Guidelines for Human Rights assessment need in contrast to be developed into simple tools with the right questions to be asked to the right people at the district level.

4) *For the Calculation of Intervention Costs*: there is evidence that these calculations are feasible based on various documentation and studies done by

experts. Clarifications on "what does an ideal program look like and how much does it cost?" (The World Bank 1999) exist at a national level, but those need to be tailored and simplified for planning purposes at the district level. The experience of the calculation of intervention costs are limited on a micro-level to projects (Ng'weshemi, Boerma et al. 1997), and remain in general an isolated effort with no benefits to other District planning exercises, or still belong to the grey (non-published) area. In addition documenting costs of interventions are favoured over the development of simple costing manuals such as the one recently developed in Primary Health Care (Creese and Parker 1994). If the latter took more than fifteen years after the Alma-Ata Declaration to address PHC issues, we may expect simple costing manual for the Local Responses to be available by the year 2015! Critical to the Local Responses planning process for managers, we have still not answered their questions on how to use economic data for district planning purposes.

5) *For Resource mobilisation*: this is a fairly new concept in the Local Responses to HIV/Aids and as such very little exists on the subject. Besides merely mobilising resources, the advantage of advocating such tools is that they allow a degree of transparency that plays to the benefit of the clients (communities and District), and their partners (public and private). The mobilisation of financial resources has been successful and is described separately (4.4 Outcomes).

6) *For the Program monitoring and evaluation*: experiences have been collected and documented in different countries more frequently by categorical areas (counselling, care...) than comprehensively, with the exception of Thailand. The complexity of the Local Responses and dimensions necessitates a multi-disciplinary team, and a mix bag of indicators. This is documented by the indicators for Formative Evaluation (ref. Section 4.4) which we developed, and were tested in Gaoua District in the last Phase 4 of the Action-Research (Flow Chart, Fig. 1.3, chap. 1).

In less than two weeks, we were able to identify almost fifty different tools that can be used for the Local Responses. Each and every expert at UNAIDS, or WHO, or any institution may come up with his/ her tool based on the individual interests and focus. A large number and spectrum of tools exist already, a couple of hundreds maybe.

The feedback I received in a presentation of the present status of the tool kit during the "UNAIDS Technical Meeting on the Facilitation of Local Responses: Training and Methodology Development" (Bulawayo, Zimbabwe, 22-25 Nov. 1999) pointed to the following limitations and potentials. The tools needed are those that share one's own paradigm, e.g. looking at communities, or understanding local institutions etc., or a combination of those. The tools may consist in a list of updated questions which one can select from, and that can match best the local situation and needs, avoiding a top-down approach. The challenge lies more in the correct selection of the most important tool(s) for a particular situation, and in asking the most important questions, and using the findings, or in a nutshell, how to make the best use of which tool at which moment? At the present time, most of the existing tools can only be used by the person who developed them, or experts in the subject, which limits as a consequence their applications and replicability.

Going back to the original image of "*The cough syrup transport system*" (Fig. 1.1), the syrup, i.e. the strategies exist, are known, and appear quite straightforward and simple (a mere syrup), as well as the apparent simple mean to deliver those (with a simple spoon). But the selection of the best mix of those, or the exact ingredients of the syrup, remains a challenge for program managers. In addition, the supportive machinery for the syrup to be delivered with a simple spoon, i.e. the various tools existing to do a situation analysis and plan the responses, is still complex under the present Local Responses, as illustrated by the cumbersome and awesome transport system. The latter can become even more complicated when efforts to develop multisectoral collaboration are pursued. Many tools still need to be adapted or refined. In addition, the best mix of tools as well needs to be selected carefully, given the frequent unique environment.

There is a need to develop and tailor simplified tools, to select the correct mix of those too, and finally be effective in delivering the "*syrup*". For this purpose, we advocate first, in the original stages that experts in different areas further develop and adapt their tools for the Local Responses in the different countries. Second, the tools can be tested and simplified in several Districts and adapted for the needs of each country. Finally, in the last stage, those can be scaled-up for use by the different countries on their own in the priority regions of each country.

In conclusion, there is no quick fix solution to the Local Responses. The state-of-the-art of the development of the existing tools and the supportive machinery to deliver those effectively, are both still limited, as well as the exact knowledge of the best mix of use of any of those. What is needed is a major financial and technical investment of different scientists from different disciplines. They should work both on the selection of the best strategies and the refinement of prevention tools to consolidate the Local Responses into commonly accepted, feasible, and successful HIV prevention strategies over the next five to ten years (5.2). This effort can be pursued as diligently as the immunologists and virologists presently are for the development of the vaccines against the HIV strains.

5.1.6 On the Development of a new Organisational Tool: the Rapid Organisational Review (ROR)

Rationale for the ROR

The Local Responses is taking place within the favourable emergence of Reforms in the Health and other Sectors as well, and accompanying structural adjustments to strengthen human and institutional capacities (ref. section 4.3.2). In the Health Sector, reforms like decentralisation or local budgeting and financing are encouraging the public sector to work hands-in-hands with the partners from the private sectors and the communities. The focus is changing to local capacity building taking stock of the wealth of experiences available locally.

In this broader context, health managers at the district or local level are increasingly responsible to plan and manage their own complex environments, including to operate with the numerous organisations, active in HIV/Aids activities or stimulate the contribution of potential ones. Two dimensions are seen as essential to tackle the various vulnerability factors of communities and larger societies to HIV/Aids. First, the improvement of the intra-sectoral collaboration in the health sector, e.g. between Departments and/ or programs (e.g. Family Planning, STD, Family Planning…). Second, the building-up of inter-sectoral partnerships between different sectors, e.g. Education, Agriculture, Interior etc. and Health, and between actors of the public and the private sectors.

The multidisciplinary approach to public health planning and programming remains largely conceptual due to the limited or lack of policy or sociological approaches available for that purpose, with rare exceptions (Soucat 1998). "Expanding partnerships in the design, implementation and evaluation of HIV/Aids-related policies and programs"(UNAIDS 1998), or as a corollary the support of the necessary tools to support such a strategy, is one of the recommended pathways to improve the responses to HIV/Aids. Bilateral agencies encompass as an approach to preventing HIV/Aids and mitigating its impact, the need to increase the capacity of non-governmental, community-based, and private sector organisations to respond to HI/Aids, such as USAID (USAID 1998) or GTZ (Hemrich G. et al. 1997) (D'Cruz-Grote 1997).

At best, projects and programs identify in their plans for activities related to HIV/ Aids most often all local private partners as Non-Governmental Organisations (NGOs), and often, group those as such. The partners' strengths and limitations, and their various roles and opinions, are often in a situation analysis either taken for granted, or not accounted for. Yet the importance and roles of institutions, systems and structures of health promotion and prevention are known (Brösskamp-Stone et al. 1998). These include the various types of NGOs (e.g. client affinity groups, social service clubs, non-profit firms, private charities), and the Community-Based Organisations (CBOs), (e.g. local associations). This renders the task of the public sector to build stock on what exists either inefficient or impossible.

Understanding those different systems and their organisations is a difficult challenge for district or local health managers. They are already burdened with numerous tasks and expectations, and usually are not from social sciences, but from medical or public health backgrounds.

In order to respond to this need, the Rapid Organisational Review (ROR) tool we developed, and presented next, aims to contribute to an improved understanding and operationalisation of the organisations functioning at the district level. It can be used as an organisational baseline as well. This allows in turn to document and understand the processes leading to improved HIV/Aids outcomes, via fostering partnerships and consensus-building.

The ROR encompasses the following three steps (situation analysis, strategies, action plan) approach illustrated in the chart "Rapid Organisational Review (ROR): Building the Organisational Plan. A Tool for Partnerships and Consensus-Building at the Local Level" (Appendix 5F). The ROR is accompanied by an "Introduction Sheet for the Users" (Appendix 5G). Finally, the next steps are detailed separately in a "Users' Guide to the ROR" (Appendix 5H).

Step 1. Situation Analysis
Illustration: *Model of the District and Communities Systems*

The Situation Analysis answers the question: *"where are we?"* The study uses a systems approach and is based on sociological and public health thinking and approaches. The units of analysis are institutions, organisations, societies, operating at the present time (or the organisational network), rather than individuals (ref. 3.2). First, systems and sub-systems are categorised and illustrated as inputs and processes in the program cycle. The inventory of the partners (sub-systems) at the local level is made for each of the three key systems illustrated in our original model (Fig. 1.4 chap. 1): the communities are placed at the centre of the model, then the public and the private sectors are reviewed. The relationships between these various partners, or the individual inter-sectoral linkages, are explored and illustrated as well at this stage. This inventory, as comprehensive as possible, allows to draw the sample of the partners involved for the review. The study uses first existing sources of data, then complements these data and identifies through questionnaires the present focus areas (strategies, interventions) for each partner reviewed, and the internal obstacles and opportunities to accomplish the present activities. Finally, as an option, in addition to the individual inter-linkages, the global co-ordinating mechanisms, needed between the three systems necessary to strengthen the partnerships, are analysed.

Step 2: Strategies

Illustration (next illustrations, and details in 4.2): *Institutional Landscape of the Partners from the Public and Private Sectors (present situation or organisational baseline)*. Originally, the team wants to know "*Where are we?*" (4.2). Then, the Strategies will answer the question: "*Where do we want to be?*" First, the review team identifies the various partners' common or diverging vision of HIV/Aids responses at a local level. Then, the team collects and discusses the partners' views to strengthen their responses in the focus areas they are presently involved in and how much (baseline), and the same in other new areas of need. Internal and external obstacles and opportunities for the future are analysed. Assumptions about the future are identified. As an option, the necessary strengthening of inter-linkages and mechanisms to facilitate the support of the future strategies are identified as well.

Step 3: Action Plan

Illustrations: *Institutional Landscape of the Partners from the Public and Private Sectors (future situation)*

We described the Situation Analysis in 1997, and the one predicted using the Strategic Planning of 1999, and projected institutional responses in a hypothetical planned scenario in 2000-2001. In addition, we distinguished the institutions involved in Preventive Strategies and those involved in Care and Support. The various scenarios were presented and discussed[136] in an overhead presentation (Appendix 5I), and are illustrated next.[137]

---

[136] UNAIDS Country Team Workshop, Gaoua, Burkina Faso, March 1999: the present researcher prepared the slide presentation. The presentation was made by the Country Broker who was present at the workshop
[137] "Public Sector" is the ministries, and the "Private Sector" encompass all other sectors, voluntary, for profit and not for profit, including NGOs, churches, CBOs

Planning and Consensus Synthesis Matrix by Objectives and Inputs
The Action Plan answers the question: *"how do we get there?"* In a follow-up workshop, for example, the partners develop a common global vision of the HIV/Aids activities in terms of the vulnerable groups to target and their needs. The main objectives to support that vision need to be outlined. Detailed strategies for each objective are spelt out. The partners' roles in relation to each of the strategies are defined based on their strengths and limitations. The action plan with priorities and calendar of implementation can be either developed immediately in the workshop, if time allows, or following the workshop with a special working group representing the various partners.

As an option again, the various parties may use the opportunity of the workshop to decide in consensus on means to strengthen the inter-linkages between partners, and mechanisms between the three key systems, i.e. communities and the private and the public sectors.

As described in details previously (chap. 4), in 1997, the general Situation Analysis (Fig. 5.2) documented in the Public Sector the involvement of the MOH and the Radio/ Communication Department, with some involvement of the political structures and the Ministry of Education, and 5 Ministries are potential actors. In the voluntary sector, 5 partners quite active, and 2 less active (PROMACO/SMC & Youth Associations). Large untapped sources remained among the private organisations (communities, Churches, NGOs).

Fig. 5.2

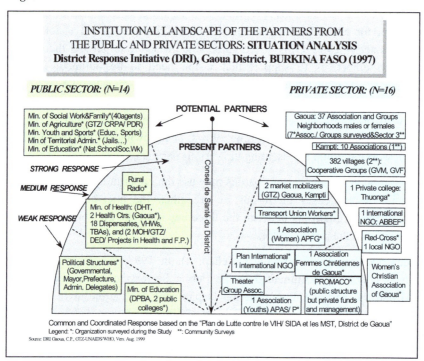

INSTITUTIONAL LANDSCAPE OF THE PARTNERS FROM
THE PUBLIC AND PRIVATE SECTORS: **SITUATION ANALYSIS**
District Response Initiative (DRI), Gaoua District, BURKINA FASO (1997)

PUBLIC SECTOR: (N=14) *PRIVATE SECTOR: (N=16)*

POTENTIAL PARTNERS

Min. of Social Work&Family*(40agents)
Min. of Agriculture* (GTZ/ CRPA/ PDR)
Min. Youth and Sports* (Educ., Sports)
Min of Territorial Admin.* (Jails...)
Min. of Education* (Nat.SchoolSoc.Wk)

PRESENT PARTNERS

Gaoua: 37 Association and Groups
Neighborhoods males or females
(7*Assoc./ Groups surveyed&Sector 3**)

Kampti: 10 Associations (1**)

382 villages (2**):
Cooperative Groups (GVM, GVF)

STRONG RESPONSE

Rural Radio*

MEDIUM RESPONSE

2 market mobilizers
(GTZ) Gaoua, Kampti

1 Private college:
Thuonga*

WEAK RESPONSE

Min. of Health: (DHT,
2 Health Ctrs. (Gaoua*),
18 Dispensaries, VHWs,
TBAs), and (2 MOH/GTZ/
DED/ Projects in Health and F.P.)

Transport Union Workers*

1 international
NGO: ABBEF*

1 Association
(Women) APFG*

Red-Cross*
1 local NGO

Plan International*
1 international NGO

1 Association
Femmes Chrétiennes
de Gaoua*

Women's
Christian
Association
of Gaoua*

Political Structures*
(Governmental,
Mayor,Prefecture,
Admin. Delegates)

Min. of Education
(DPBA, 2 public
colleges*)

Theater
Group Assoc.

PROMACO*
(public structure
but private funds
and management)

1 Association
(Youths) APAS/ P*

Conseil de Santé du District

Common and Coordinated Response based on the "Plan de Lutte contre le VIH/ SIDA et les MST, District de Gaoua"
Legend: *: Organization surveyed during the Study **: Community Surveys
Source: DRI Gaoua, C.P., GTZ-UNAIDS/WHO, Vers. Aug. 1999

As illustrated next, another useful dimension and analysis of the landscape allow to detect that the bulk of organisations active intervened in prevention strategies (Fig. 5.3) . In contrast, for the care and support strategies (Fig. 5.4), those were largely left out with the MOH active only, and one large NGO (Plan International Burkinabé), but in a limited geographical area (ref. chap. 4).

Fig. 5.3

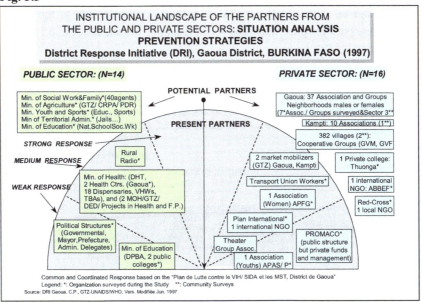

INSTITUTIONAL LANDSCAPE OF THE PARTNERS FROM
THE PUBLIC AND PRIVATE SECTORS: **SITUATION ANALYSIS**
PREVENTION STRATEGIES
District Response Initiative (DRI), Gaoua District, BURKINA FASO (1997)

PUBLIC SECTOR: (N=14)   *PRIVATE SECTOR: (N=16)*

POTENTIAL PARTNERS

Min. of Social Work&Family*(40agents)
Min. of Agriculture* (GTZ/ CRPA/ PDR)
Min. Youth and Sports* (Educ., Sports)
Min of Territorial Admin.* (Jails…)
Min. of Education* (Nat.SchoolSoc.Wk)

Gaoua: 37 Association and Groups
Neighborhoods males or females
(7*Assoc./ Groups surveyed&Sector 3**

PRESENT PARTNERS

Kampti: 10 Associations (1**):

382 villages (2**):
Cooperative Groups (GVM, GVF)

STRONG RESPONSE

Rural Radio*

MEDIUM RESPONSE

2 market mobilizers
(GTZ) Gaoua, Kampti

1 Private college:
Thuonga*

WEAK RESPONSE

Min. of Health: (DHT,
2 Health Ctrs. (Gaoua*),
18 Dispensaries, VHWs,
TBAs), and (2 MOH/GTZ/
DED/ Projects in Health and F.P.)

Transport Union Workers*

1 international
NGO: ABBEF*

1 Association
(Women) APFG*

Red-Cross*
1 local NGO

Political Structures*
(Governmental,
Mayor,Prefecture,
Admin. Delegates)

Plan International*
1 international NGO

Min. of Education
(DPBA, 2 public
colleges*)

Theater
Group Assoc.

1 Association
(Youths) APAS/ P*

PROMACO*
(public structure
but private funds
and management)

Common and Coordinated Response based on the "Plan de Lutte contre le VIH/ SIDA et les MST, District de Gaoua"
Legend: *: Organization surveyed during the Study   **: Community Surveys
Source: DRI Gaoua, C.P., GTZ-UNAIDS/WHO, Vers. Modifiée Jun. 1997

Fig. 5.4

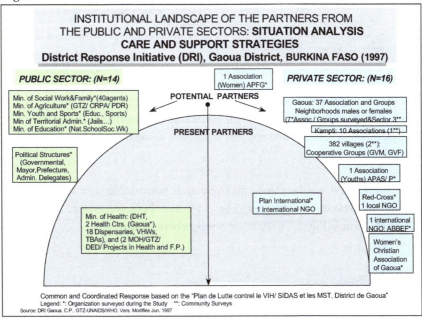

INSTITUTIONAL LANDSCAPE OF THE PARTNERS FROM
THE PUBLIC AND PRIVATE SECTORS: **SITUATION ANALYSIS**
CARE AND SUPPORT STRATEGIES
District Response Initiative (DRI), Gaoua District, BURKINA FASO (1997)

PUBLIC SECTOR: (N=14)

1 Association
(Women) APFG*

PRIVATE SECTOR: (N=16)

POTENTIAL PARTNERS

Min. of Social Work&Family*(40agents)
Min. of Agriculture* (GTZ/ CRPA/ PDR)
Min. Youth and Sports* (Educ., Sports)
Min of Territorial Admin.* (Jails…)
Min. of Education* (Nat.SchoolSoc.Wk)

Gaoua: 37 Association and Groups
Neighborhoods males or females
(7*Assoc./ Groups surveyed&Sector 3**

PRESENT PARTNERS

Kampti: 10 Associations (1**)

382 villages (2**):
Cooperative Groups (GVM, GVF)

Political Structures*
(Governmental,
Mayor,Prefecture,
Admin. Delegates)

1 Association
(Youths) APAS/ P*

Plan International*
1 international NGO

Red-Cross*
1 local NGO

Min. of Health: (DHT,
2 Health Ctrs. (Gaoua*),
18 Dispensaries, VHWs,
TBAs), and (2 MOH/GTZ/
DED/ Projects in Health and F.P.)

1 international
NGO: ABBEF*

Women's
Christian
Association
of Gaoua*

Common and Coordinated Response based on the "Plan de Lutte contrel le VIH/ SIDAS et les MST, District de Gaoua"
Legend: *: Organization surveyed during the Study   **: Community Surveys
Source: DRI Gaoua, C.P., GTZ-UNAIDS/WHO, Vers. Modifiée Jun. 1997

Two years later, in 1999, the Strategic Planning (Fig. 5.5) aimed to have in the Public Sector all new partners or 5 new partners involved, and in the Private Sector 4 new partners plus numerous Associations in Gaoua and Kampti towns.

Fig. 5.5

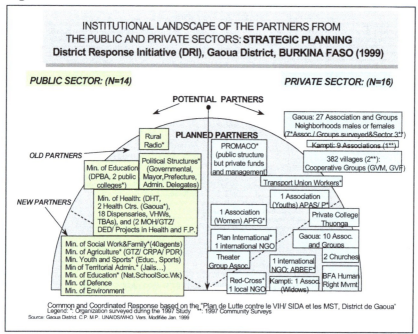

In 1999, the Strategic Planning aims to have in the Public Sector 7 new partners involved (4 in preventive strategies, and 3 in care and support). In the Private Sector, 8 new partners are involved, including Associations (18 in preventive strategies, and 16 in care and support strategies, some of them involved in both strategies).

As illustrated next, a substantial improvement is now visible with 4 new partners involved in preventive strategies (Fig. 5.6), and 11 new partners in care and support strategies (Fig. 5.7), some involved in both strategies.

Fig. 5.6

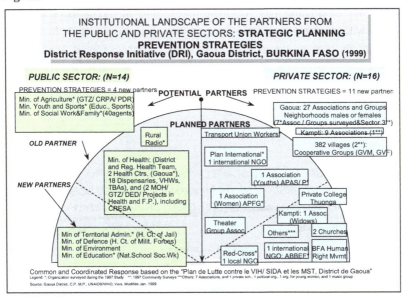

INSTITUTIONAL LANDSCAPE OF THE PARTNERS FROM
THE PUBLIC AND PRIVATE SECTORS: **STRATEGIC PLANNING**
PREVENTION STRATEGIES
District Response Initiative (DRI), Gaoua District, BURKINA FASO (1999)

PUBLIC SECTOR: (N=14)   *PRIVATE SECTOR: (N=16)*

PREVENTION STRATEGIES = 4 new partners POTENTIAL PARTNERS   PREVENTION STRATEGIES = 11 new partner

Min. of Agriculture* (GTZ/ CRPA/ PDR)
Min. Youth and Sports* (Educ., Sports)
Min. of Social Work&Family*(40agents)

Gaoua: 27 Associations and Groups
Neighborhoods males or females
(7*Assoc./ Groups surveyed&Sector 3*)

PLANNED PARTNERS

Kampti: 9 Associations (1**)

OLD PARTNER

Rural
Radio*

Transport Union Workers*

382 villages (2**):
Cooperative Groups (GVM, GVF)

Plan International*
1 international NGO

Min. of Health: (District
and Reg. Health Team,
2 Health Ctrs. (Gaoua*),
18 Dispensaries, VHWs,
TBAs), and (2 MOH/
GTZ/ DED/ Projects in
Health and F.P.), including
CRESA

1 Association
(Youths) APAS/ P*

NEW PARTNERS

1 Association
(Women) APFG*

Private College
Thuonga

Kampti: 1 Assoc
(Widows)

Theater
Group Assoc

Others***

2 Churches

Min. of Territorial Admin.* (H. Ct. of Jail)
Min. of Defence (H. Ct. of Milit. Forces)
Min. of Environment
Min. of Education* (Nat.School Soc.Wk)

Red-Cross*
1 local NGO

1 international
NGO: ABBEF

BFA Human
Right Mvmt

Common and Coordinated Response based on the "Plan de Lutte contre le VIH/ SIDA et les MST, District de Gaoua"
Legend: *: Organization surveyed during the 1997 Study   **: 1997 Community Surveys ***Others: 7 Associations, and 1 private sch., 1 political org., 1 org. for young women, and 1 music group
Source: Gaoua District, C.P. M.P., UNAIDS/WHO, Vers. Modifiée Jan. 1999

Fig. 5.7

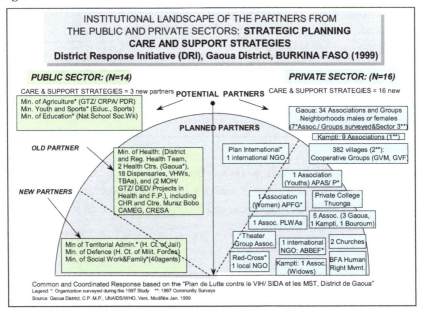

INSTITUTIONAL LANDSCAPE OF THE PARTNERS FROM
THE PUBLIC AND PRIVATE SECTORS: **STRATEGIC PLANNING**
CARE AND SUPPORT STRATEGIES
District Response Initiative (DRI), Gaoua District, BURKINA FASO (1999)

PUBLIC SECTOR: (N=14)   *PRIVATE SECTOR: (N=16)*

CARE & SUPPORT STRATEGIES = 3 new partners POTENTIAL PARTNERS   CARE & SUPPORT STRATEGIES = 16 new

Min. of Agriculture* (GTZ/ CRPA/ PDR)
Min. Youth and Sports* (Educ., Sports)
Min. of Education* (Nat.School Soc.Wk)

Gaoua: 34 Associations and Groups
Neighborhoods males or females
(7*Assoc./ Groups surveyed&Sector 3**)

PLANNED PARTNERS

Kampti: 9 Associations (1**)

OLD PARTNER

Min. of Health: (District
and Reg. Health Team,
2 Health Ctrs. (Gaoua*),
18 Dispensaries, VHWs,
TBAs), and (2 MOH/
GTZ/ DED/ Projects in
Health and F.P.), including
CHR and Ctre. Muraz Bobo
CAMEG, CRESA

Plan International*
1 international NGO

382 villages (2**):
Cooperative Groups (GVM, GVF)

1 Association
(Youths) APAS/ P*

NEW PARTNERS

1 Association
(Women) APFG*

Private College
Thuonga

5 Assoc. (3 Gaoua,
1 Kampti, 1 Bouroum)

1 Assoc. PLWAs

Theater
Group Assoc.

1 international
NGO: ABBEF

2 Churches

Min. of Territorial Admin.* (H. Ct. of Jail)
Min. of Defence (H. Ct. of Milit. Forces)
Min. of Social Work&Family*(40agents)

Red-Cross*
1 local NGO

Kampti: 1 Assoc.
(Widows)

BFA Human
Right Mvmt.

Common and Coordinated Response based on the "Plan de Lutte contre le VIH/ SIDA et les MST, District de Gaoua"
Legend: *: Organization surveyed during the 1997 Study   **: 1997 Community Surveys
Source: Gaoua District, C.P. M.P., UNAIDS/WHO, Vers. Modifiée Jan. 1999

315

Ultimately, the planned scenario for Years 2000-2001 (Fig. 5.8) in a situation of Monitoring and Evaluation may document that among the old partners, those are responding with a strong or a medium responses given their means. In turn, the new partners are responding, at least, with weak responses (are at least active). Finally, there is now within five years of the original baseline, a new balance between preventive and care and support strategies, meeting the original needs collected in the Situation Analysis at the community level (chap. 4).

Fig. 5.8

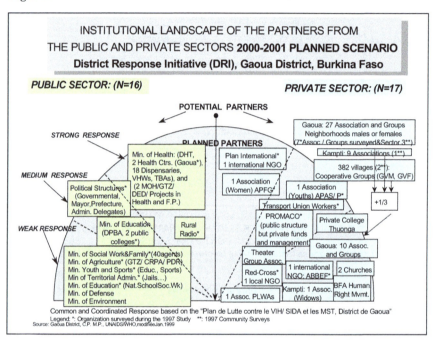

Strategic Planning documents in Gaoua District (Lamboray and M'Pele 1999). We recommend using new units of analysis, i.e. organisations and institutions as markers of the HIV/Aids Responses, and incorporating those as standard output indicators of HIV/Aids programs.

5.1.7 On the Applications and Limitations: the Case of Migrants as a Specific Vulnerable Group

Despite the above mentioned existing tools, and their developments, the application and limitation of those can be better comprehended looking at the case of migrants as a specific vulnerable group addressed by the Local Responses (Pervilhac and Kielmann 1999).[138]

HIV and Migration in West Africa

The origins of migration in West Africa can be traced back to medieval times when an extensive network of trade routes connected the region to the Mediterranean and Middle East (Davidson 1968). The slave trade and the conquest of the region by the Felani empire from the north and the European colonial armies from the south were the major determinants of population migration in the 18th and 19th century. In the early 20th Century, the European colonialists established their cocoa and sugar plantations on the coast of the Gulf of Guinea with forced labour from the Sahel, thereby laying the foundations for a migration pattern that persists until today.

Despite the many international borders established through European colonial geo-politics of the early 20th century, West Africa remains an economic and social unit in which people circulate freely while maintaining their ties to the region of origin for social or religious reasons (Lalou and Piché 1994). Almost all West African borders divide ethnic and linguistic groups, and residents of border regions move easily between countries. New social situations created through rapid urbanisation or migration are known to increase the vulnerability to HIV (Gilks, Floyd et al. 1998), and the association of migration with the spread of Aids in East, Central, and Southern Africa (the "Aids Belt") is well known (Brockerhoff and Biddlecom 1998).

Several studies (Brockerhoff 1995; Caldwell, Anarfi et al. 1997), including studies in agriculture (FAO 1997) (FAO 1997) (Baier 1997) have linked labour mobility to the spread of HIV in Africa due to new social environments inducing high risk sexual behaviors, and new sexual networks, with more recent similar findings in the West Africa sub-Region (Anarfi 1992) (Decosas, Kane et al. 1995) (French 1996) (Equipe du Burkina Faso 1998). The observed profile of the HIV epidemic in West Africa can to a large degree be explained by the pattern of circular migration between the cities and plantations along the Gulf of Guinea and the rural areas of the Sahel (Decosas 1998).

---

[138] This section is based on the draft of an article written with Joseph Decosas to be submitted for publication

Côte d'Ivoire is one the main poles of attraction for labour migrants in West Africa. The 1988 national census reported that 25 percent of the Ivoirian population was of foreign origin (FAO 1997), about half of them from Burkina Faso (Decosas 1998). About sixty percent of men from the arid Mossi Plateau west of Ouagadougou travel abroad to find work at least once in their life (Traore and Ouango 1994). Migrant workers in Côte d'Ivoire are predominantly male and come from rural areas. However, the proportion of women migrants is reported to be increasing steadily. At the origins of the migration behaviour is the short farming season and insufficient agricultural yield in the Sahel. The Sahelian farmers are thus forced to complement their incomes with additional revenues earned in the off-seasons in plantations, factories, or service jobs on the coast (FAO 1997). A pattern of long term migration taking place over several years is becoming increasingly more important, although the main pattern continues to be seasonal migration.

Thomas Painter recently evaluated twenty-one United States supported projects for Aids prevention among mobile populations in Sub-Saharan Africa (Painter 1998). The projects focused on the large and heterogeneous group of migrants represented by labor migrants, itinerant traders, migrant sex workers, mine workers, soldiers, long distance truckers, bus and boat conductors and crews, pastoralists, and refugees. The majority of the interventions targeted female sex workers and long-distance truck drivers. The vulnerability to HIV of these groups is well known and the groups are easy to identify. Only three interventions were conceived in a multi-country framework, and only one intervention targeted residents of border communities. This latter group deserves special attention because it represents a large proportion of the total migrant population, and it is relatively invisible, yet often socio-economically disadvantaged. International mobility among border populations is high, presumably translating into high vulnerability to HIV.

Despite the fact that Burkina Faso is one of the countries most severely affected by the HIV epidemic in West Africa, it receives relatively little international attention. At the 12th World AIDS Congress in Geneva in 1998, for example, 242 presentations documented different research projects and interventions in Uganda, whereas only 18 presentations documented those in Burkina Faso, none addressing the issue of migration.

HIV and AIDS related to Migration in Gaoua District

The importance of the migration factor is illustrated by the village of Banlo, one of the four communities.

Banlo has a population of about 1,000 of whom 200, particularly the youth, were working in Côte d'Ivoire at the time of the study. The push factors which determine the out-migration of young men from Banlo include poor harvests, poor soils, insufficient or irregular rainfalls, insufficient agricultural equipment, lack of storage and milling facilities for crops, lack of potable water, poor conditions of schools, lack of access to health care, and the need to raise money for the payment of dowry (Sanon 1997). We estimated that about one fourth of the population of Gaoua District, or 50,000 or more people experience a similar migration pattern as found in Banlo. The survival of these communities depends on seasonal or long-term migration of young people to Côte d'Ivoire and Ghana. The pull factors are the long term, more permanent, economic benefits and opportunities offered by the countries of destination. They have been described in detail in a recent economic theory of African rural-urban migration (Todaro 1997).

Through key informant interviews and group discussions, we ascertained the following determinants of vulnerability to HIV in these communities (4.1.2). The factors documented next are more related to the issue of migration and are grouped in three categories: behaviours and beliefs, weakness of services and programs, and social organisation and the societal impact of Aids.

Factors of vulnerability to HIV related to *behaviours and believes* reflect the fear of Aids and a lack of accurate information.

> *"AIDS is caused by men because there are some who come from Côte d'Ivoire with AIDS and negotiate with the girl once in the room, and refuse to use the condom."*
>
> (a young woman from Kampti)

Vulnerability factors related to *weaknesses of services and programs* in the study communities include poor access to and poor quality of condoms. Shopkeepers do not store condoms under appropriate conditions, and supplies break down. At the village level condoms are not available and the cost is too high for some youths, particularly when condoms are sold in packets of three rather than as a single unit. Services for information and treatment of STD are lacking but highly desired, and sources of information about Aids are not available in the villages. Previously, Aids information activities (theatre, market stalls, local conferences, and video showings) were conducted in Kampti and were highly appreciated but the program has been discontinued.

> *"We are at the border and many of our brothers are in Côte d'Ivoire, the country most hit in the region, and the bus comes every Friday from Abidjan. We need to have people do the test and help the sick people."* (a young man from Kampti)

The ascertained vulnerability factors related to *social organisation and the societal impact of HIV* include high mortality among the youth clustered in some neighbourhoods or villages and associated with return migration. The financial and labour costs of caring for Aids patients weigh heavily on their families, while the reduction of remittances by migrant workers and the loss of productivity by young people at home is showing an overall negative development impact on the villages. Social security for the elderly which was once assured through the labour of young people is failing; widows and young girls can no longer depend on the male migrants' remittances and have started to migrate to Côte d'Ivoire to find jobs; and the stigmatisation of returned migrants with Aids or suspected to be infected with HIV is tearing down the fabric of traditional village solidarity.

> *"Today girls are not serious. They can go to Gaoua to get their identity cards and leave to Côte d'Ivoire where they can get AIDS before coming back to get a spouse in their village."* (a young man from Banlo)
>
> *"It is particularly due to the girls. They think they are aware, do not listen to their parents and go to Côte d'Ivoire. As they are taken care of by men who have AIDS...*
>
> (a young men from Banlo)

Based upon the study findings, and the participants' knowledge of the local situation and priority needs, a consensus was reached on where to target interventions based on the identification and ranking of vulnerable groups. International migrants were ranked second as a specific vulnerable group after STD patients and followed by orphans, soldiers, truckers, prisoners, people living with Aids and sex workers. The issue of border migration emerged as one of the most important social factor of vulnerability to HIV, despite the fact it had not received much attention previously. The process of the study combined with the workshop was recognised as an important means to focus attention on programs targeting these border migrants.

Opportunities for the Responses to HIV and AIDS among Migrants

Border communities, especially out-migrating communities, like the villages and towns of Gaoua District are receiving relatively little attention in the national and international responses to Aids for a number of reasons related to: population issues, paradigmatic and epidemiological reasons, program conception and design, organisational and institutional issues, political and economic issues. These reasons and the opportunities they offer are detailed next.

Population issues

The international migration of border communities, particularly across the divisive borders of the post-colonial African states, follows historically established patterns of population movement. It may gradually increase in volume due to population pressures, drought, or unequal economic development, but in comparison to the dramatically visible movement of refugees it remains a largely silent phenomenon. The mobility of border migrants appears relatively organised and is of little concern to the countries of origin since these populations are not economically active at home; nor is it a priority in the countries of destination, because the individuals concerned are not country nationals. Border migrants thus tend to fall through the social safety nets in both their country of origin, and the one of destination.

Paradigmatic and epidemiological reasons

The understanding of HIV epidemics is largely based on epidemiological data derived from sentinel serological surveys. In many countries, the rather loose networks of national sentinel survey sites miss the important local epidemics in remote areas where most of the border migrants are found. Furthermore, the focus on numbers and rates precludes efforts to understand determinant factors of vulnerability to HIV which require information of a more qualitative nature. It is precisely this qualitative information which is needed to stimulate and design appropriate strategies for the reduction of vulnerability.

District strategies for the responses to Aids are largely based on the presumption that rural districts are inhabited by the "general" or a homogenous population. Interventions are therefore conceived within the very broad framework of "general population interventions" (Sumartojo, Carey et al. 1997) with little attention to specificity and targeting. Border districts such as Gaoua, however,

321

are part of a system of circulatory migration. They have specific needs related to the migration behaviour of their young population such as an increased need for young women to be able to negotiate safe sexual practices, or an increased focus on the promotion of condom use for extramarital sexual relationships. They would, in addition, benefit from targeted program support.

Prioritisation techniques that exist for the control of outbreaks such as Cholera and Meningitis are not applied for HIV programming, and mapping techniques (Long 1998) to identify and collect detailed information about communities and social networks are just being developed.

Program conception and design
Because targeted interventions may stigmatise some groups, national policies have tended to pursue general population interventions (Taverne 1996). Targeted interventions on a restricted scale (Sumartojo, Carey et al. 1997), on the other hand, have been a mainstay of HIV prevention for many years. Education materials, strategy manuals, and other tools have been developed for many different groups. Yet, very little has been developed specifically for migrants despite the fact that migrants have specific needs related to their cultural identity and level of literacy (Lalou and Piché 1994). Furthermore, wherever these materials exist, they are almost exclusively designed for migrants at their destination points. The important role of the communities of origin has not yet been explored from a programmatic perspective, and the necessary partnership with these communities is not yet part of the standard responses to Aids.

The communities themselves have many urgent and essential needs for survival which are at the basis of their dependence on out-migration. Lessons which were learned by the Primary Health Care movement on prioritisation through community participation have not yet been fully appreciated by the National AIDS Programs and their international supporters who tend to determine priorities at the international or national levels, and not at the community level. The challenge lies in establishing the relative priority of the responses to Aids in border communities such as those found in Gaoua District. The communities need to have ownership of the prioritisation process in order to establish a functional hierarchy of priorities.

Organisational and institutional issues

The fundamental and multi-faceted structural problems of poor and remote border communities and their chronic and largely silent adaptive responses of seasonal migration preclude short-term project aid as a viable support strategy. Sustainable assistance needs to be planned with a long horizon and a broad focus. This is generally very difficult for international aid agencies. Furthermore, the migration pattern itself, together with the high mortality from Aids (M'Boa, N'Dah et al. 1998), weakens local community organisations who could serve as partners for an intervention. Finally neither national governments nor international organisations working primarily in partnership with governments are well organised to address migrant communities on both sides of a border, at the origin and the destination of their migration. This, however, is one of the key requirements of an appropriate and effective program (Long 1998). International Non-Governmental Organisations generally have greater flexibility in this area.

Political and economic issues

The first and still the most prevalent responses to the issue of HIV and migration is deportation and the closure of borders (Decosas, Kane et al. 1995). The prevailing image is that of the migrant as a vector carrying disease. This charges the issue of HIV and migration with political explosives used by many different sources for their own means. The main public health discourse, the discussion of the factors that link the social phenomenon of migration to greater vulnerability to HIV, is often lost. There is an understandable hesitation by public health professionals to develop and expose the theme of migration through targeted programming, in order to avoid that it be captured and instrumentalised by political forces promoting xenophobia and racism.

The fora where inter-country health issues such as the issue of HIV and migration are discussed usually in international scientific meetings or regional consultative bodies without an executive capacity or role. Consensus on issues may be reached such as the inter-country meeting of Ministries (June 1997) on creating new cross-borders "solidarity" in West Africa to combat emerging diseases such as Meningitis, Cholera, and Aids. Agreements on program approaches may even be signed, but they rarely trickle down to the implementation level. Occasionally a functional executive inter-country program for a specific disease is established (e.g. Onchocerciasis), but in most cases the regional institutions are consultative and advisory and have little impact on actual program delivery.

African Governments are under enormous internal and international pressure to reform their health and social systems, and to increase the quality of social services while controlling costs. Cost versus benefit analysis rules the public social services. There is no issue which raises the question of "whose cost and whose benefit?" more blatantly than health and social programs for circulatory migrants. It can be argued that decreasing the vulnerability in the migrants' environment has benefits for all, but this argument is complex and politically inexpedient. Investing scarce public resources in services for a foreign population temporarily working in the country is difficult to defend politically, as would be the investment of resources in another country to provide services to their expatriate workers. International agencies are subjected to the same pressures because most donor agencies negotiate the use of their resources with the national Governments.

Burkina Faso has recently developed a new strategic plan (Lamboray and M'Pele 1999) using the UNAIDS planning tool (UNAIDS 1998) which includes a specific strategy to target programs for truckers as a vulnerable group. Future interventions may address interventions for the border migrants but the opportunities analysed previously need to be further exploited. Striving towards resolving the issues raised will contribute to prioritising strategies addressing the vulnerability of border migrants in Burkina Faso, and in sub-Sahara Africa. Effective and feasible interventions would already be possible in Gaoua District by concentrating efforts in and close to the communities with international migrants, such as: health promotion to youth before departing their communities through peer education, making condoms accessible and accepted, availability of outreach services and mobile counsellors, strengthening health services with quality STD services, facilitating HIV voluntary testing and counselling for returnees and their families. Further work is required locally to develop a more precise social profile of migrating communities. Internationally, the issue of border migration requires more attention by organisations capable of developing and implementing programs that span beyond and across borders. There is a need for institutional structures to address migrant workers' needs through interventions in their communities of origins, along the migration pathways, and at their destinations.

In conclusion to this section on the development of tools and their applications (5.1.5 to 5.1.7), we have documented the large potential but also the limitations of existing tools that can be used for the Local Responses. New ones, such as the Rapid Organisational Review (ROR), can be developed, or refined and further tested, for the Local Responses specific use at little additional cost. The large spectrum of issues and barriers documented for the case of border migrants as a vulnerable group show that the ultimate success of implementing an expanded responses may also lie in overcoming other barriers or constraints as well. This brings another dimension of complexity to succeed in the Local Responses approach in addition to the mere development of the ideal tool kit that we are presently striving for.

5.1.8 On the limitations of the study

The study has several overall limitations due to the nature of the study design, the limited implementation time and low coverage, the lack of epidemiological and behavioural evidence, an incomplete systems analysis, and the lack of a multi-country evidenced-based prevention study.

Study design

The present set-up of the study design of the local responses which follows the "pre-experimental design" before and after prospective intervention study described earlier is poor in comparison to the last two more valid and forceful potential designs of a true experimental design or a quasi-experimental design (3.2). In addition the "X" or interventions (Fig. 1.1) are not carefully singled out and their direct effects cannot be monitored. The Local Responses in general has not yet received the attention it merits in terms of a careful and sound systems research design. It cannot compete with, and is little convincing to the scientific community, in comparison to the well-financed and better-designed research of the bio-medical field. for example, the well-designed study of the vaccine development field trials of the synthetic malaria vaccine SPf66 (Alonso and al. 1994; Alonso P. et al. 1994) in Tanzania,[139] a practical similar field-testing of vaccine. It contrasts to the present almost improvised form of field-testing of the HIV/Aids prevention in Burkina Faso (ref. last para. On *"Lack of multi-country evidenced-based prevention study"*).

There are current debates raised on "how to promote multidisciplinary research without 'biomedicalizing' prevention," acknowledging the value of "quasi-experimental, ethnographic, and other kinds of behavioural information and social research" (Auerbach 1998) to test highly active anti-retroviral therapy (HAART). Such discussion has not yet trickled over to the domain of systems

---

[139] the researcher coordinated the Ifakara research Centre in Tanzania where this biomedical trial took place at the time the trial

research in HIV/Aids prevention such as the present Local Responses experiment.

In a nutshell, the findings of the present Local Responses country case studies in general cannot yet either document carefully the impact of the interventions and their causal factors, or receive the attention they deserve in the scientific audiences (ref. poster session in Durban (M'Pele, Pervilhac et al. 2000)). As a consequence those, largely anecdotal for a strict scientist and conservative audience, can only and unfortunately for the time being be more taken at face value.

Limited implementation time, low coverage
The implementation time (half a year for Phase 3) was too short, with as a consequence a review too much based on processes, and insufficient time to evaluate outputs and outcomes, and to measure the sustainability of the approach.

The coverage was low (Gaoua and Kampti towns and approximately twenty communities) making essential recommendations for scaling-up still missing.

Lack of epidemiological and behavioural evidence

2nd generation surveillance for HIV combining behavioural data to validate the biological data collected (MAP (Monitoring the AIDS Pandemic Network) 2000) have not yet reached Gaoua District. Behavioural surveillance was never set up, and the impact of the Local Responses on a reduction of HIV prevalence, based on the sero-prevalence surveillance, may only be visible in five to ten years from now.

Research priorities for the Future (5.2.3) need to address those in order to validate further this study, and replicate such a model for other Local Responses study trials.

Incomplete systems analysis
For the sake of the present study constrained by time, money and technical inputs, the present research was limited to HIV/AIDS in Reproductive Health, excluding other Sexually Transmitted Infections (STI), or family planning components. In addition, the original "systems analysis" designed originally (1.3 and Fig. 1.3) could not be fully comprehended and answer the essential

question: which part(s) of the system is or are essential in influencing the outputs and having an impact on the outcome?

Lack of a multi-country evidenced-based prevention study
Although the Local Responses, or District expanded Response Initiative, was originally designed to encompass three districts in each of the five countries, the countries met and discussed only once in the preliminary stages of the study for the original situation analyses (Appendix 1 A, May 1998: Technical Workshop, UNAIDS/WHO the multi-country study teams). No lessons were learned systematically based on the compared experiences of how to move into the planning at the local level, nor to prioritise, nor to implement on a small and large scale within a District, or within a country. Is the approach similar in high and low prevalence areas? We are still hard press to prove scientifically that Local Responses are part of a larger valid way to go to implement effective local responses. The positive results of the Gaoua case study may originate from its unique experience, and cannot unfortunately be substantiated by any other several multi-country evidence-based prevention studies.

5.1.9 On the Overall Results and Hypotheses

The present research documents the early stages of an innovative approach called the *Local Responses to HIV/Aids* to stimulate HIV/Aids activities in a rural district of Africa with a high epidemic of HIV/Aids, and measure its early outcomes (4.4).

Based on the above four objectives, the present operations research was broken down into **three hypotheses** (ref. chap. 1) which were tested in different Phases (chap. 1, Fig. 1.3). We highlight the essential findings and limitations for each, for the purpose of replicating the approach in other contexts. Further research priorities are highlighted separately in the Conclusions (next section 5.2)

- **First (phase 1), the feasibility of using a systems approach to analyse the situation at a local level (district and communities)**
We documented in the situation analyses carried out at the community level the essential determinants of the epidemic at the community level (4.1), and at the district level (4.2), and the different existing partners' inputs, and potential ones, from the public and voluntary sectors. A rapid appraisal method has been developed and applied to assist district and communities in determining their options for approaches to meeting social and development challenges of the

HIV/Aids epidemics at the District level, giving evidence that tools and techniques are available.

However, the earlier tool used was largely focused on prevention aspects. One year later a complementary study of three weeks (supported by UNAIDS) highlighted other aspects related to care and counselling. The fact the epidemic is already high may have facilitated the mobilisation of partners. The development of a simple comprehensive rapid assessment participatory method to capture the full spectrum of prevention to care and counselling, and policies, and which can be used by the local partners in the district, merits further development and research. In addition, the approach needs still to be tested in other settings with a lower prevalence of HIV.

- **Second (phase 2), the possibility, based on the findings of the situation analysis, to design and stimulate well tailored priority interventions**

Based on the aforementioned situation analyses, essential strategies and priority activities to respond to the HIV/Aids epidemics could be designed and stimulated in a planning process (4.3).

The strategic planning approach used by UNAIDS has shown its limitations in terms the complexity and length of the approach, the need for an outside expert to carefully drive the local team through the process (5.1.4). The further development of a simple planning framework for local applications may also be a future challenge and merits further development and research too.

- **Third (phase 3), to give evidence that as a consequence, a number of activities can be implemented successfully over a short period of time by taking stock of the existing and potential partners**

Following the planning exercise, within less than one year, several priority activities have already taken place to set the ground of Local Responses (4.4), even if it is too early to detect any direct impact such as a decrease in the incidence or prevalence of HIV.

"Changing organizational behavior is a harder, more time-consuming, and slower process and requires more scarcely available skills than changing individual attitudes, even among group of individuals" (Vladeck 1993).

Despite the known difficulties, and using these activities as proxy indicators of organisational changes, the findings of the Local Responses give strong evidence that local organisations can be within a short time period mobilised and involved in HIV/Aids.

Yet, the process was largely supported by the external country broker's inputs and the original enthusiasm of a new project bringing in extra funding. In addition, it remains to be seen what will be the more specific outcomes and impact of the different interventions in the communities in general, as well as on specific groups (e.g. the many barriers to overcome in order for migrants to respond to HIV/Aids). The nature and long term results of a locally owned and sustainable process cannot yet be assessed. A three to five year follow-up will allow to evaluate these essential questions to validate further the added-value of the Local Responses approach.

In conclusion, in addition to taking into consideration the limitations of the study which still need to be overcome (5.1.8), much research is still needed to ground further the Local Responses (next section 5.2). Yet, the recent UNAIDS Press Release (ref. following abstract) of the International AIDS Conference (Durban, July 2000), is a solid convincing argument validating the present approach used to stimulate the HIV/Aids with three different country examples, including Gaoua District, Burkina Faso. It summarises in a nutshell the concepts and achievements of the Local Responses agenda which has improved tremendously and become more focused over the past two years.

> **"People, not technology, drive AIDS responses**
>
> *Local partnerships on ideas for dealing with HIV/AIDS, practices and sharing effective approaches may be the key to scaling-up what we know works to slow down the spread of HIV and minimise the impact of the pandemic.*
>
> *During the opening day of the conference several countries shared their experiences and agreed on these conclusions:*
>
> *It is people who drive the response to AIDS. Technology and information facilitate, but do not substitute for people-driven responses.*
>
> *In an increasing number of countries, real progress is being made because communities acknowledge that HIV/AIDS is affecting everyone.*
>
> *As a result, they are developing local partnerships that enable them to effectively deal with the pandemic and its consequences.*
>
> *United in local partnerships, people are gradually building societies that live positively with AIDS.*
>
> *Improvements in quality of life, the acceptance of People Living with AIDS (PLWA) in communities and the participation of groups of PLWA in activities can all be seen as indicators of the success of local responses.*
>
> *To achieve this the AIDS community needs to change its mindset. We need to put ourselves in a learning, rather than a teaching mode.*

The Local Responses may become in the near future the basis of a well-known approach for a successful control of the HIV/Aids epidemic in the Africa region in the XXI century.

5.2 Conclusions

This three years action-research study (1.1) leads to many more questions than answers. To move the Local Responses approach beyond a mere fad, into a visible, credible, feasible, replicable and sustainable program, much research remains to be done addressing methodological (5.2.1) and policy (5.2.2) issues, and research priorities (5.2.3) as well, which we review next as conclusions.

5.2.1 Methodology Conclusions

Based on a recent "**UNAIDS Technical Meeting on the Facilitation of Local Responses: Training and Methodology Development**" (Bulawayo, Zimbabwe, Nov. 22-25 1999, in C. Pervilhac, 3.12.1999) several practical answers for a phased-approach to the Local Responses were formulated. This meeting can be seen an important technical benchmark of the Local Responses initiative which started three years ago, and described in the present research work in more details for the case study of Burkina Faso from early 1997 to mid-2000 (Appendix 1 A Chronological Benchmarks).

The findings of this meeting can be summarised in the following five key points. Those highlight the overall status of development of the Local Responses and the limitations of the approach still.

First, in less than three years the Local Responses have expanded geographically as documented with the ten countries presently involved, and several countries which are already replicating the approach in different districts. There is strong evidence that the Local Responses process which started in different countries, has in turn stimulated many districts to be proactive in Aids, whereas originally they were barely addressing HIV/Aids as an issue, as documented in the present case study of Gaoua (4.5). In addition, the launching of the 'International Partnership against AIDS in Africa is setting a positive environment for such initiative with a vision that within five years, African nations will be implementing large scale, sustained and effective national responses to HIV and Aids. The partnership aims to mobilise vastly more resources with and for the African countries together with seven UNAIDS cosponsors and secretariat, bilateral development agencies (including GTZ), Non-Governmental Organisations (NGOs), and the private sector. A larger mobilisation of the public, and voluntary and private sectors, is at the heart of the Local Responses as documented in this research (chap. 4).

Second, within the same limited time span, both the concepts and values of the Local Responses, and mechanisms to implement the scheme have been clarified. One of the key concept to stimulate and have an Aids competent society is to listen and involve all stakeholders, from individuals to Ministries, via different sectors, to make them competent to participate to the responses. The agreed denomination of the "Local Responses" supports the nature of the responses at a "local level", i.e. sub-district (vs. the "District responses"), and not of an administrative nature (vs. the "Government responses"). A number of basic steps, recently documented under the form of a *Technical Note* (Appendix 1 B), have been identified to facilitate the process which can be implemented sequentially or in parallel, and in different order than listed next:

- Appointment of a national facilitator of local learning ("the country broker")
- Establishment of Local Responses support teams of local learning
- Situation/ responses analysis
- Identification of key social groups
- Common vision of all partners
- Definition of institutional relationships and determining the Local Responses structures
- Planning
- Development of local partnerships
- Mobilisation of resources and implementation
- Monitoring and evaluation
- Learning from action.

Third, the Local Responses need to grow from a mere approach to become a more marketable approach, or a full-fledged strategy, but the nature of the process often precludes clear goals and hard objectives (e.g. how to measure health reforms? How to measure changes in community participation to HIV/Aids?). Such limitations need to be quickly addressed for international partners to buy the product.

Fourth, at this stage, we are at the cross-road of the development of the Local Responses with a number of questions which remain to be answered. Following this research, in my opinion, the answers to those may be the following:

- Should we move the Local Responses along with more control or with the facilitation of the process only? – Yes, Local Responses need to be further nurtured with more control. This can be explained because one cannot hope the communities can act and react on their own initiatives, particularly in the case of heterosexual transmission in Africa, in comparison to the some of the original vulnerable groups found in Europe, e.g. homosexuals or Intra-Venous Drug Users (IVDUs). In addition, in the African context, other scourges and priorities, combined with scarce resources, generally do not allow local communities to organise themselves on their own against HIV/Aids, or to perceive the epidemic as a priority.
- Is it a movement or a program? – It is both a movement and a program. It is a movement, or an approach, because by nature as we explained earlier (section 1.2.1) we found the Local Responses is the forgotten PHC concept

adapted to the reality of HIV/Aids. In complement, it is a program because its final goals are the reduction of HIV/Aids prevalence both among the general population and some vulnerable groups, with objectives and priorities going beyond the mere statements of classical indicators of interventions. The program avoids to be caught up in a constraining "project" cycle and allows with the existing flexibility to have any partner or communities join into the effort any time.

- How should the country/ district selection or participation process be dealt with? The original generic "District Responses Initiative Protocol for Field Assessments and District Case studies" (UNAIDS January 1997) proposed approaches focusing more on generalised epidemic approaches, and selecting three districts per country. Based on the past three years, districts at any stage of the epidemic, generalised, concentrated, or nascent may join the Local Responses with different strategies tailored for the circumstance. It is well known that locations with a nascent epidemic need to promote early on already prevention strategies. Furthermore, the Local Responses wishes not to embark on similar negative past experiences of investing in expensive pilot studies that have no chance of being sustained, replicated, or expanded. It is foreseen that the urgency of setting Local Responses, at any stage of the epidemic and anywhere, leaves a chance to any partner to join in the effort.

- What are the teaching or learning processes involved? The experiences documented up to now show that thanks to the national Aids theme groups that the Local Responses experiences are known and being shared within countries. The whole process is now challenged on how to institutionalise the teaching and learning process both nationally and internationally (next para.).

Fifth, the technical meeting identified a number of solutions to formalise the Local Responses, and legitimise the approach:

- involving and supporting more sub-regional experiences (UNAIDS regional offices, SADEC…),
- documenting case studies, diffusing information via videos, and sharing the state-of-the-art and papers related to different steps of the process, and spreading best practices,
- facilitating the sharing of successful experiences between countries, and learning from others in-countries and through site tours, and involve training organisations, particularly with open walls,
- mobilising resources,

- monitoring the process,[140]
- spreading information through Conferences (Satellite meeting of the 13th World AIDS Conference in Durban on the subject).

1) Research design and documentation of the process

Carefully designed action research (ref. chap. 3) has not yet permeated systems research, at least for the Local Responses to HIV/Aids, in comparison to any bio-medical research, e.g. AIDS vaccine trials. The crossover design already documented in a recent quasi-experimental design of an education program would have the advantage of intervening in an index site, and later, given the ethical aspects, a replication (control) site (expanding the response) receives the intervention at a latter stage (Skinner, Arfken et al. 2000). The findings of the Bulawayo technical meeting, just mentioned, overlooked this aspect. As a consequence, the present research design and presentation of findings for Burkina Faso, building on carefully designed systems research, remain an exception rather than a rule, despite the intention in the original protocol to do so (UNAIDS 1996). As a consequence, three years into the process, the findings are still soft, too anecdotal, and not sufficiently convincing to the broader scientific community. At least, efforts are being made in year 2000-on to have the processes documented carefully. Our study shows the added value to ground the Local Responses findings on a scientific quasi-experimental research design, even if it is not the most powerful one. Well-designed community studies, such as a cross-sectional design with repeated sampling over time in matched intervention and comparison communities, seem to be the luxury of industrial countries, and have been recently carried out for HIV/Aids (The CDC AIDS Community Demonstration Projects Research Group 1999) (Lauby, Smith et al. 2000). More financial resources for Local Responses may allow such developments in the near future, or pairing up with projects funded for this purpose (e.g. USAID funded "*Measure*" project)

2) Situation analysis at the community level

A thorough understanding of the community is at the heart of any situation analysis for the Local Responses as documented in the original systems Model (chap. 1, Fig. 1.4), and to plan and build the bottom-up approach through an improved understanding of their determinants and their structures. The study at the community level (chap. 4) using some of the latest qualitative methods

---

[140] UNAIDS Technical Meeting on Measuring Progress of Local Responses, Mwanza, Tanzania, 5-7 June 2000, and "How do communities measure progress on Local Responses to HIV/AIDS" (Technical Note 3, Aug. 2000)

brings forth data that could not have been collected ten years ago. Post-facto, we think that the present gap of interventions addressing vulnerable groups (5.1.7) can and should be overcome by focusing on those identified in the original situation analysis as well (e.g. migrants, truck drivers).

3) Situation analysis at the district level and the Rapid Organisational Review (R.O.R.)

The study revealed the wealth of existing and potential partners existing at a local level, namely at the district level and their communities, using an innovative sociological method, the Rapid Organisational Review (ROR) tool we designed for the circumstance. Organisations are often synonymous to bureaucracies, in the narrow definition of the theories of Max Weber. We adapted a broad definition of organisations as both formal and informal organised structures or groups, e.g. community-based organisations to Non-Governmental Organisations (NGOs). Much attention has been paid over the years to the individual responses. Yet, an understanding of the institutional or organisational responses lacks using those as a unit of analysis (ref. Susser's "eco-epidemiology" in 3.2), and working with directly with organisations, without understanding them fully, is often the standard way to operate. As a consequence, the institutions at a local level have been largely left out of the process and can explain as a major contributing factor inefficient responses as we documented in the situation analyses at the community and district levels (chap. 4). The present inventory and task sharing of the partners from the public and voluntary sectors, combined with the improved understanding and agreement of their roles towards a common vision, foster more effective Local Responses (4.4 and 4.5) which we hope will be sustainable too.

4) Combination of different approaches

The complex problem calling for different solutions explains why different approaches are necessary to understand and respond to the HIV/Aids epidemic at the local level. The present research had too high ambitions with limited means and time (chap. 3), and focused in the end on anthropological and sociological approaches only. Yet, epidemiological, policy, and economics approaches are necessary to have a full picture of the environment in which the virus proliferates. The Local Responses would benefit from the expertise of different specialists working in the same geographical location together to tackle the responses from different angles. This in turn would help contribute to the design of responses that may be better replicated or adapted in different geographical areas of a national context.

5.2.2 International Policy Conclusions

1) HIV/Aids Local Responses as the HIV prevention and Aids mitigation vaccine

HIV/Aids Local Responses approach outlined in the present research must be accepted by all institutions in a united front. Presently, not all agencies, including within UNAIDS, are behind the approach, mainly because of the lack of documented success still.

Considering the aforementioned epidemiology and impact of HIV/Aids in the communities (chap. 1), and the search for more effective interventions, the Local Responses ought to be recognised as an innovative and leading strategy to prevent HIV and mitigate Aids. To this effect, it requires well funded and designed cross-country trials, just as vaccine trials or multi-drug therapies benefit from. The present development of the multi-preventive and mitigation responses in public health to combat HIV and Aids is part of the development of a systemic prevention vaccine (C. Pervilhac 1997). It needs to be considered as an important approach in public health, as the development of the vaccine to prevent Aids, or the multi-drug therapy to combat Aids, are in the bio-medical sciences. Despite this, it is not yet recognised as such but three years is still a short time to gain credibility in the public health field.

2) Focus at the local level

The focus at the local level is an essential and feasible ingredient of the responses to HIV/Aids. Burkina Faso illustrates the value of bottom-up approaches vs. other former top-down, or national to district, blueprint approaches. National strategic plans should be based on aggregated findings from district plans, and not the opposite. The situation analyses need to combine a balanced improved understanding of the determinants of HIV/Aids among the various communities, the different vulnerable groups, and the institutional partners from the public and voluntary sectors.

3) National and international support mechanisms and procedures
Efforts at the local level are sustainable and can be replicated only if the national level supports the Local Responses through support mechanisms and procedures. The experience of Burkina Faso has allowed such developments through an early and on-going information and participation of decision-makers from the national level to the local processes, either through the National AIDS Commission, or field visits and meetings. National policy can set guidelines for the country-specific Local Responses approach, but specific key national policy questions (ref. conclusion to 4.2.3) need to be addressed. We have illustrated with the "Cough Syrup Transport System" (1.1), the necessity to simplify the support mechanisms and procedures for what should be in a reality a relatively simple operation (the mere delivery of the syrup with the spoon).

The role of international agencies to support the local level mechanisms and procedures, for example through the important concept development and refinement, needs in turn to be defined taking the example of the recent UNAIDS inputs through the country broker in Burkina Faso and the Local Responses team in Geneva.

4) Country specific approaches
The recent findings of an inventory and review of HIV Prevention Policies in Europe (Weilandt, Pervilhac et al. 2000) document how European countries have either developed or adapted for their own country the HIV prevention strategies and interventions with the supportive policies. In Europe, some of the core strategies (e.g. condom distribution and use, clean and free syringes for IVDUs) are the same in appearance. The key to their success may lie in what is the best constellation or mix of those, and how have they been adapted to the different country cultures or sub-cultures. Similarly, for the countries in Africa, the Local Responses may need a core set of strategies, accompanied by similar individual flexibility for each country, with local managers confronted with the large set of choices illustrated by the coloured barrels presented earlier (Fig. 5.1). The combination of the ingredients to success is learning by doing, recognising and correcting errors, and exchanging within and between countries.

5.2.3 Research Priorities for the Future

The present research priorities have two main aims: first, to support the development of the methodologies necessary to strengthen (5.1.8 and 5.2.1 and 5.2.2), document and disseminate (para. 4.5) the Local Responses, and second, to combat the present scepticism that may deter organisations to join the approach. Some countries have already shown successful results in handling the epidemic (e.g. in Uganda the prevalence of HIV has decreased among the youth) but these trends were visible before the setting of the Local Responses. Nevertheless, in Uganda, like in Thailand, all the ingredients of the Local Responses could be found already before the present initiative that takes stock of past experiences.

At the recent XIII International AIDS Conference, P. Piot, Executive Director at UNAIDS, suggested two paths of research which can form the two prone research strategy for the Local Responses:

- *"Applied research: what works best in various contexts?*
- *"Basic research: what are the most effective tools and interventions?"*(Piot 2000)

1) Local Responses with improved study design and methodology
Despite the present study design, the Burkina Faso results based on the local partners' contribution may have been confounded by heavy technical inputs and additional financial support received (4.3.2). The necessity to address improved study design and the methodology of the Local Responses is compelling (5.2.1). In addition to processes and outputs, outcomes must be measured in addition (reduction in HIV prevalence accompanied by changes in behaviours). To validate the Local Responses biological markers need to go in pair with sexual behaviour markers and measure the outcomes. For this purpose, for example, a similar design than the recent findings of the "Triangulation of biological markers and quantitative and qualitative responses in sexual behaviour research with adolescents in rural Tanzania" (Plummer, Todd et al. 2000) could be adapted and tested widely using different tools and interventions. Standards need to be set as high for the development of this prevention vaccine as high as the ones in the bio-medical field.

Inter-country comparative Local Responses studies, funded by the E.U. or other international agencies, similar to the ones we carried out in Europe on HIV Prevention Policies (Weilandt, Pervilhac et al. 2000) could stimulate research specific areas. The support of country collaborators who know the country and have access to information is fairly simple and effective to document the work.

There is a need for an improved understanding of how to take the best advantage of the local capacities to support the process, and to determine the gaps. This will allow to identify what outside support is necessary for local ownership, sustainability and replicability purposes.

2) Cost-effectiveness

Apart from the overall worthiness of the approach, agencies do want to know how much the Local Responses costs, and whether it is cost effective in comparison to other approaches, for example more vertical approaches to HIV/Aids services delivery. Simple cost analysis methods can be set up to plan and monitor costs. Further research might focus on the cost effectiveness of the Local Responses in other districts than Gaoua in comparison to other more traditional classical strategies.

3) Links and effects between the Local Responses and the Health Sector Reform

The Local Responses takes advantage and at the same time stimulates the Health Sector Reform. Yet, the links between the two processes merit further study to understand how the Local Responses stimulates the Health Sector Reform, and in turn how much the Health Sector Reform facilitates the implementation of the Local Responses. In Burkina Faso, on one hand, the Local Responses has allowed the local Governments (Region and Districts) to play fully their roles in setting up the co-ordinating structures and participating to those, or in earmarking locally a budget line to HIV/Aids, for example. The Health Sector Reform, on the other hand, has permitted the local level to take full responsibility of the new HIV/Aids plans and activities, and to get the necessary support from national and international partners.

4) Refining the tool kit for the Local Responses

The Local Responses is no quick fix but a set of tools that can be used and applied depending of the local needs. Presently, there exists a mere incomplete inventory of those with applications on a small scale or experimental basis (5.1.5). Carefully documented research needs to test, document, and illustrate the experiences of the different tools used in each setting, coming from different sciences, and applications on a national scale. As an example to a local application, we described for Burkina Faso the situation analyses (chap. 4) at the community level of an anthropological nature, and district level of a sociological nature with for the latter the development of the Rapid Organisational Review

(ROR) tool (5.1.6). New tools, such as risk behaviour mapping (Nyonyo, Mayunga et al. 2000), are being now being shared to wider audiences.

5) Planning: determining and using the vulnerability determinants to identify priorities and selecting and improving responses

The rationale for planning is the selection of the best mix of strategies, or as illustrated earlier in the "Cough Transport System" (chap. 1), or what is the best syrup? The tools used are powerful enough to identify the different vulnerability determinants. Research needs to focus more, based on the vulnerability determinants, how to identify local priorities, or how to address and overcome negative factors, and how to take advantage of the positive ones, in order to select and design improved interventions.

In addition as part of priority setting, the mix share between interventions for general and vulnerable population needs to be determined which is another necessary area of research. In Burkina Faso, we noticed the difficulty to identify, and as a consequence to work with the vulnerable groups in the local environment when they are still stigmatised (ref. 5.1.7 with migrants). Countries of western and southern Europe, ironically, are struggling presently as well to find better paths to respond to the mobile populations' needs. In addition with stigmatisation, there is a parallel between Africa and the situation in Europe ten to fifteen years ago. In Africa, there is a wide and diffuse vision of how to go about responding to HIV/Aids linked to the nature of the problem due to the large heterosexual transmission of the virus. This may render the task of overcoming stigmatisation even more difficult than in Europe which has an epidemic largely concentrated in vulnerable groups transmission (e.g. homosexual, IVDUs).

Finally, if we discourage the use of strategic planning as a method to plan the Local Responses (5.1.4), research needs to test and select better options still.

6) Simplifying the supportive machinery for the Local Responses

As simple as the medication can be, i.e. the syrup in our original illustration of the "Cough Transport System" (chap. 1), the Local Responses carried out in Burkina Faso, and which we described in more details for the four different successive phases, is cumbersome and heavy. The supportive machinery for the Local Responses needs to be simplified in order to be more appealing to the local and international partners. Research needs to focus on how to simplify the process. A distinction should be drawn between the original efforts and trials in individual countries that are automatically more complex (time-consuming, costly, difficult) in the original Local Responses, and the next stages of dissemination which should be more straightforward.

7) Monitoring and selection of the best indicators
The Local Responses necessitates the monitoring of the process to take on-going corrective actions. In addition, to measure the effect of the Local Responses a set of best indicators needs to be identified. Different Local Responses efforts need to join efforts to select the best indicators to measure the Local Responses along the indicators classification (inputs, process, outputs, and outcome). In Burkina Faso, the recent review (4.4) and use of indicators to measure progress is a first attempt to do so. The last UNAIDS technical meeting (Mwanza, Tanzania, June 2000) on the subject shows the urgency to exchange the experiences on the measurement of the Local Responses and improving the monitoring of those.[141]

In conclusion, following these early stages of development over the past three years of what we identified as the HIV prevention and Aids mitigation vaccine development, the various research areas identified above show that much work remains to be accomplished for an international recognition and application of the Local Responses to HIV/Aids. Based on the recent rapid and positive developments of the approach reported and described in this study, I foresee a breakthrough of the Local Responses in the next five to ten years as a standard and effective approach to respond to the HIV/Aids epidemic and implement HIV/Aids activities in different parts of the world.

---

[141] the present researcher is presently producing a Technical Note no. 3 on the subject (expected publication in Aug. 2000)

References

Alonso, P. et. al. (1994). "Randomized trial of efficacy of SPf66 vaccine against P. falciparum malaria in children of southern Tanzania." Lancet **344**: 1175-1181.

Alonso P. et al. (1994). "A trial of SPf66, a synthetic malaria vaccine, in Kilombero (Tanzania). Rationale and Design." Vaccine **12**: 181-187.

Anarfi, J., Ed. (1992). Sexual Networking in Selected Communities in Ghana and the Sexual Behaviour of Ghanaian Female Migrants in Abidjan, Côte d'Ivoire. Sexual Behaviour and Networking: Anthropological and Socio-Cultural Studies on the Transmission of HIV. Liege, Derouaux-Ordina Editions.

Auerbach, J. D. (1998). Current Research on HIV Prevention and its Application for Effective and Sustainable Interventions. 2nd International Symposium on HIV Prevention, Geneva.

Baier, E. (1997). De l'impact du VIH/ SIDA sur les familles/ communautés rurales et de la nécessité de concevoir des stratégies multisectorielles en vue de prévenir la pandémie et d'en atténuer les effets dans les zones rurales (Orientation: Afrique). Rome, FAO.

Brockerhoff, M. (1995). "Fertility and Family Planning in African Cities: The Impact of Female Migration." Journal of Biosocial Science **27**: 347-358.

Brockerhoff, M. and A. Biddlecom (1998). Migration, Sexual Behavior, and HIV Diffusion in Kenya. New York, Population Council.

Brösskamp-Stone U. et al., "Institutionen, Systeme und Strukturen der Gesundheitsförderung und Prävention", in Schwartz, F. W., B. Badura, et al., Eds. (1998). Das Public Health Buch Gesundheit und Gesundheitswesen. München-Wien-Baltimore, Urban & Schwarzenberg.

Caldwell, J., J. Anarfi, et al., Eds. (1997). Mobility, Migration, Sex, STDs, and AIDS: An Essay on Sub-Saharan Africa with Other Parallels. Sexual Cultures and Migration in the Era of AIDS. New York, Oxford University Press.

Creese, A. and D. Parker, Eds. (1994). Cost analysis in primary health care A training manual for programme managers. Geneva, World Health Organization.

Davidson, B. (1968). Africa in History. New York, MacMillan Publishing Co., Inc.

D'Cruz-Grote, D. (1997). Prevention of sexual transmission of HIV/ STD in developing countries. Experiences and concepts. Eschborn, GTZ.

Decosas, J. (1998). Labour migration and HIV epidemics in Africa. 12th World AIDS Conference, Geneva, Merck & Co., Inc.

Decosas, J., F. Kane, et al. (1995). "Migration and AIDS." The Lancet **346**: 826-828.

Equipe du Burkina Faso (1998). Etude Régionale Migration Internationale Santé Sexuelle MST/SIDA couvrant le Burkina Faso, le Ghana et le Togo. Ouagadougou, Ministère de la Santé.

FAO (1997). Impact du VIH/SIDA sur les systèmes d'exploitations agricoles en Afrique de l'Ouest. Roma, FAO.

FAO (1997). Les populations rurales d'Afrique face au SIDA: un défi au développement (Synthèse des travaux de la FAO sur le SIDA). Rome, FAO.

French, H. (1996). Migrant Workers Take AIDS Risk Home to Niger. New York Times. New York: 3.

Gilks, C., K. Floyd, et al. (1998). Sexual Health and Health Care: Care and Support for People with HIV/ AIDS in Resource-Poor Settings. Liverpool, Department for International Development.

Hemrich G. et al. (1997). HIV/ AIDS as a cross-sectoral issue for Technical Cooperation. Eschborn, GTZ.

Kahrmann, C. (1997). "Survival in the Sahel Problems with Applying Participatory Methods." Development and Cooperation **5**: 22-24.

Kenis, P. and B. Marin (1997). Managing AIDS. Organizational Responses in six European Countries. Aldershot, Ashgate Publishing Company.

Lalou, R. and V. Piché (1994). Migration et SIDA en Afrique de l'Ouest. Un état des connaissances. Laval, Canada, Université de Laval.

Lamboray, J. L. and P. M'Pele (1999). Planification stratégique et réformes pour une Réponse élargie face au VIH/SIDA dans un district sanitaire Gaoua-Burkina Faso Documentation des processus et des résultats Rapport Intermédiaire. Geneva, ONUSIDA/PSR/HRHIV.

Lauby, J., P. Smith, et al. (2000). "A Community-Level HIV Prevention Intervention for Inner-City Women: Results of the Women and Infants Demonstration Projects." AJPH **90**(2): 216-222.

Long, L. (1998). Empowerment Strategies with Highly Mobile Populations. 2nd International Symposium on HIV Prevention, Official Satellite Meeting of the 12th World AIDS Conference, Geneva, Merck & Co., Inc.

MAP (Monitoring the AIDS Pandemic Network) (2000). The Status and Trends of The HIV/AIDS Epidemics In the World. XIII International AIDS Conference, Durban, South Africa, UNAIDS.

M'Boa, L., N. N'Dah, et al. (1998). The Supervision of Income-Generating Projects by PWA Support Groups in West Africa. 12th World AIDS Conference, Geneva, Merck & Co., Inc.

Mintzberg, H. (1982). Structure et dynamique des organisations. Paris, Les éditions d' organisation.

Mintzberg, H. (1989). Mintzberg on Management Inside our Strange World of Organizations. New York, the Free Press.

Mintzberg, H. (1994). The Rise and Fall of Strategic Planning. New York, The Free Press A Division of Macmillan Inc.

M'Pelé, P., C. Pervilhac, et al. (2000). The impact of a local response to HIV/AIDS in a rural district of Burkina Faso. 13th AIDS International Conference, Durban, South Africa.

Ng'weshemi, J., T. Boerma, et al., Eds. (1997). HIV Prevention and AIDS Care in Africa. A district level approach. Amsterdam, Royal Tropical Institute.

Nyonyo, V., D. Mayunga, C. Pervilhac, J. Ng'weshemi, and G. Mwaluko. (2000). Process Approach Guide to HIV/AIDS risk behaviour mapping Magu District experience 1996-1998, (TANESA), Tanzania. 13 th International AIDS Conference (High Transmission Area Workshop), Durban, South Africa.

Painter, T. (1998). A Review of HIV/ AIDS interventions for people on the move in Sub-Saharan Africa. 12th World AIDS Conference, Geneva, Merck & Co., Inc.

Pervilhac, C. and K. Kielmann (1999). Mid-Term Review HIV/ STD Prevention (Social Marketing) Ministry of Health Republic of Rwanda KfW. Heidelberg, University Hospital Ruprechts-Karls-Universität of Heidelberg Department of Tropical Hygiene and Public Health.

Pervilhac, C., W. Kipp, et al. (1997). Report on the District Expanded Response Initiative (DRI) UNAIDS/WHO/GTZ Case-Study of Kabarole District the Republic of Uganda. Bonn and Alberta and Kampala, GTZ.

Piot, P. (2000). HIV Non-intervention: a Costly Option. XIII International AIDS Conference, Durban, South Africa.

Plummer, M., J. Todd, et al. (2000). Triangulation of Biological Markers and Quantitative and Qualitative Responses in Sexual Behaviour Research with Adolescents in Rural Tanzania. XIII International AIDS Conference, Durban, South Africa.

Porter, M. (1987). "Corporate Strategy: The State of Strategic Thinking." The Economist 303(7499): 17.

Reeler, A. (1999). Health Reform and HIV. Geneva, Health Access International.

Sanon (1997). Rapport Provisoire du Diagnostic Participatif à Banlo, Kalambira, Zinka, Sibera, pour le compte du Projet PDR-PONI, Diébougou, GTZ. Gaoua, GTZ.

Skinner, C. S., C. Arfken, et al. (2000). "Outcomes of the Learn, Share & Live Breast Cancer Education Program for Older Urban Women." AJPH 90(8): 1229-1234.

Soucat, A. (1998). HIV and Health Care Reform: Making Health Care Systems Respond Effectively to HIV and AIDS. A tool for local assessment, analysis and action by and for peripheral managers and communities. Office of Health Care Reform-AIDS Division, Ministry of Public Health, Thailand-UNAIDS. Geneva, UNAIDS.

Sumartojo, E., J. Carey, et al. (1997). "Targeted and general population interventions for HIV prevention: towards a comprehensive approach." AIDS 11: 1201-1209.

Taverne, B. (1996). "SIDA et Migrants au Burkina Faso: l'Illusion d'une Prévention Ciblée." Médecine d'Afrique Noire 43(1): 31-35.

Taverne, B. (1996). "Stratégie de communication et stigmatisation des femmes: lévirat et sida au Burkina Faso." Sciences Sociales et Santé 14(2): 87-106.

The CDC AIDS Community Demonstration Projects Research Group (1999). "Community-Level HIV Intervention in 5 Cities: Final Outcome Data From the CDC AIDS Community Demonstration Projects." AJPH 89(3): 336-345.

The World Bank (1999). Intensifying Action Against HIV/AIDS in Africa: Responding to a Development Crisis. Washington D.C., The World Bank.

Todaro, M. (1997). Urbanization, Unemployment, and Migration in Africa: Theory and Policy. New York, The Population Council.

Traoré, F. and J. Ouango (1994). Femmes, migration et SIDA. Actes du Symposium.

UNAIDS (1996). Expanding the Response. Geneva, UNAIDS.

UNAIDS (1998). Consensus régional sur l'amélioration de la surveillance comportementale et de la sérosurveillance face au VIH: Rapport d'une conférence régionale tenue en Afrique orientale. Geneva, UNAIDS.

UNAIDS (1998). Expanding the global response to HIV/ AIDS through focused action. Reducing risk and vulnerability: definitions, rationale and pathways. Geneva, UNAIDS.

UNAIDS (1998). Guide to the strategic planning process for a national response to HIV/ AIDS. Strategic plan formulation. Geneva, UNAIDS.

UNAIDS (1998). Guide to the strategic planning process for a national response to HIV/AIDS Introduction. Geneva, UNAIDS.

UNAIDS (1998). Looking deeper into the HIV epidemic: A questionnaire for tracing sexual networks. Geneva, UNAIDS.

UNAIDS (1999). A review of household and community responses to the HIV/AIDS epidemic in the rural areas of sub-Saharan Africa. Geneva, UNAIDS.

USAID (1998). USAID Responds to HIV/ AIDS A Strategy for the Future. To increase use of improved effective and sustainable responses to reduce HIV transmission and to mitigate the impact of the HIV/ AIDS pandemic. Washington D.C., USAID.

Vladeck, B. C. (1993). "Editorial: Beliefs vs Behaviors in Healthcare Decision Making." AJPH 83(1): 13.

Weilandt, C., C. Pervilhac, et al. (2000). HIV Prevention in Europe: A Review of Policy and Practice Summary Report. Bonn-Berlin, WIAD and SPI.

Wiggins, S. and D. Shields (1995). "Clarifying the 'logical framework' as a tool for planning and managing development projects." Project Appraisal 10(1): 2-12.

CHAPTER SIX:
BIBLIOGRAPHY

AIDSCAP, The Francois Xavier Bagnoud Center for Health and Human Rights of the Harvard School of Public Health, et al. (1996). The Status and Trends of the Global HIV/ AIDS Pandemic. XI International Conference on AIDS, Vancouver.

Alonso, P., et. al. (1994). "Randomized trial of efficacy of SPf66 vaccine against P. falciparum malaria in children of southern Tanzania." Lancet **344**: 1175-1181.

Alonso, P., et. al. (1994). "A trial of SPf66, a synthetic malaria vaccine, in Kilombero (Tanzania). Rationale and Design." Vaccine **12**: 181-187.

Anarfi, J., Ed. (1992). Sexual Networking in Selected Communities in Ghana and the Sexual Behaviour of Ghanaian Female Migrants in Abidjan, Côte d'Ivoire. Sexual Behaviour and Networking: Anthropological and Socio-Cultural Studies on the Transmission of HIV. Liège, Derouaux-Ordina Editions.

Auerbach, J. D. (1998). Current Research on HIV Prevention and its Application for Effective and Sustainable Interventions. 2nd International Symposium on HIV Prevention, Geneva.

Baier, E. (1997). De l'impact du VIH/ SIDA sur les familles/ communautés rurales et de la nécessité de concevoir des stratégies multisectorielles en vue de prévenir la pandémie et d'en atténuer les effets dans les zones rurales (Orientation: Afrique). Rome, FAO.

Barker, C. and M. Turshen (1986). "Primary Health Care or Selective Health Strategies." A Review of African Political Economy **36**: 78-85.

Barnett, T. and A. Whiteside (1999). "HIV/AIDS and Development: Case Studies and a Conceptual Framework." The European Journal of Development Research **11**(2): 200-234.

Bererr, M. and S. Ray (1993). Women and HIV/ AIDS. London, Pandora Press.

Bjaras, G. (1991). "A new approach to community participation assessment." Health Promotion International **6**(3): 199-206.

Blumenfeld, S. (1985). Operations Research Methods: A General Approach in Primary Health Care. Chevy Chase, Maryland, Center for Human Services.

Borman, K., et. al. (1986). "Ethnographic and Qualitative Research Design and Why It Doesn't Work." American Behavioral Scientist **30**(1): 42-57.

Brannstrom, I., et. al. (1994). "Towards a framework for outcome assessment of health intervention Conceptual and methodological considerations." European Journal of Public Health **4**: 125-130.

Brockerhoff, M. (1995). "Fertility and Family Planning in African Cities: The Impact of Female Migration." Journal of Biosocial Science **27**: 347-358.

Brockerhoff, M. and A. Biddlecom (1998). Migration, Sexual Behavior, and HIV Diffusion in Kenya. New York, Population Council.

Brösskamp-Stone U. et al., "Institutionen, Systeme und Strukturen der Gesundheitsförderung und Prävention", in Schwartz, F. W., B. Badura, et al., Eds. (1998). Das Public Health Buch Gesundheit und Gesundheitswesen. München-Wien-Baltimore, Urban & Schwarzenberg.

Burton, A. et. al. (1998). "Provisional country estimates of prevalent adult human immunodeficiency virus infections as of end 1994: a description of the methods." International Journal of Epidemiology **27**: 101-107.

Caldwell, J., J. Anarfi, et al., Eds. (1997). Mobility, Migration, Sex, STDs, and AIDS: An Essay on Sub-Saharan Africa with Other Parallels. Sexual Cultures and Migration in the Era of AIDS. New York, Oxford University Press.

Campbell, D., et. al (1963). Experimental and Quasi-Experimental Designs for Research. Chicago, Rand McNally College Publishing Company.

Caraël, M., A. Buvé, et al. (1997). "The making of HIV epidemics: what are the driving forces?" AIDS **11**(suppl B): S23-31.

Caraël, M. and B. Schwartländer (1998). "Demographic Impact of AIDS." AIDS **1998** 12 (Supplement 1).

Cassels, A. (1995). "Health sector reform: key issues in less developed countries." Journal of International Health Development **7**(3): 329-349.

Cassels A. et al. (1998). "Better Health in Developing Countries: Are Sector-Wide Approaches the Way of the Future?" The Lancet **352**: 1777-1779.

Chabot, J. (1984). "Primary Health Care will fail if we do not change our approach." The Lancet (August 11 1984): 340-1.

Chambers, R. (1981). Rapid Rural Appraisal: Rationale and Repertoire. Sussex, University of Sussex.

Chambers, R. (1992). Rural Appraisal: Rapid, Relaxed, and Participatory. Brighton, University of Sussex Institute of Development Studies.

Ching-Bunge, P. (1995). Report of the Questionnaire Survey on the Use of Combined Messages and the Integration of AIDS/ STD Information into Family Planning Programs in Developing Countries. Eschborn, GTZ.

Cohen, B. and J. Trussell, Eds. (1996). Preventing and Mitigating AIDS in Sub-Saharan Africa. Washington D.C., National Academy Press.

Creese, A. and D. Parker, Eds. (1994). Cost analysis in primary health care A training manual for programme managers. Geneva, World Health Organization.

Cros, M. (1994). Araignée-sida et politique de santé en pays lobi burkinabè. Le Burkina entre la révolution et démocratie. R. Otayek, F. M. Sawadogo and J.-P. Guingane. Paris, Editions Karthala.

Cros, M. (1995). "Quête thérapeutique burkinabè en temps de SIDA De la capture du double à l'écoute du médicament." Champ Psychosomatique **2/3**: 89-101.

Cros, M., P. Msellati, et al. (1997). Faire dire, dessiner et narrer le sida Un vivier de sens en pays Lobi Burkinabè. Le sida en Afrique Recherches en sciences de l'homme et de la societé. Paris, ANRS ORSTOM.

Davidson, B. (1968). Africa in History. New York, MacMillan Publishing Co., Inc.

D'Cruz-Grote, D. (1997). Prevention of sexual transmission of HIV/ STD in developing countries. Experiences and concepts. Eschborn, GTZ.

De Cock K. (1996). "Editiorial: Tuberculosis Control in Resource-Poor Settings with High Rates of HIV Infection." AJPH **86**(8): 1071-73.

Decosas, J. (1998). Labour migration and HIV epidemics in Africa. 12th World AIDS Conference, Geneva, Merck & Co., Inc.

Decosas, J., F. Kane, et al. (1995). "Migration and AIDS." The Lancet **346**: 826-828.

Denzin, N., Ed. (1994). Handbook of Qualitative Research. London, Sage Publications.

Desconnets, S. and B. Taverne (1997). Annuaire des Associations et O.N.G. intervenant dans la lutte contre le sida au Burkina Faso, installées à Ouagadougou et Bobo-Dioulasso, 1996-1997. Ouagadougou, ORSTOM et CNLS.

Donabedian, A. (1973). Aspects of Medical Care Administration. Cambridge, Mass., Harvard University Press.

Equipe du Burkina Faso (1998). Etude Régionale Migration Internationale Santé Sexuelle MST/SIDA couvrant le Burkina Faso, le Ghana et le Togo. Ouagadougou, Ministère de la Santé.

European Commission (1999). Development -HIV/ AIDS action in developing countries. Brussels, European Community.

FAO (1997). Impact du VIH/SIDA sur les systèmes d'exploitations agricoles en Afrique de l'Ouest. Roma, FAO.

FAO (1997). Les populations rurales d'Afrique face au SIDA: un défi au développement (Synthèse des travaux de la FAO sur le SIDA). Rome, FAO.

Feinleib, M. (1996). "Editorial: New Directions for Community Intervention Studies." AJPH 86(12): 1696-1698.

Fishbein, M., et. al. (1996). "Editorial: Great Expectations, or Do We Ask Too Much from Community-Level Interventions?" AJPH 86(8): 1075-76.

Foltz A.-M. et al. (1996). Decentralization and Health Systems Change: Burkina Faso Case Study. Geneva, WHO.

French, H. (1996). Migrant Workers Take AIDS Risk Home to Niger. New York Times. New York: 3.

Frenk, J. (1994). "Dimensions of Health System Reform." Health Policy 27: 119-134.

Gilbert, L. K. (1999). "The female condoms in the US: Lessons Learned A Literature Review." AJPH 89(6): 1-28.

Gilks, C., K. Floyd, et al. (1998). Sexual Health and Health Care: Care and Support for People with HIV/ AIDS in Resource-Poor Settings. Liverpool, Department for International Development.

Girma, M. and H. Schietinger (1998). Discussion Papers on HIV/ AIDS Care and Support. Integrating HIV/ AIDS Prevention, Care, and Support: A Rationale. Arlington, USAID, Health Technical Services Project.

Grodos, D. and Xavier de Béthune (1988). "Les interventions sanitaires sélectives: un piège pour les politiques de santé du tiers monde." Social Science and Medicine 26(9): 879-889.

GTZ and ITHÖG (1989). Indicators for District Health Systems. Eschborn, GTZ and IHTÖG.

Hemrich G., et al. (1997). HIV/ AIDS as a cross-sectoral issue for Technical Cooperation. Eschborn, GTZ.

Hopkins, D. (1985). "Au-delà de l'Eradication de la Variole." Carnets de l'Enfance **69/72**: 229-237.

Hoth-Guechot, M. (1996). "Mais laissons donc l'Afrique respirer." Croissance **396**: 12-13.

Hunter Susan and J. Williamson. (n.d.). Children on the Brink. Strategies to Support Children Isolated by HIV/ AIDS. Arlington, USAID.

Jaffre, B. (1999). "Un journaliste face au pouvoir Le Burkina Faso ébranlé par l'Affaire Zongo". Le Monde Diplomatique. Paris: 21.

Janovsky, K., Ed. (1996). Health policy and systems development An agenda for research. Geneva, World Health Organization.

Jefremovas, V. (1995). Qualitative Research Methods An Annotated Bibliography, IDRC.

Kahn, J. (1996). "The Cost-Effectiveness of HIV Prevention Targeting: How Much More Bang for the Buck?" American Journal of Public Health **86**(12): 1709-1712.

Kahrmann, C. (1997). "Survival in the Sahel Problems with Applying Participatory Methods." Development and Cooperation **5**: 22-24.

Keeley, J. (1999). "Community-Level Interventions Are Needed to Prevent New HIV Infections." AJPH **89**(3): 299-301.

Kenis, P. and B. Marin (1997). Managing AIDS. Organizational Responses in six European Countries. Aldershot, Ashgate Publishing Company.

Kikwawila Study Group (1994). Qualitative Research Methods: Teaching Materials from a TDR Workshop. Geneva, UNDP/ World Bank/ WHO TDR.

Kikwawila Study Group (1995). WHO/TDR Workshop on Qualitative Research Methods Report on the Field Work. Geneva, WHO.

Krauss, M., E. Steffan, et al. (1998). Border Crossing HIV/ AIDS Prevention in Different European States -A Comparison. The "Umbrella Network". 12 th World AIDS Conference, Geneva, Merck & Co., Inc.

Krenz, C., et. al. (1986). "What Quantitative Research Is and Why It Doesn't Work." American Behavioral Scientist **30**(1): 58-69.

Lalou, R. and V. Piché (1994). Migration et SIDA en Afrique de l'Ouest. Un état des connaissances. Laval, Canada, Université de Laval.

Lamboray, J. L. and P. M'Pelé (1999). Planification stratégique et réformes pour une Réponse élargie face au VIH/SIDA dans un district sanitaire Gaoua-Burkina Faso Documentation des processus et des résultats Rapport Intermédiaire. Geneva, ONUSIDA/PSR/HRHIV.

Lamptey P. et al. (1997). "Prevention of sexual transmission of HIV in sub-Saharan Africa: lessons learned." AIDS **11**(suppl B): S63-S77.

Lauby, J., P. Smith, et al. (2000). "A Community-Level HIV Prevention Intervention for Inner-City Women: Results of the Women and Infants Demonstration Projects." AJPH **90**(2): 216-222.

Lawson, J., et. al. (1996). "The Future of Epidemiology: A Humanist Response." AJPH **86**(7): 1029.

Long, L. (1998). Empowerment Strategies with Highly Mobile Populations. 2nd International Symposium on HIV Prevention, Official Satellite Meeting of the 12th World AIDS Conference, Geneva, Merck & Co., Inc.

Luger, L. (1998). HIV/AIDS prevention and 'class' and socio-economic related factors of risk of HIV infection. Berlin, WZB.

Maier, B., et. al., Eds. (1994). Assessment of the District Health System Using Qualitative Methods. London, The Macmillan Press Ltd.

Mann, J., D. Tarantola, et al., Eds. (1992). AIDS in the World: The Global AIDS Policy Coalition. Cambridge, MA, Harvard University Press.

Mann, J. and D. Tarantola (1998). "AIDS - die globale Bilanz." Spektrum der Wissenschaft: 34-35.

Mann J. et al., Ed. (1992). Assessing vulnerability to HIV infection and AIDS. AIDS in the World. Cambridge, Harvard University Press.

MAP and the AIDS Pandemic (MAP) Network (2000). The Status and Trends of The HIV/AIDS Epidemics In the World. XIII International AIDS Conference, Durban, South Africa, UNAIDS.

Mayhew, S. (1996). "Integrating MCH/ FP and STD/ HIV services: current debates and future directions." Health Policy and Planning **11**(4): 339-353.

M'Boa, L., N. N'Dah, et al. (1998). The Supervision of Income-Generating Projects by PWA Support Groups in West Africa. 12th World AIDS Conference, Geneva, Merck & Co., Inc.

Mertens T. et al. (1993). "Evaluating National AIDS Programmes: New Core Indicators." AIDS Health Promotion Exchange **4**: 13-16.

Mhalu, F. (2000). The Disaster of the HIV Infection/AIDS Epidemic in sub-Saharan Africa: Who will be accountable for the many lost opportunities for prevention and control brought about by silence and denial? Stockholm, International AIDS Society (AIDS).

Mills, A. (1994). "Decentralization and accountability in the health sector from an international perspective: what are the choices?" Public Administration and Development **14**: 281-292.

Mintzberg, H. (1982). Structure et dynamique des organisations. Paris, Les éditions d' organisation.

Mintzberg, H. (1989). Mintzberg on Management Inside our Strange World of Organizations. New York, the Free Press.

Mintzberg, H. (1994). The Rise and Fall of Strategic Planning. New York, The Free Press A Division of Macmillan Inc.

Moore, M. (1996). Public Sector Reform: Downsizing, Restructuring, Improving Performance. Geneva, WHO.

M'Pelé, P., C. Pervilhac, et al. (2000). The impact of a local response to HIV/AIDS in a rural district of Burkina Faso. 13th AIDS International Conference, Durban, South Africa.

Murray, C. and A. Lopez, Eds. (1996). The Global Burden of Disease A comprehensive assessment of mortality and disability from diseases, injuries, and risk factors in 1990 and projected to 2020. Boston, Harvard University Press.

Mutangadura, G., H. Jackson, et al. (1999). AIDS and African Smallholder Agriculture. Harare, Southern Africa AIDS Information Dissemination Service (SAfAIDS).

Nakamura, Y., et. al. (1996). "Qualitative assessment of community participation in health promotion activities." World Health Forum **17**: 415-417.

Nana, L. M. and I. Sanogo (1998). Rapport de l'Atelier de Pré-Planification et de Consensus des Partenaires des Secteurs Public, Privé et Communautaire sur la Réponse Elargie au VIH/ SIDA au niveau du District de Gaoua, Burkina Faso. Ouagadougou, Ministère de la Santé, S.G., DGSP.

Newell, K. (1988). "Selective Primary Health Care: The Counter Revolution." Social Science and Medicine **26**(9): 903-906.

Ngoutara, A. and Yayo (1996). Revue Documentaire Analytique sur la Santé de la Reproduction au Burkina Faso. Ouagadougou, Population Council. WHO.

Ng'weshemi, J., T. Boerma, et al., Eds. (1997). HIV Prevention and AIDS Care in Africa. A district level approach. Amsterdam, Royal Tropical Institute.

Nordberg, E. (1995). Health care planning under severe constraints Development of methods applicable at district level in sub-Saharan Africa. Department of International Health and Social Medicine. Stockholm, Kongl Carolinska Medico Chirurgiska Institutet: 58.

Nyonyo, V., D. Mayunga, C. Pervilhac, J. Ng'weshemi, G. Mwaluko (2000). Process Approach Guide to HIV/AIDS risk behaviour mapping Magu District experience 1996-1998, (TANESA), Tanzania. 13 th International AIDS Conference (High Transmission Area Workshop), Durban, South Africa.

Oulai D. et al. (1993). The Impact of HIV/ AIDS on Education. Paris, UNESCO.

Painter, T. (1998). A Review of HIV/ AIDS interventions for people on the move in Sub-Saharan Africa. 12th World AIDS Conference, Geneva, Merck & Co., Inc.

PANOS Dossier (1988). AIDS and the Third World. London, The Panos Institute.

Pervilhac, C. (1998). "The Role and Approaches of the European Schools of Public Health in Improving Public Health Managerial Skills of the Human Resources from Developing Countries: Challenges into the Years 2000." Zeitschrift fur Gesundheitswissenschaften Journal of Public Health 6(Heft 3): 283-288.

Pervilhac, C. and J. Decosas (2000). "The Response to HIV and AIDS for Border Migrants and their Communities in West Africa: Issues and Opportunities from Gaoua District, Burkina Faso." to be submitted.

Pervilhac, C. and K. Kielmann (1999). Mid-Term Review HIV/ STD Prevention (Social Marketing) Ministry of Health Republic of Rwanda KfW. Heidelberg, University Hospital Ruprechts-Karls-Universität of Heidelberg Department of Tropical Hygiene and Public Health.

Pervilhac, C., W. Kipp, et al. (1997). Report on the District Expanded Response Initiative (DRI) UNAIDS/WHO/GTZ Case-Study of Kabarole District the Republic of Uganda. Bonn and Alberta and Kampala, GTZ.

Pervilhac, C. and W. Seidel (1995). Training for better District Health Management. First European Conference on Tropical Medicine, Hamburg, Public Health Promotion Centre DSE Berlin.

Pervilhac C. et al. (1997). Rapport d'Initiative ONUSIDA/ OMS/ GTZ de Riposte Elargie au Niveau du District. Etude de Cas du Burkina Faso. Bonn, GTZ.

Pervilhac C. et al. (1998). Rapport de Synthèse de l'Atelier sur l'Initiative de la Réponse Elargie au VIH/ SIDA: District de Gaoua, Burkina Faso. Bonn, GTZ.

Piot, P. (1997). "Executive Director of UNAIDS outlines challenges ahead and some of achievements so far". Press Release. Nairobi: 2.

Piot, P. (1998). Current Sate of HIV Prevention -Advances and Challenges. 2nd International Symposium on HIV Prevention, Geneva, the Swiss AIDS Federation.

Piot, P. (1999). UNAIDS Appeals for more Funds in International AIDS Fight. Geneva, UNAIDS.

Piot, P. (2000). HIV Non-intervention: a Costly Option. XIII International AIDS Conference, Durban, South Africa.

Piot P. et al. (1990). "The global epidemiology of HIV infection: Continuity, heterogeneity, and change." Journal of Acquired Immune Deficiency Syndrome 3(4): 403-412.

Plummer, M., J. Todd, et al. (2000). Triangulation of Biological Markers and Quantitative and Qualitative Responses in Sexual Behaviour Research with Adolescents in Rural Tanzania. XIII International AIDS Conference, Durban, South Africa.

Porter, M. (1987). "Corporate Strategy: The State of Strategic Thinking." The Economist 303(7499): 17.

Reeler, A. (1999). Health Reform and HIV. Geneva, Health Access International.

Reich, M. (1994). Political Mapping of Health Policy A Guide for Managing the Political Dimensions of Health Policy, Harvard School of Public Health.

Rifkin, S. et. al, Eds. (1991). Using Rapid Appraisal for Data Collection in Poor Urban Areas. Primary Health Care. Bombay, Tata Institute of Social Sciences.

Rifkin, S. and G. Walt (1988). "The Debate on Selective or Comprehensive Primary Health Care." Social Science and Medicine 26(9): 877-977.

Rohrer, J. (1996). Planning for Community-Oriented Health Systems. Baltimore, United Book Press, Inc.

Salla, R., P. Sebgo, C. Pervilhac et al. (1998). District Response Initiative (DRI): Fostering Partnership in HIV/ AIDS Control. Situation Analysis in Burkina Faso. 12 th World AIDS Conference, Geneva, Merck & Co., Inc.

Sanon (1997). Rapport Provisoire du Diagnostic Participatif à Banlo, Kalambira, Zinka, Sibera, pour le compte du Projet PDR-PONI, Diébougou, GTZ. Gaoua, GTZ.

Sayagues, M. (1999). "AIDS Hits Uganda's Villages." Africa Recovery in Development and Cooperation(5): 18.

Schmidt D. et al. (1996). "Measuring Participation: its Use as a Managerial Tool for District Health Planners Based on a Case-Study in Tanzania." International Journal of Health Planning and Management 11: 345-358.

Silva Saavedra, M. (1996). AIDS and the Developing World. In HIV-Ausbreitung und Prävention. Alexander Krämer and Christiane Stock (Hrsg.). Weinheim und München, Juventa Verlag: 147-160.

Simonnet, D. (1998). Pr. Luc Montagnier "Le sida devient la maladie de pays pauvres". L'Express.

Skinner, C. S., C. Arfken, et al. (2000). "Outcomes of the Learn, Share & Live Breast Cancer Education Program for Older Urban Women." AJPH 90(8): 1229-1234.

Some, L. (1997). Disparition de sexes à Ouagadougou Des victimes témoignent... Quotidien Ouest Africain d'information Le Journal. Ouagadougou: 1-3.

Soucat, A. (1998). HIV and Health Care Reform: Making Health Care Systems Respond Effectively to HIV and AIDS. A tool for local assessment, analysis and action by and for peripheral managers and communities. Office of Health Care Reform-AIDS Division, Ministry of Public Health, Thailand-UNAIDS. Geneva, UNAIDS.

St. Louis M. et. al. (1997). "Editorial: Janus Considers the HIV Pandemic - Harnessing Recent Advances to Enhance AIDS Prevention." American Journal of Public Health 87(1): 10-12.

Starfield, B. (1996). "Public Health and Primary Care: A Framework for Proposed Linkages." AJPH 86(10): 1365-1369.

Stein, Z. (1996). "Editorial: Family Planning, Sexually Transmitted Diseases, and the Prevention of AIDS-Divided We Fail?" AJPH 6: 783-4.

Sumartojo, E., J. Carey, et al. (1997). "Targeted and general population interventions for HIV prevention: towards a comprehensive approach." AIDS **11**: 1201-1209.

Susser, M. (1995). "The tribulations of trials-intervention in communities." AJPH **95**: 156-158.

Susser, M. (1996). "Some Principles in Study Design for Preventing HIV Transmission: Rigor or Reality." American Journal of Public Health **86**(12): 1713-16.

Swiss AIDS Federation (1998). HIV Prevention Symposium Report. 2nd International Symposium on HIV Prevention, Geneva, Swiss AIDS Federation.

Tanbanjong, A., Piyanat, et al. (1998). HIV and Health Care Reform in Phayao From Crisis to Opportunity. Bangkok, UNAIDS and PAAC.

Taverne, B. (1996). "SIDA et Migrants au Burkina Faso: l'Illusion d'une Prévention Ciblée." Médecine d'Afrique Noire **43**(1): 31-35.

Taverne, B. (1996). "Stratégie de communication et stigmatisation des femmes: lévirat et sida au Burkina Faso." Sciences Sociales et Santé **14**(2): 87-106.

Taylor, C. (1987). "Ten Years after Alma-Ata: Health Progress, Problems and Future Priorities." International Health News (September).

Tesch, R. (1990). Qualitative Research: Analysis Types and Software Tools. New York, The Falmer Press.

Testa J. et al. (1996). "Evaluation d'une Action d'Information et d'Education sur le SIDA chez des Chauffeurs Routiers du Burkina Faso." Médecine d'Afrique Noire **43**(1): 25-29.

The CDC AIDS Community Demonstration Projects Research Group (1999). "Community-Level HIV Intervention in 5 Cities: Final Outcome Data From the CDC AIDS Community Demonstration Projects." AJPH **89**(3): 336-345.

The Lancet (1998). "AIDS, the unbridgeable gap." The Lancet **351**(9119): 1825.

The World Bank (1993). World Development Report 1993: Investing in Health. Washington D.C., World Bank.

The World Bank (1997). Confronting AIDS Public Priorities in a Global Epidemic. Washington D.C., Oxford University Press.

The World Bank (1999). Intensifying Action Against HIV/AIDS in Africa: Responding to a Development Crisis. Washington D.C., The World Bank.

357

Todaro, M. (1997). Urbanization, Unemployment, and Migration in Africa: Theory and Policy. New York, The Population Council.

Topouzis, D. and J. D. Guerny (1999). Sustainable Agricultural/Rural Development and Vulnerability to the AIDS Epidemic. Geneva, FAO and UNAIDS.

Traore, F. and J. Ouango (1994). Femmes, migration et SIDA. Actes du Symposium.

UNAIDS (1996). Expanding the Response. Geneva, UNAIDS.

UNAIDS (1996). Fact about UNAIDS. UNAIDS an overview. Geneva, UNAIDS.

UNAIDS (1997). Children with AIDS: a Crisis Mature. Geneva, UNAIDS.

UNAIDS (1997). Community Mobilization and AIDS. Geneva, UNAIDS.

UNAIDS (1997). Mother-to-child transmission of HIV. Geneva, UNICEF UNDP UNFPA UNESCO WHO World Bank.

UNAIDS (1997). The Orphans of AIDS: Breaking the Vicious Circle Children Living in a World with AIDS. Geneva, UNAIDS.

UNAIDS (1997). Report on the Global HIV/ AIDS Epidemic. Geneva, UNAIDS-WHO.

UNAIDS (1997). Sexually transmitted diseases: policies and principles for prevention and care. Geneva, UNAIDS.

UNAIDS (1997). Tuberculosis and AIDS. Geneva, UNAIDS.

UNAIDS (1998). Consensus régional sur l'amélioration de la surveillance comportementale et de la sérosurveillance face au VIH: Rapport d'une conférence régionale tenue en Afrique orientale. Geneva, UNAIDS.

UNAIDS (1998). Epidemiological Fact Sheets, Africa Region. Geneva, UNAIDS.

UNAIDS (1998). Expanding the global response to HIV/ AIDS through focused action. Reducing risk and vulnerability: definitions, rationale and pathways. Geneva, UNAIDS.

UNAIDS (1998). Guide to the strategic planning process for a national response to HIV/ AIDS Response Analysis (Vol. 2). Geneva, UNICEF UNDP UNFPA UNESCO WHO World Bank.

UNAIDS (1998). Guide to the strategic planning process for a national response to HIV/ AIDS. Situation Analysis. Geneva, UNAIDS.

UNAIDS (1998). Guide to the strategic planning process for a national response to HIV/ AIDS. Strategic plan formulation. Geneva, UNAIDS.

UNAIDS (1998). Guide to the strategic planning process for a national response to HIV/AIDS Introduction. Geneva, UNAIDS.

UNAIDS (1998). Looking deeper into the HIV epidemic: A questionnaire for tracing sexual networks. Geneva, UNAIDS.

UNAIDS (1998). The public health approach to STD control. Geneva, UNAIDS.

UNAIDS (1998). Relationships of HIV and STD declines in Thailand to behavioural change A synthesis of existing studies. Geneva, UNAIDS.

UNAIDS (1999). Communications programming for HIV/ AIDS: An annotated bibliography. Geneva, UNAIDS.

UNAIDS (1999). A review of household and community responses to the HIV/AIDS epidemic in the rural areas of sub-Saharan Africa. Geneva, UNAIDS.

UNAIDS (2000). HIV and health-care reform in Phayao *From crisis to opportunity*. Geneva, UNAIDS.

UNAIDS (2000). National AIDS Programmes A Guide to Monitoring and Evaluation. Geneva, UNAIDS, WHO, Measure Evaluation Project.

UNAIDS (2000). Report on the global HIV/AIDS epidemic June 2000. Geneva, UNAIDS.

UNAIDS and PennState (1999). Communications Framework for HIV/AIDS A New Direction. Geneva, UNAIDS and PennState.

UNAIDS and The Prince of Wales Business Leaders Forum (1997). The Business Response to HIV/AIDS: Innovation and Partnership. Geneva, UNAIDS.

UNDP (1997). Human Development Report 1997. New York, Oxford University Press.

Unger, J.-P. and J. R. Killingsworth (1986). "Selective Primary Health Care: A Critical Review of Methods and Results." Social Science and Medicine **22**(10): 1001-1013.

UNICEF (1998). "AIDS breitet sich unter Jugendlichen aus". Frankfurter Rundschau. Frankfurt.

USAID (1998). USAID Responds to HIV/ AIDS A Strategy for the Future. To increase use of improved effective and sustainable responses to reduce HIV transmission and to mitigate the impact of the HIV/ AIDS pandemic. Washington D.C., USAID.

Vaughan, J. P. and R. H. Morrow, Eds. (1989). Manual of Epidemiology for District Health Management. Geneva, World Health Organization.

Vladeck, B. C. (1993). "Editorial: Beliefs vs Behaviors in Healthcare Decision Making." AJPH **83**(1): 13.

Vlassof, C. et. al (1992). "The relevance of rapid assessment to health research and interventions." Health Policy Planning **7**: 1-9.

Walsh, J. (1988). "Selectivity within Primary Health Care." Social Science and Medicine **26**(9): 899-902.

Walsh, J. A. and K. S. Warren (1979). "Selective Primary Health Care: an Interim Strategy for Disease Control in Developing Countries." New England Journal of Medicine **301**(18): 967-974.

Walt G. and J.P. Vaughan. (1981). An Introduction to Primary Health Care Approach in Developing Countries. London, Ross Publication.

Walt, G. (1994). Health policy: an introduction to process and power. People, governments and international agencies -who drives policy and how it is made. London, Zed Books.

Warren, K. (1988). "The evolution of selective primary health care." Social Science and Medicine **26**(9): 891-898.

Weilandt, C., C. Pervilhac, et al. (2000). HIV Prevention in Europe: A Review of Policy and Practice Summary Report. Bonn-Berlin, WIAD and SPI.

WHO (1978). Declaration of Alma Ata. International Conference on Primary Health Care, Alma Ata, World Health Organization.

WHO (1980). Discussion Paper Selected Primary Health Care Interventions (Field Test Version). Geneva, WHO.

WHO (1991). Epidemiological and Statistical Methods for Rapid Health Assessment. Geneva, WHO.

WHO (1991). <u>Report on a Meeting on the Application of Rapid Assessment Methods to Tropical Diseases</u>. Rapid Assessment Methods, Baroda, India, WHO.

WHO (1994). Qualitative Research for Health Programmes. Geneva, Division of Mental Health.

WHO (1995). <u>Achieving evidence-based health sector reforms in Sub-Saharan Africa. Background paper for an inter-country meeting</u>, Arusha, WHO.

WHO (1995). Decentralisation and Health Systems Change: A Framework for Analysis. Geneva, WHO.

WHO (1995). Interventions and Policies. National AIDS Programme Management. A Training Course. Geneva, WHO. Global Programme on AIDS.

WHO (1996). Catalogue on Health Indicators A selection of important health indicators recommended by WHO Programmes. Geneva, WHO.

WHO (1996). Integration of Health Care Delivery Report of a WHO Study Group. Geneva, WHO.

WHO (1998). "Criteria for selection of indicators." <u>Progress in Human Reproduction Research</u> **45**(www.who.int/hrp/progress/45): 1-2.

WHO-GPA (1995). HIV/ AIDS Care and Social Support. Geneva, WHO.

WHO-GPA (1995). HIV/ AIDS Problem, Control Activities and Target Populations for Prevention. Geneva, WHO.

WHO-GPA (1995). Interventions and Policies. Geneva, WHO/ GPA. **3**.

WHO-GPA (1995). Interventions and Policies. A Training Course. Geneva, WHO.

Wiggins, S. and D. Shields (1995). "Clarifying the 'logical framework' as a tool for planning and managing development projects." <u>Project Appraisal</u> **10**(1): 2-12.

Wisner, B. (1988). "GOBI vs PHC? Some dangers of selective primary health care." <u>Social Science and Medicine</u> **26**(9): 963-969.

Zerbo, P. J. (1998). Projet Canadien d'Appui à la Lutte contre le SIDA en Afrique de l'Ouest. Abidjan.

APPENDIX 1A
CHRONOLOGICAL BENCHMARKS OF THE DEVELOPMENT OF THE HEALTH SECTOR REFORM AND LOCAL RESPONSE: GENERAL EVENTS AND PERSONAL CONTRIBUTIONS (Jan. 1997- Aug. 2000)

DATE:	GENERAL EVENTS:	PERSONAL CONTRIBUTIONS:
January 1997	District Response Initiative (DRI) First Working Draft Protocol for Field Assessments and District Case Studies (UNAIDS/ WHO, Jan. 97)	
March 1997	UNAIDS, WHO, and GTZ representatives meeting on the GTZ's involvement and contribution in Uganda and Burkina-Faso (BFA)	Participated, GTZ, Eschborn (1 day)
April 1997		Adaptation of the study protocol for the District Expanded Response Initiative Case-Studies in Uganda and Burkina-Faso
May 1997		Visits to UNAIDS Geneva, and to the GTZ/ RAP Office, Accra, Ghana
May- June 1997		**Original situation analyses Case-Study in Gaoua, 14 May- 6 June**
June 1997	UNDP Human Development Against Poverty (launching) with special section on AIDS and the links to Poverty	Participated, Bonn, 12-13 June
Sept. 1997	UNAIDS Technical Meeting	Presentation of the BFA findings and Uganda study protocol; UNAIDS, Geneva (1 day)
Sept.- October 1997		District Expanded Response Initiative Case-Study in Uganda, 17 Sept. to 8 October
March 1998		**Pre-Planning and Consensus Workshop in Gaoua, 1-12 March**
	DRI Meeting, GTZ Regional AIDS Programme for W. and C. Africa: Ghana and BFA Experiences	Participated, Accra, 16-17 March
May 1998	Technical Workshop, UNAIDS/ WHO of the multi-country study teams	Participated, Dar-es-Salaam, 6-8 May

June 1998	Health Reform and HIV Workshop: an Agenda for Health Reform and HIV, UNAIDS/ WHO and co-sponsors 2nd Symposium on HIV Prevention (Satellite Meeting of the 12th World AIDS Conference), Geneva, 27-28th June	Participated, Geneva, 24-26 June
July 1998	12th World AIDS Conference, "Bridging the Gap," Geneva	2 posters presentations: (1 July) - DRI: Fostering Partnership in HIV/ AIDS Control. Situation Analysis in Burkina Faso. - The DRI: Missing Link in HIV/ AIDS Control. A Situation Analysis in Uganda
July-Aug. 1998	**Situation Analysis and Response focusing on Care and Counseling**, Gaoua, UNAIDS Consultant "Country Broker", Burkina Faso (27 days)	

DATE:	GENERAL:	PERSONAL CONTRIBUTION:
Sept. 1998	VII Entwicklungsmedizinischen Forum, "Migration innerhalb und aus Entwicklungsländern", Bonn	Paper presentation "HIV/ AIDS for Border Migrants in West Africa: Hidden Problems and New Perspectives from the Gaoua District Case-Study, Burkina Faso"
Sept. 1998	Local synthesis of results of the previous situation analysis and response, Gaoua, UNAIDS Consultant "Country Broker", Burkina Faso (7 days)	
Nov. 1998	**Workshop of feedback and consensus on priority areas and objectives with 57 participants** (4 days)	
Dec. 1998	Strategic planning writing with local participants (9 days, including 77 participants for a 4 day workshop)	
January	**Strategic Planning Gaoua (finalisation of Plan and budgeting)** and UNAIDS	

1999	Consultant "Country Broker", Burkina Faso, 2 days GTZ-UNAIDS Meeting: Health Sector Reform and the Expanded Response	 Participated, GTZ, Eschborn, 8 January
February 1999		Identification and simplification of key tools to be used in facilitating the Health Reform and HIV Agenda in various national settings, UNAIDS, Geneva, 4-19 Feb.
March 1999	The Health Reform and HIV Country Team Workshop for the West Africa Region, Gaoua, BFA, 15-19 March 1999	Prepared Overhead Presentation of Landscapes (1997, 1999, 2000-2001) for UNAIDS Workshop
May 1999	Operational Priority Gaoua Plan for June to Dec. 1999 (4 days) UNAIDS Consultant "Country Broker", Burkina Faso	
June 1999	**Implementation of the priority plan** (2nd semester 1999) by the local actors	**Development of a Formative Evaluation Framework** (submission of proposed draft to UNAIDS country office and broker): Measurement of progresses using Inputs, Process, Outcomes and indirect benefits Indicators
June-July 1999	Elaboration of Plan of Activities for Gaoua/ Strategic Planning Process and Results documentation, and International Partner Meeting in Ouagadougou (Jun.25th) for financial commitments, UNAIDS Consultant "Country Broker", Burkina Faso	Institutional Landscapes incorporated as baseline and benchmarks
July 1999	Setting of local coordinating structures for the follow-up of the implementation of the Plan and Meeting of the Provincial Administrative Heads (45) for whole of Burkina Faso, UNAIDS Consultant "Country Broker", Burkina Faso	
Aug. 1999	Contact with Muraz Center in Bobo-Dioulasso, and Meetings of the Mayors of Burkina Faso, UNAIDS Consultant "Country Broker", Burkina Faso. Implementation of the Strategic Plan.	
Nov. 1999	UNAIDS Technical Meeting on the Facilitation of Local Responses: Training and Methodology Development,	- Participated: Presentation of the Gaoua District, Burkina Faso Local Level Response, by P. M'Pele, country

	Bulawayo, Zimbabwe, 22 to 25 Nov. 1999	facilitator
		- Presentation of the status of the tool kit for the local level response (ref. Feb. 1999) by C. Pervilhac, and of the preliminary findings of the E.U. funded research on HIV Prevention Policies in Europe
Jan. 2000	**1st Formative Evaluation (O3)** **by external review team**	**Measurement of progresses** using Inputs, Process, Outcomes and indirect benefits Indicators
April 2000	Setting-up of the Local Responses library, UNAIDS, Geneva	Comprehensive review of fifty documents related to the Local Responses
May 2000	"Local Responses to HIV/AIDS in Burkina The Gaoua Experience, a Health District in the Poni Province": presentation at the OAU Ministers of Health of the Africa Region Conference, Ougadougou	

June 2000	Measuring Progress of Local Responses to HIV/AIDS, Mwanza, UNAIDS Technical Meeting, 5-7 Jun. 2000	Editing of the new Technical Note 3 on the subject.
	Ms. Karidia Kyere, Director of Social Affairs, Gaoua Province, presents the **"Progress of Local Responses 1997-2000 and their Indicators in Gaoua District, Burkina Faso"** (among a dozen other country presentations)	Designing and editing the TANESA tool on a "Step Approach Guide to HIV/AIDS risk behaviour mapping: Magu District experience (TANESA), Tanzania
July 2000	13th International AIDS Conference, Durban	- Design of an improved "Progress Report on activities in the field" of Local Responses to HIV/AIDS in 8 countries and collection of information.
		- Participation to the Satellite meeting on "Local Responses" organized by UNAIDS Local Responses team, and to a poster presentation on **"The impact of a local response to HIV/AIDS in a rural district of Burkina Faso"** by P. M'Pelé, C. Pervilhac, J.L. Lamboray et al.
Aug. 2000	Gaoua District: Lessons learned from the Local Responses over the past 3 years with P. M'Pelé, ex-country broker, UNAIDS Abidjan Office. (1 week visit)	Final compilation of the lessons learned from Gaoua District to be published in the **UNAIDS** *Best Practice* **Collection.** **"UNAIDS Case-Study Gaoua District Local Responses:** *The Burkina Faso approach"*

COMPILATION OF POTENTIAL KEY INFORMANTS AT THE COMMUNITY LEVEL IN BURKINA FASO

LISTE DES INFORMANTS-CLES RECENSES

PRIORITAIRES HOMMES:

1. Chef du Village
2. Délégué Administratif (village) ou Chef de Quartier ou Concessions (ville)
3. Responsables d'Associations de Cultures (Groupements, Associations Coopératives...)
4. Enseignant (instituteur) de l'Ecole
5. Encadreur d'Agriculture de Zone (élevage, développement rural) (village) ou Animateurs "GRAP" SIDA/ P.P.I. (ville)
6. Tradipraticiens

Autres hommes:
- Chefs religieux (marabouts, imams, catéchistes...)
- Agents de Santé Villageois
- Commerçants
- Agent de Santé de la Formation Sanitaire la plus proche

PRIORITAIRES FEMMES:
7. Responsables de Groupements ou Associations Féminines (tontines...)
8. Commerçantes ("Dolo"...) (village) ou Animatrices "GRAP" SIDA/ P.P.I. (ville)
9. Responsables de Groupements Coopératives (coton, arachides...) (village), action sociale/ promotion féminine (ville)
10. Accoucheuse Traditionnelle

Autres femmes:
- Responsables de groupements religieux
- Groupes artistiques traditionnels (des 2 sexes)
- Enseignantes (rares)
- Accoucheuse villageoise formée
- Exciseuse

PRIORITAIRES JEUNES:

11. Groupes Coopératifs "Associations de Cultures" (jeunes hommes)
12. Président de l'Association des Parents d'Elèves

Autres jeunes hommes:
- Groupe Danse musique (mixte)
- Groupes de thé
- Associations de sports
- Club musique (mixte)
- "Leaders naturels"
- Vacanciers

Autres jeunes femmes:
- Equipe de Football (villes)
- Vendeuses
- Club musique (mixte)
- Tontines
- Groupes professionnels
- Vacancières

APPENDIX 3B

Units of Analysis and Sample Checklist of Specific Problems related to District Systems

* required component for each district analysis

District Health System

Units of analysis	Specific Questions
Health Committees or equivalent*	1. Poor representation (women, powerful leaders etc.) 2. Role of committee too passive (say always yes) 3. No quorum reached
DHMT*	1. Leadership of in charges (DMO, program mangers etc.) 2. Delegation of responsibility, if yes to which degree? Team spirit? Satisfaction of work 3. Financial accountability
Projects/donor support*	1. Does donor know government (district policy)? 2. Does donor execute activities agreed upon in coordinating meetings? 3. Planning not integrated in DH plan
Different programs • HIV/AIDS*	1. Planning process weak (planning national level) 2. Critical limit of manpower, new types of workers not available (counselors etc.) 3. Multisectoral approach difficult ("others" do not see AIDS as a problem) 4. No clear policy (e.g. condom use etc.)
• MCH*	1. Non national plan or guidelines existing 2. Often too vertical, no interest in AIDS 3. See activities not as their duties (taking blood for HIV testing etc.)
• FP*	1. No joint program planning between FP and AIDS 2. Different messages for public (e.g. condom promotion)

	3. Offices in different locations.
• TB*	1. Very vertical program
	2. Limited interest in AIDS control
	3. TB coordinator not part of DHT (physically office, mentally)
• EPI	1. Little interest in AIDS problems
	2. Managed as national program (limited cooperation)
	3. Limited knowledge of staff about HIV
• Other Comm. Diseases (malaria, CDD, ARI etc.)	
• others as relevant	
Support services	1. Old-fashioned system of accounting
• Finance*	2. Limited supervision and control by higher authorities
	3. Misuse of public funds was considered as normal
• Personnel*	1. Extreme shortage of staff
	2. No personnel plan existing
	3. Remuneration low, staff can put in less hours (40-60%)
• Training*	1. Training not tailored towards real training needs of staff
	2. Training not integrated
	3. Training results not evaluated at later stages (I month, 1 year etc.)
• HIMS*	1. Data not fed back to communities
	2. Data not fully used for planning
	3. Feed back of data to health units existed, but data not explained by supervisor
• Logistics*	1. No demand oriented supply system
	2. Supervision visits to health units not fully used for

369

(supply, transport, storage, maintenance etc.)	supplying 3. No updates of inventories, no yearly inventory done
• Health education/ IEC*	1. Done in old fashioned and negative way (example condoms) 2. Department, other health workers felt not responsible for it 3. Traditional communication not fully utilized
Health infrastructures/ personnel • district hospital	1. Role between MS and DMO not clear 2. Hospital did not participate enough in field work and supervision of health units 3. No community oriented spirit, not client focused
• peripheral health units*	1. Shortage of qualified staff 2. Little attractive of remote corners in the district 3. In charges often weak, no supervision of subordinate staff
PHC workers • VHWs*	1. Overrepresentation of males, selection 2. Few efforts to create small scale income for them, other wise drop out high 3. Concept of VHW not understood by health workers, VHW and communities
• TBAs*	1. Willingness to learn new things limited (age) 2. Resistance to participate in FP/HIV
• Trad. healers*	1. Differentiation between "true" TH and quacks sometimes difficult 2. Promote unsafe practices and make dangerous promises (AIDS is curable) 3. Not open about their work

Community Organization System

Units of analysis	Specific Problems
Local village committees/ groups	
• political*	1. Health/AIDS was not priority 2. Personality problems blocked decisions for a long ti 3. Weak in manpower decisions 4. Health worker did not understand importance of getting political support
• health*	1. Good leadership missing (however existing) 2. Do not understand their role 3. Not enough technical basic background
• gen. development	Did not exist
• agriculture*	No information (health worker do not know about it). If they exist, no links with HW or VHC
• women groups*	1. Poor skills for designing realistic income generating schemes, poor proposal writing, what makes sense 2. Poor accounting of funds 3. Links to other groups weak or not existing
• youth groups* • others	1. Only few existed (boy scouts), more on paper, not active 2. Many youth did not grasp concept of peer education 3. Leadership within groups almost absent
AIDS patients* (if possible)	1. Accessibility to care difficult 2. Stigmatization (family breaks apart) 3. Widows have no right on property

Caretakers	
• relatives*	1. Often refuse to care for relatives with AIDS
	2. Can be overburdened with orphans
	3. AIDS patient in family seems to increase stigmatization and prejudice
• friends neighbors	1. Are sometimes main caregiver
	2. Tend to be not included in care plan by staff (home based care staff), if caregiver
	3. Neighbor support traditional?
• profes-sionals*	1. Fear of HIV infection
	2. Lack of compassion (moral aspects)
	3. Lack of confidentiality
Support groups for HIV infected persons*	1. Still too much in secrecy
	2. Fear of publicity
	3. Some skills (counseling) within groups missing, understanding of role of group in individuals weak
Persons at high risk of HIV infection* (if possible)	
Local church groups* (care, counseling etc.)	1. Refused to participate in condom promotion
	2. FP and sexual health not welcomed topics fc discussions
	3. Information and coordination with PH department insufficient
NGO support groups (care, counseling etc.)*	1. Own agenda, planning outside district plan
	2. Activities can be counterproductive to PH government
	3. Budgets not open to government officials

Private Health Systems

Units of analysis	Specific Problems
NGO groups*	see above
Church groups*	see above
Social marketing condoms/ contraceptives	
• institution in charge (DHT)*	1. Little involvement of private enterprise 2. Initially reluctant to include private providers in training 3. sometime arrogant attitude
• pharmacies*	1. Poor network 2. Potential for IEC of pharmacists not recognized by DHT 3. Offer products without any quality control
• shopowners*	1. Thought selling condoms would negatively affect their business 2. Participate only if profits are made 3. Not clear which information they give to customers
• other distributors*	
Private praxis	
• clinics*	1. Quality can be poor, no quality control, sometimes not licensed 2. Reluctant to give information to DHT 3. do not want to be supervised by DMO
• home based*	1. Very difficult to supervise, QA control 2. Sometimes exploit patients (easy for AIDS patients) 3. Poor training, no upgrading, low knowledge and skills
Pharmacies*	1. Rather laymen, few have trained pharmacist 2. Sell products without QA control, some drugs may be only placebo 3. Sell antibiotics without prescription

Local Government System

Units of analysis	Specific Problems
District development committee*	1. Under representation of women 2. Focus on budgetary issues rather than technical or policy issues 3. Role as supervisory board not fully understood, few actions taken
PHC committee health specific committees)*	see above
Other committees	
• education*	1. Did it exist? 2. No information available
• agriculture*	1. Did it exist? 2. No information available
• community development etc.*	1. Did not exist
District officials*	1. Accountability of funds was not enforced 2. AIDS was seen as problem for DHT 3. Limited outreach (transport, per diems, too lazy)
Political parties/ officials*	1. Do not have awareness of full impact of AIDS 2. Weak support in controversial public discussions for DHT (e.g. condom issue, HE on sex in schools) 3. Decentralization in party different from administration, party too much dependent on national groups)

Education System

Units of analysis	Specific Problems
District education team (Min. of education)*	1. No real team existing (team spirit) 2. Reluctant to include sexual health education in school health curricula 3. Very limited resources for program development and outreach (staff, budget, transport) 4. Do not use modern methods for communication 5. External technical support limited
Health education/ school health (Min. of Health)*	1. Negative approach to design of messages 2. Coordination with health messages from DET weak or not existing (different messages-big problem-community confused) 3. Professional competence of DHE (DHT) weak
Parents association	1. Main task to collect money 2. Not involved in curriculum development or other technical issues 3. No official role in AIDS control activities
Teachers association	1. Only certain teachers were part of it 2. Teachers did not like it (how many?) 3. Very "invisible"
Church/private schools	1. Concentrate on abstinence, no info on safe sex practices 2. Limited authority of government to enforce curriculum 3. DEO did not supervise church schools
School children male	1. No information about sex from parents 2. Early start of sexual activities 3. No legal framework for sexual abuse of children existing? If existing, is it enforced
School children female*	1. Cultural difficult to say no to sexual offers 2. Accessibility to counseling services-FP services of

| | young girls (pregnant or non pregnant difficult (geographically, provider bias) |
| | 3. Limited information about prevention of STDs |

Out of school youths*	1. Difficult to reach
	2. More prone to unsafe sex and sexual abuse due to lower educational status?
	3. Less likely to be part of youth organizations

Media coverage

• radio*	1. Coverage still low
	2. Radio listeners are more adults than adolescents
	3. Limited coverage due to language problems

• TV	1. No coverage in rural areas, can be replaced by video presentations with projector
	2. Most available videos in English
	3. TV and rural populations-evaluation of effects, cost effective

Traditional communication

• theater	1. Not always appropriate messages
	2. Costs-can groups be organized in a sustainable way (commercial performances etc.)?
	3. Technical advice and supervision of groups not easily available

• puppet shows	1. HIV presented as monster
	2. Technology for building puppets not easily available and costly
	3. Presentation not adopted enough to the understanding of young people (adult presentations)
	4. No systematic evaluation done (valid for all traditional ways of IEC

• oral traditions*	1. Little efforts by HE and other DHT members/officials/health workers to include them into IEC
	2. Some are lost during cultural shifts
	3. Limited interest of young people

Agriculture System

Units of analysis	Specific Problems
Agriculture district team*	1. No team spirit, weak DAO 2. No coordination, no meetings within head of departments 3. Lack of technical competence
Agriculture extension programs*	1. No systematic planning, no plans available (monthly, yearly) 2. Coverage of activities not district wide 3. Advice not tailored towards needs of farmers 4. No special program for AIDS affected families
Extension workers*	1. Not familiar with modern methods due to lack of training (not upgraded for years) 2. Not accepted by many farmers 3. Redundancy created lack of motivation 4. Promotion of dangerous pesticides
Farmers' groups* Women groups*	1. Emphasis on handicrafts 2. Agricultural "needs" of AIDS affected families not recognized 3. Resistant to new ideas
Cooperatives Small scale farmers	1. Exist. Some supported by Ag. Sector 1. Unknown

APPENDIX 3C
Descriptive Table of the various Types of Studies (Purposes) and Tools

APPROACHES:	TASKS/ STUDIES:	REFERENCE TOOLS: (see Biblio. Ref. and Attachments in Appdx.)	UNITS OF ANALYSIS:	METHOD USED:
1. Epidemiology, Economics	1. Assessment of the present performance of each system	- classical evaluation tools (from GTZ PfK etc.) (if exists, open to any specific suggestion ex.: for 1.5. "Health Information Sub-System Issue Framework" in WHO, SCHIU/ DHSTA, "Guidelines for The Assessment of National Health Information Systems", 1996)	- programme managers	- key informant interviews
2. Anthropology, Policy	2. Self-analysis of roles from different District System Leaders (in complement with Specific Problems (Appdx. C)	- Position Mapping (Reich's "Position Map" from "Political Mapping") combined with qualitative research methods (WHO/ TDR "Key informant interviews")	- opinion leaders - programme managers	- group discussion
3. Policy	3. Stakeholder Analysis for an improved response	- Stakeholder Analysis and Policy Network Map and Transitions Assessment (Reich's "Stakeholder Analysis" from "Political Mapping")	- opinion leaders - programme managers (different systems organizations or individuals)	- group discussion
4. Sociology	4. Categorization of the types of organizations running each system	- Organizational Analysis (Mintzberg's classification from "Mintzberg on Management")	- opinion leaders - programme managers (different systems organizations or individuals)	- combined observations from 1 to 3
5. Anthropology	5. Assessment of the community managed response	- Qualitative Research Methods from WHO/ TDR "Workshop on Qualitative Research Methods" - S. Rifkin's and et al. "Community Participation Assessment"	- males, females adults - children	- key informants (political, health, agriculture, education…) - focus groups

378

KEY INFORMANTS QUESTIONNAIRE AT THE COMMUNITY LEVEL

CADRE D'ANALYSE NIVEAU DU DISTRICT
(GRILLE D'ENQUETE)
QUESTIONNAIRES NIVEAU DES COMMUNAUTES
(\comburkq)
1. QUESTIONNAIRE GENERAL D'INFORMANTS-CLES
(Vers. 25.05.97)

VILLAGE OU VILLE (QUARTIER):
INFORMANT-CLE:
TITRE (respecter l'anonymat):
SYSTEME (ne pas remplir):

1.1. Quelles structures (formelles ou organisées de l'extérieures, i.e. Gouvernements, Projets... et communautaires ou organisations propres aux villageois) existent à présent pour réaliser au village des activités de développement dans des domaines tels que agriculture (agents), éducation (écoles), santé (Postes de Santé Primaires, agents de santé si ils existent...), autres?

Préciser la ou les activités pour chaque structure identifiée.

1.2. Il y a 10 ou 15 ans, est-ce que ce village s'est organisé pour mettre en place les Postes de Santé Primaires ("Opération 1 Village: 1 Poste de Santé Primaire"), c'est-à-dire formations de comités de santé, agents de santé communautaires, accoucheuses traditionnelles formées, caisses de médicaments etc.?

Si oui, comment est-ce que ce village s'est organisé (est-ce que cela a fonctionné longtemps ou non, est-ce que ça marche encor ou non etc.)? Préciser bienfaits pour la communauté et réussites ou échecs?

1.3. Est-ce que le SIDA est considéré comme un problème au village? Si oui: grave ou non? Pourquoi "grave"? (pas seulement les aspects médicaux)

1.4. A présent concernant le SIDA, est-ce que le village a pris des initiatives à partir de ses propores structures communautaires et/ ou a été associé par des structures de l'extérieur (contribution) ou a vu faire (observation seulement) des mesures particulières? Lesquelles (discussion, activités, organisation...)? Comment? Depuis combien de temps ces mesures ont été prises? Progrès et réussites? Echecs et leurs causes?

1.5. Lesquelles parmi ces structures communautaires et/ ou de l'extérieure pourraient être utiles dans le actions futures de lutte contre le SIDA? Préciser la ou les activités pour chaque structure identifiée.

2. QUESTIONNAIRE DETAILLE D'INFORMANTS-CLES
(Vers. 25.05.97)
VILLAGE OU VILLE (QUARTIER):
INFORMANT-CLE:
TITRE (respecter l'anonymat):
SYSTEME (ne pas remplir):
EVALUATION DES BESOINS:

2.1. Y-a-t-il eu des besoins identifiés ou évalués sur un aspect quelconque de développement (agriculture, éducation, santé...) au niveau du village par des structures intérieures ou par des structures externes?

2.2. En fonction de ces différents besoins qui a conçu les activités à mener: de structures intérieures ou communautaires ou de l'extérieur? Pourquoi?

2.3. Y-a-t-il eu des besoins identifiés ou évalués concernant le problème du VIH/ SIDA au niveau du village?

APPRECIATION GENERALE:

BON   OK   FAIBLE

PERSONNES INFLUENTES:
2.4. Quelles sont les personnes influentes dans le village? (noter hommes et femmes)

2.5. Ces personnes ont-elles de l'influence sur quels groupes? (très réduits, larges... préciser du groupe normal d'influence, en dehors du groupe direct de l'informant-clé)

2.6. Est-ce que les décisions des personnes influentes au village ou dans les quartiers sont prises en général en groupes ou bien autrement? Préciser comment avec 2 ou 3 exemples.

2.7. Comment (ou moyens utilisés?) les personnes influentes mobilisent-t-elles la communauté pour entreprendre des actions dans le village?

2.8. Est-ce que les personnes influentes ont fait mener des actions? Si oui, Lesquelles? Est-ce que certains groupes ont été lésés? Dans quels sens (pourquoi)?

2.9. Est-ce que d'après vous, les personnes influentes du village jouent-elles un rôle contre le problème du SIDA au village? Lequel?

2.10. Qui pourrait-être d'après vous la personne la plus influente pour trouver des solutions aux problèmes du SIDA au village et suivre les activités? Pourquoi cette personne?
APPRECIATION GENERALE:
BON   OK   FAIBLE

ORGANISATION: (Comment les buts sont-ils achevés?)
(Vers. 25.05.97)

2.11. Est-ce qu'il a une organisation communautaire qui existe ou se met en place quand il y a des problèmes graves de santé au village?
2.12. Pour le problème du SIDA, est-ce que le village a une organisation communautaire spécifique? Et en dohors du village, avec quelles structures externes travaillent les villageois?

Comment la structure communautaire a-t-elle vu le jour?

2.13. Comment la ou les organisation(s) présente(s) est ou sont-elle(s) financée(s)?

2.14. Quels groupes (par sexes, par tranches d'ages, par religions...) de la communauté sont impliqués dans cette organisation? Les membres du groupe sont-ils payés?

2.15. A-t-on besoin d'une structure (comité, agents, autres...) spéciale pour le SIDA au niveau du village? Si oui, préciser pourquoi?

APPRECIATION GENERALE:

BON   OK   FAIBLE

GESTION: (Comment est-ce que l'organisation communautaire réalise son but?)

2.16. Quelles sont les principales activités que votre communauté a accompli concernant le VIH/ SIDA et principaux obstacles?

2.17. Comment est-ce que celles-ci ont été accomplies: initiative propre, associé à d'autres de l'extérieur, imposées de l'extérieur, etc.?

Comment est-ce que l'on décide de l'allocation de ressources internes ou externes pour les activités du SIDA (par les personnes influentes, par des groupes, par des comités etc.)?

2.19. Est-ce que les agents communautaires (Agents de Santé Communautaires, Animateurs/ trices Action Sociale, Animateurs Villages...) participent à ces activités de lutte contre le SIDA? Si oui, comment?

2.20. Y-a-t-il des agents communautaires formés en VIH/ SIDA? Si oui, qu'est-ce qu'ils/ elles font?

APPRECIATION GENERALE:
BON   OK   FAIBLE

MOBILISER DES RESSOURCES:

2.21. Est-ce qu'il existe un moyen dans le village pour générer des ressources par les villageois pour leurs propres bénéfices (puits, eau, route, école, poste de santé etc.)?

Donner des exemples et quand (approximatif: année)?

2.22. Est-ce que les réalisations découlant de ces ressources profitent à tout le monde? (inégalités, de malentendus...)

2.23. Y-a-t-il des activités communautaires génératrices de ressources spécifiques à certains groupes du village? Quels groupes? Quelles activités?

2.24. Y-a-t-il un système pour aider les indigents (10% de collecte par exemple)?

2.25. En cas d'un problème grave au village (maladies, décès...) et de manque de moyens par la personne frappée, quelles ressources sont mises en jeu? (chercher type de solidarité existante: famille, proches, amis, écoles, religion, clans, aucun i.e. juste famille etc.)

2.26. Un père vient de mourir de SIDA. Sa femme élève actuellement toute seule ses 4 enfants, et elle a besoin d'aide pour plusieurs mois pour s'en sortir (culture de son champ, se rendre à l'hôpital, acheter des médicaments acheter des livres pour l'école...).
Est-ce que la communauté va l'aider? Si oui, comment? Si non, pourquoi pas?

APPRECIATION GENERALE:
BON   OK   FAIBLE

FOCUS GROUPS QUESTIONNAIRE FOR THE YOUTH
AT THE COMMUNITY LEVEL

QUESTIONNAIRE D'EVALUATION DES COMPORTEMENTS
PAR DISCUSSION DE GROUPES DIRIGEE:
(Vers. 25.05.97)
POUR LES JEUNES GARÇONS (16 A 25 ANS) ET JEUNES FILLES (16 A 25 ANS):

3.1. Quels sont les principaux problèmes de santé que vous rencontrez dans le village?

3.2. Classez les par ordre de priorité (ou "il faut faire quelque chose tout de suite") d'après vous.

3.3. Est-ce que dans le village, vous pensez que le SIDA constitue un problème important?

3.4. Si oui, pourquoi le SIDA constitue-t-il un problème important?

3.5. Que peut-on faire d'autres pour éviter le SIDA? (citer)

3.6. Est-ce que le problème du SIDA est dû aux surtout aux comportements des jeunes hommes ou des jeunes femmes?

3.7. Est-ce que les garçons au village ont changé leurs comportements sexuels depuis la connaissance du SIDA? Si oui, en quoi faisant?
Et les filles? (même question)

3.8. Est-ce que l'utilisation de capotes lors de relations sexuelles est un bon moyen d'éviter le SIDA?

3.9. Est-ce que dans le village les jeunes utilisent ces capotes? Problèmes ou difficultés rencontrées (timidité, honte de demander, difficulté d'utilisation: lesquelles etc.)?

3.10. Est-ce qu'il est facile ou difficile d'avoir (d'acheter?) des capotes? Problèmes ou difficultés rencontrées (pas d'approvisionnement, pas de disponibilité, problème de coûts...)

3.11. Est-ce que des jeunes cherchent les informations sur les problèmes du SIDA, ou bien des Malaides Sexuellement Transmissibles, ou bien de Planning Familial? Est-ce qu'ils les trouvent disponibles? Auprès de qui (personnes? structures?)? Ont-ils des difficultés pour les obtenir? Lesquelles?

3.12. Quelle structure ou personne est la mieux adaptée d'après vous pour vous fournir des informations sur le SIDA que vous cherchez?

VULNERABILITY FACTORS: ORIGINAL FINDINGS

FACTEURS DE VULNERABILITE PERSONNELLE

CONNAISSANCE DES MOYENS DE PREVENTION:
RURAL:
- "Il faut éviter le vagabondage sexuel et rester fidèle à sa femme" (un jeune homme de Banlo)
- "Si tu n'es pas fidèle à ton partenaire, c'est sûr que tu vas avoir le SIDA" (une jeune femme de Banlo)
- "Pour moi, il y a beaucoup de moyens qui peuvent permettre d'éviter le SIDA: il faut éviter d'utiliser les lames déjà utilisées par d'autres personnes, lorsque les ciseaux du coiffeur sont couverts de sang il faut les faire bouillir ou les brûler avant un autre usage, il faut porter les capotes pendant les rapports sexuels" (un jeune homme de Banlo)
- "... Pour moi, ce qu'il vient de dire c'est vrai parce qu'on ne peut pas cesser de faire la cour aux femmes donc il vaut mieux porter les capotes" (un jeune homme de Banlo)
- "En enjambant les urines d'un malade du SIDA on peut avoir le SIDA... et si un porc mange les selles d'un malade du SIDA et que l'on consomme sa viande, on peut avoir le SIDA" (une jeune femme de Banlo)
- "Celui qui utilise la capote, si elle est bonne c'est un bon moyen pour éviter le SIDA." (une jeune femme de Sidimoukar)

URBAIN:
- "Il faut éviter d'exciser plusieurs personnes avec le même matériel, éviter de recevoir du sang non examiné." (une jeune femme de Kampti)
- "(Le préservatif) c'est un bon moyen pour celui qui sait l'utiliser" (une jeune femme de Kampti)
- "C'est un bon moyen, mais il faut aussi un préservatif pour les femmes." (un jeune homme de Kampti)
- "Il faut s'abstenir" (une jeune femme de Gaoua)
- "Pour les accouchements, il faut faire attention et avoir tout son matériel nécessaire (gants, plastiques...) pour couvrir la table." (une jeune femme de Gaoua)

RECHERCHE D'INFORMATIONS DE PREVENTION:
RURAL:
- "C'est quand on a la maladie qu'on cherche des informations" (une jeune fille de Banlo)

URBAIN:
- "Il faut que l'on sensibilise la population sur l'utilisation des condoms. Avant nos parents de la brousse ignoraient le SIDA, mais avec la sensibilisation du PPI, ils se méfient actuellement des filles." (un jeune homme de Kampti)

CHANGEMENTS DE COMPORTEMENTS POSITIFS:
RURAL:
- "Ils (les jeunes hommes) ont changé de comportements parce qu'ils utilisent les capotes maintenant" (un jeune homme de Banlo)
- "Les jeunes filles ont changé leurs comportements, elles sont devenues fidèles…" (une jeune femme de Banlo)
- "Les jeunes hommes portent la capote parce que les filles l'exigent" (une jeune fille de Banlo)
- "Pour éviter le SIDA, moi je resterai fidèle." (un jeune homme de Sidimoukar)
- "J'accuse les garçons et les filles, car les deux se valent et sont frivoles. Certains garçons ne sont pas aussi fidèles et fréquentent plusieurs filles à la fois." (un jeune homme de Sidimoukar)
- "Moi j'accuse les grands aussi car certains ne suivent que les petites filles." (un jeune homme de Sidimoukar)
- "Moi j'ai changé de comportements: je reste fidèle à ma copine." (un jeune homme de Sidimoukar)
- "J'ai remarqué chez les jeunes qui ont reçu des conseils de comportements, que ceux qui "draguaient" à droite et à gauche ont arrêté par crainte de la maladie." (un jeune homme de Sidimoukar)

URBAIN:
- "Certains ont changé, d'autres pas: ceux qui ont changé ont peur et ont un seul partenaire, les autres s'en foutent du SIDA." (une jeune femme de Kampti)
- "Beaucoup ont changé de comportements. Quand nous étions petits, nos aînés disaient que le bon jeune c'est celui qui fait la cour à beaucoup de

filles. On disait même qu'un vrai jeune doit contracter la gono. De nos jours ce n'est plus le cas. (un jeune homme de Gaoua)

- "C'est un bon moyen, sauf si c'est mal utilisé." (une jeune femme de Gaoua)

CHANGEMENTS DE COMPORTEMENTS NEGATIFS ET CROYANCES NEGATIVES:

RURAL

- "Les jeunes hommes n'ont pas changé, ils ne peuvent même pas changer" (une jeune femme de Banlo)
- "... d'autres garçons n'ont pas changé du tout" (un jeune homme de Sidimoukar)
- "Certaines filles n'ont pas laissé leur infidélité parce qu'elles ne croient pas au SIDA." (une jeune fille de Sidimoukar)
- "Je n'ai pas confiance aux condoms car ce sont les blancs qui les fabriquent et ils peuvent y introduire la maladie qu'on peut contracter en les utilisant." (un jeune homme de Sidimoukar)

URBAIN

- "Actuellement nous n'avons plus confiance à nos copines, on a peur du mot SIDA." (un jeune homme de Kampti)
- "C'est une femme qui a introduit le SIDA dans le monde en couchant avec un singe. Les femmes construisent des chambres noires qui augmentent le SIDA." (une jeune femme de Kampti)
- "C'est dû aux hommes parce qu'il y a des hommes qui viennent de la Côte d'Ivoire atteints du SIDA et qui négocient une fille une fois dans la chambre, et refusent d'utiliser le préservatif." (une jeune femme de Kampti)
- "Une femme ne négocie pas un homme, c'est l'homme qui le fait et si il ne te dit pas qu'il est Sidéen qu'est-ce que tu vas faire?" (une jeune femme de Kampti)
- "Selon moi, c'est tout le monde, car certains ne sont pas sérieux et font le vagabondage sexuel" (un jeune homme de Kampti)
- "Il y a même des papas qui ont des femmes partout et des mamans qui ont des hommes partout: si on sensibilise ceux-ci, nous (les jeunes) nous serons aussi sensibilisés." (un jeune homme de Kampti)
- "Certains garçons disent que si tu ne meurs pas de SIDA, c'est que tu n'es pas beau." (une jeune fille de Kampti)
- "Je trouve que l'infidélité règne beaucoup ici et j'accuse les filles car

aujourd'hui elles sont avec toi et demain ailleurs." (un jeune homme de Kampti)

- "Beaucoup ne l'utilisent pas parce qu'ils trouvent que la fille est sérieuse." (une jeune femme de Kampti)

- "Seuls quelques uns l'utilisent ici." (une jeune femme de Kampti)

- "Elles n'ont pas du tout changé. A l'approche des fêtes, si une fille veut 10 paquets de mèche, elle fait la prostitution." (un jeune homme de Gaoua)

- "C'est surtout les garçons qui sont infidèles." (une jeune femme de Gaoua)

- "Certains hommes et certaines femmes ne veulent pas de capotes." (une jeune femme de Gaoua)

- "Les filles n'aiment pas utiliser la capote. Certaines filles pensent qu'avec la capote il n'y a pas de goût" (une jeune femme de Gaoua)

- "C'est dû aux comportements des filles qui disent qu'avec la capote, elles ne reçoivent pas tout le sperme car c'est le sperme qui met la fille en forme et que la capote fatigue seulement." (une jeune femme de Gaoua)

- "Garçons et filles, les deux sont infidèles" (une jeune femme de Gaoua)

- "C'est les deux sexes, car les hommes ne savent pas s'abstenir et les femmes non plus." (une jeune femme de Gaoua)

MAUVAISES EXPERIENCES:
RURAL:
- "Ce n'est pas tout à fait un bon moyen car il peut se percer, il faut donc s'abstenir" (un jeune homme de Banlo)

- "Il y en a qui utilisent la capote et tombent enceintes, alors pourquoi tu n'attraperas pas le SIDA si tu l'utilises?" (une jeune femme de Sidimoukar)

- "Selon moi ceux qui l'utilisent ne font pas une bonne chose. On voit des gens qui l'utilisent mais malgré cela leurs copines contractent une grossesse. Qu'est-ce qui prouve que le condom empêche le SIDA?" (un jeune homme de Sidimoukar)

URBAIN:
- "Les filles n'ont pas changé, car si un homme vient de l'extérieur avec une 404 et leur donne un rendez-vous puisque c'est l'argent qu'elles veulent, si cet homme est atteint de SIDA, elle sera également atteinte: c'est ce que l'on voit à Kampti." (un jeune homme de Kampti)

- "On a des problèmes pour le mettre car il pète souvent, certains le mettent à l'envers, d'autres disent qu'une fois placé il peut sortir" (un jeune homme de Kampti)

- "Moi j'ai fait beaucoup de démonstrations sur le port du condom pendant les sensibilisations, mais en l'utilisant une fois elle s'est éclatée avec moi." (un jeune homme de Gaoua)

- "J'ai fait une expérience. En mettant de l'eau dans une capote et lorsque j'ai attaché le bout de la capote et que je l'ai déposé sur un miroir, le lendemain j'ai trouvé des gouttelettes d'eau entre la capote et le miroir. Donc elle est perméable." (un jeune homme de Gaoua)

- "En mettant le doigt dans du piment, si on remt ce doigt dans la capote et qu'on la passe devant les yeux, le piment vous pique, donc elle est perméable." (un jeune homme de Gaoua)

FACTEURS DE VULNERABILITE EN RELATION AUX SERVICES ET PROGRAMMES

FAIBLESSE DES SERVICES:
RURAL:
- "La capote constitue le seul remède contre le SIDA, mais il faut attirer l'attention des commerçants sur les conditions de conservation car ils sont parfois exposés au soleil" (un jeune homme de Banlo)
- "Je ne sais pas si c'est bien ou pas parce que je ne l'ai pas utilisé. Je n'ai plus confiance aux condoms car ils sont adaptés aux climats des pays qui les fabriquent et non les nôtres: la température peut les détériorer." (un jeune homme de Sidimoukar)
- "... il faut seulement qu'on évite les ruptures de stock" (un jeune homme de Banlo)

URBAIN:
- "Nous sommes à la frontière et beaucoup de nos frères sont en Côte d'Ivoire, le pays le plus touché de la région, et le car vient chaque vendredi d'Abidjan. Il faut que les gens fassent des test et qu'on aide les malades." (un jeune homme de Kampti)
- "Oui il est utilisé ici, parfois même il y a un manque de préservatifs dans les boutiques parce que les gens l'achètent beaucoup et ça finit." (un jeune homme de Kampti)
- "Il n'a pas de coins pour les MST, c'est uniquement sur le SIDA ici à Kampti." (un jeune homme de Kampti)
- "...Actuellement je suis plus informé sur le SIDA que la gonoccocie dont je ne connais même pas toutes les voies de transmission. (un jeune homme de Kampti)

ACCESSIBILITE AUX SERVICES D'INFORMATIONS SUR LE VIH/ SIDA:
RURAL:
- "Le lieu d'informations est loin, ce n'est pas facile: il serait souhaitable qu'on nous envoie quelqu'un qui nous donne ces informations ici" (une jeune femme de Banlo)
- "Il serait intéressant qu'on vienne nous apprendre comment porter la capote" (parce que certains ne savent pas comment l'utiliser) (un jeune homme de Banlo)

- "Les jeunes ne cherchent pas d'informations sur le SIDA et les MST, parce q'ils ne savent pas à quelle structure s'adresser" (un jeune homme de Sidimoukar)
- "Nous nous informons entre jeunes pour le moment en attendant d'avoir au village des personnes qui sont en mesure de nous informer." (un jeune homme de Sidimoukar)
- "Nous ne connaissons pas d'autres personnes en dehors des agents de santé pour nous offrir des informations sur le SIDA." (un jeune homme de Sidimoukar)
- Il faut que quelqu'un vienne d'ailleurs pour nous informer." (une jeune femme de Sidimoukar)

URBAIN:
- "C'est un problème important parce qu'on veut s'informer mais on ne sait pas où le faire." (une jeune femme de Kampti)
- "Le problème est très sérieux parce que la sensibilisation est moindre, surtout pour nos soeurs." (un jeune homme de Kampti)
- "Il y a des fois des infirmiers qui viennent nous sensibiliser sur le SIDA." (un jeune homme de Kampti)
- "Je ne cherche pas d'informations parce que je ne sais pas à qui les demander." (une jeune femme de Kampti)
- "Les jeunes cherchent des informations sur le SIDA car beaucoup lisent à Kampti le livret SIDA-STOP" (un jeune homme de Kampti)
- "On a participé à une Conférence organisée par les jeunes où on a abordé le SIDA avec quelqu'un venu de Ouagadougou." (un jeune homme de Kampti)
-"Si ou projette un film vidéo sur le SIDA, les jeunes y affluent" (un jeune homme de Kampti)
- "Il a y une place vers le Marché de Kampti, où on pouvait avoir des informations usr le SIDA, j'y voyais beaucoup de jeunes." (un jeune homme de Kampti)
- "Je ne suis pas d'accord pour le cas du Docteur car nos parents des villages n'ont pas le courage de s'adresser à un Docteur. Donc il faut des agents de sensibilisation qui parcourent tous les villages. De plus le Docteur n'est pas disponible, il a son travail." (un jeune homme de Kampti)
- "Il faut quelqu'un de Kampti pour nous sensibiliser parce que tout le monde le connaît" (un jeune homme de Kampti)
- "Avant il y avait un groupe de théâtre chargé de la sensibilisation contre le

SIDA donc il faut que ce groupe revive" (un jeune homme de Kampti)
- "Quand elles vont dans les SMI, les jeunes cherchent des informations."
(une jeune femme de Gaoua)- "Les jeunes cherchent des informations entre
amies à l'école." (une jeune femme de Gaoua)
- "Les Docteurs ou les infirmiers, et là on peut croire." (une jeune femme de
Gaoua)
- "Ce sont les infirmiers qui connaissent ça très bien." (une jeune femme de
Gaoua)

ACCESSIBILITE GEOGRAPHIQUE A LA PREVENTION (préservatifs, tests):
RURAL:
- "Il est facile à avoir, dans la ville il y a un boutiquier qui le vend" (un jeune
homme de Banlo)
- "Il faut aller à Bouroum-Bouroum pour l'avoir" (une jeune femme de
Banlo)
- "Il y en a plein ici au PSP." (un jeune homme de Sidimoukar)

URBAIN:
- "Ici les gens ne font pas de test pour savoir si ils ont la maladie, il n'existe
pas un Centre pour ça" (un jeune homme de Kampti)
- "Si on part dans les boutiques pour l'acheter, certains trouvent qu'on est
trop jeune et on est obligé de mentir que c'es pour notre frère." (un jeune
homme de Kampti)
- "Si on va pour l'acheter en boutique, on se gêne car les boutiquiers sont
nos parents, et on a des problèmes pour le payer" (un jeune homme de
Kampti)
- "Souvent il est facile de l'avoir, souvent il est difficile, quand ça manque
le réaprovisionnement se fait lentement car les condoms viennent de Gaoua
ou Ouagadougou." (un jeune homme de Kampti)
- "Certains font le traffic de condoms sur la Côte d'Ivoire parce que là-bas il
coûte plus cher. Si on pouvait ouvrir un centre ici, cela pourrait diminuer le
problème de ruptures. (une jeune homme de Kampti)
- "Oui, c'est facile d'en avoir, on en trouve dans les boutiques." (une jeune
femme de Gaoua)

ACCESSIBILITE FINANCIERE A LA PREVENTION (ACHAT DU CONDOM):
RURAL:
- "Le prix est abordable…" (un jeune homme de Banlo)
- "Il est cher, le paquet fait 50 fr. et lorsque tu n'as pas d'argent, tu restes toujours exposé" (un jeune homme de Banlo)
- Mon inquiétude c'est qu'il y des jours où l'on n'est pas en mesure de l'acheter par manque d'argent" (un jeune homme de Banlo)
- "Ce n'est pas un problème de femmes (que d'acheter les condoms) je n'ai aucune idée du prix" (une jeune femme de Banlo)
- Comme la femme ne porte pas de capotes, je ne connais pas le prix" (une jeune femme de Banlo)
- "… et ce n'est pas cher, environ 15 F CFA l'unité." (un jeune homme de Sidimoukar)
- "C'est disponible pour ceux qui en ont besoin mais c'est cher, 50 F. CFA (le paquet) (une jeune femme de Sidimoukar)

URBAIN:
- "Le jour de la sensibilisation, les jeunes luttent pour l'avoir gratuitement." (un jeune homme de Kampti)
- "Avant on le vendait au détail (10 f/ l'unité) et maintenant on vend plus que le paquet à 50 f. et pour quelqu'un qui n'a pas 50f., c'est dur." (un jeune homme de Kampti)
- "Pour moi on devrait diminuer le prix pour que beaucoup de gens puissent l'avoir, même à 5 f. je suis d'accord" (un jeune homme de Kampti)
- "Si on diminue le prix, ça peut encourager les gens à l'acheter beaucoup, ce n'est pas à ma portée, on peut le faire à 25 f. le paquet" (un jeune homme de Kampti)
- "Il faut diminuer le prix du paquet à 25 au lieu de 50 f." (une jeune femme de Gaoua)
- "En tout cas pour ce fléau qui est en train de ravager le monde, il doit être distribué gratuitement." (un jeune homme de Gaoua)

ACCESSIBILITE FINANCIERE AUX SOINS:
RURAL:

- "Si on n'a pas d'argent, on ne peut pas se soigner dans un service de santé: la pauvreté en elle-même est une maladie" (une jeune femme de Banlo)

FACTEURS SOCIAUX ET ECONOMIQUES
IMPACT MORTEL DE LA MALADIE:
RURAL:
- "C'est un problème important parce qu'il a tué beaucoup de jeunes dans le village: au moins 5 personnes" (un jeune homme de Banlo)
- "Lorsqu'on a le SIDA, on est condamné à mourir" (une jeune femme de Banlo)
- "Tous ceux qui ont eu le SIDA en sont morts" (une jeune femme de Banlo)
- "Le SIDA a tué beaucoup de gens dans le village: femmes comme hommes (une jeune femme de Banlo)
- "C'est un problème parce que j'ai vu des Sidéens ici et si ça continue nous sommes foutus. J'ai connu 5 personnes mortes de SIDA à Sidimoukar." (un jeune homme de Sidimoukar)
- "Il (le SIDA) a tué 3 hommes et 4 femmes" (une jeune femme de Sidimoukar)
- "Le SIDA n'est pas bien parce qu'on ne peut le soigner." (une jeune femme de Sidimoukar)

URBAIN:
- "On trouve ici beaucoup de malades du SIDA, il fait souffrir les gens, il les fait maigrir." (un jeune homme de Kampti)
- "Le SIDA est grave à Gongone (quartier enquêté de Kampti), il y en a beaucoup qui sont morts de SIDA, il y en aura encore parce qu'il y a beaucoup de malades actuellement." (une jeune femme de Kampti)
-"…A Loropéni (un village à quelques kms. de Kampti), il y une soixante de cas de SIDA." (un jeune homme de Kampti)
- "C'est un problème de santé au niveau du Secteur 3 à Gaoua, parce que ça a fait beaucoup de décès." (une jeune femme de Gaoua)

IMPACT FINANCIER DE LA MALADIE:
RURAL:
- "Tu dépenses ta fortune avant de mourir" (une jeune femme de Banlo)
- "C'est une maladie qui amène aussi la pauvreté parce que quand ces gens sont malades, leurs parents bien portants ne peuvent plus travailler" (un jeune homme de Banlo)

URBAIN:
- "A Cause du SIDA certains bras valides ont disparu alors qu'ils constituaient des éléments importants pour leurs familles et la société." (un jeune homme de Banlo)

IMPACT SUR LA POPULATION:
RURAL:
- "le SIDA diminue le nombre de la population car il tue les jeunes qui sont appelés à faire des enfants" (une jeune femme de Banlo)

IMPACT SUR LE DEVELOPPEMENT:
RURAL:
- "Le SIDA et un problème de santé ici parce que ce sont les jeunes qui sont chargés de développer le village et ce sont eux qui sont les plus frappés par la maladie: alors qui va cultiver les champs? Qui développera le village?" (un jeune homme de Sidimoukar)
- "Ce sont les jeunes qui ont des idées pour le village et ils meurent. Notre village ne se développera pas." (un jeune homme de Sidimoukar)

IMPACT SUR LE SOUTIEN FAMILIAL TRADITIONNEL:
RURAL:
- "le SIDA tue beaucoup de jeunes qui sont les travailleurs des vieux" (un jeune homme de Banlo)

URBAIN:
- "C'est dangereux le SIDA car le jeune qui l'a abandonne ses enfants avec leurs mères qui a de la peine à s'occuper de ceux-ci" (un jeune homme de Kampti)

IMPACT DE SOUFFRANCE HUMAINE:
RURAL:
- "Si le SIDA attrape quelqu'un, il souffre beaucoup avant de mourir et la famille souffre aussi parce qu'elle voit leurs parents mourir." (une jeune femme de Sidimoukar)

URBAIN:
- "C'est un problème important parce que nos frères et soeurs viennent de

Côte d'Ivoire et meurent du SIDA sous nos yeux impuissants" (une jeune femme de Kampti)
- "C'est un vrai problème, j'avais des amis qui ne sont plus, quand je pense à cela ça me travaille." (un jeune homme de Gaoua)

NORMES CULTURELLES ET SEXISME:
RURAL:
- "Aujourd'hui les filles ne sont pas sérieuses, elles peuvent se rendre à Gaoua pour établir leurs pièces d'identité et partir pour la Côte d'Ivoire où elles peuvent avoir le SIDA avant de reveni le transmettre à ceux qui les épousent au village." (un jeune homme de Banlo)
- "C'est surtout (dû aux comportements des) filles, elles se croient éveillées, n'écoutent pas leurs parents et se rendent en Côte d'Ivoire, comme elles y sont entretenues par des hommes qui ont le SIDA…" (un jeune homme de Banlo)
- "C'est une maladie qui passe de la femme à l'homme." (un jeune homme de Sidimoukar)

URBAIN:
- "Ce sont surtout les filles car elles 'servent' trop, c'est-à-dire qu'elles ne sont pas fidèles." (un jeune homme de Kampti)
- "Ce sont surtout les filles qui maigrissent et qui vomissent tout le temps." (un jeune homme de Kampti)
- "La plupart du temps le garçon est fidèle, mais les filles se vendent et propagent le SIDA." (un jeune homme de Gaoua)

AUTRES NORMES:
RURAL:
- "Certains disent qu'ils ont honte de l'utiliser mais je pense que c'est parce qu'ils ne savent pas l'utiliser…" (un jeune homme de Banlo)
- "Pour moi c'est une maladie des jeunes: ce sont eux qui se promènent et vont en Côte d'Ivoire et donc à eux de s'informer" (un jeune homme de Banlo)

FORCES SOCIALES ET STIGMATISATION:
RURAL:

- "…au village ici les filles se moquent des malades du SIDA donc il faut tout faire pour ne pas l'avoir" (une jeune femme de Banlo)
- "Il ne faut pas manger avec un Sidéen." (une jeune femme de Sidimoukar)
- "Il faut éviter de manger la nourriture qu'un Sidéen a préparé parce qu'il peut mettre ses urines ou ses selles dans le repas." (une jeune femme de Sidimoukar)
- "Personne n'ose remarier une veuve du SIDA." (un jeune homme de Sidimoukar)
URBAIN:
- "Il faut s'éloigner du Sidéen." (une jeune femme de Kampti)

APPENDIX 4D

GENERAL QUESTIONNAIRE AT THE DISTRICT LEVEL

Key Approaches, Purposes, and General Sample Questions for the Local Level
(Vers. 21.04.97)

1. Assessment of the present performance of each system

1.1 Auto assessment by each system of its own performance, based on documents and available information, using existing indicators

1.2 External review of the above assessment, using the above and other existing external evaluations or reports (only for health and community organization)

1.3 Assessment of the existing capacity and the tools used to carry out cost analysis, e.g. cost-effectiveness analysis. If not, existing what is the potential for setting up a costing system?

1.4 If cost-effectiveness analysis exists, what are the tools used to carry out sustainability analysis? If not done, what is the potential to set up such a system?

1.5 Assessment of the monitoring system for behavioral changes and evaluation of the existing capacity to set up such a system

2.   Position Map with the self-analysis of and other organizations roles from different district systems' leaders opinions

(questions based on the findings of new policy decisions relating to an improved HIV/ AIDS response at a district level; a sample checklist of specific problems)

(based on M. Reich's "Political Mapping of Health Policy", Jun. 1994)

2.1   What has been your role for the past five years in response to the HIV/AIDS in the district?

2.2   What is your present role in response to HIV/AIDS in the district? If positive, what are the main enabling factors?

2.3   How do you foresee your role (and strategies) to an improved response to HIV/AIDS in your district for the next 3-5 years? (probe for each system, if necessary)

2.4 Do you think you can achieve this, if not what are the main constraints?

2.5 What is your organization's position on the proposed decision: support, opposition, or non-mobilized?

2.6 How strong is your organization's position on the proposed decision: high, medium, or low?

2.7 Which organizations are supporting the proposed decision? (high, medium, and low opposition)

2.8 Which major organizations have not taken positions on the proposed decision (non-mobilized)?

3. **Stakeholder analysis for an improved response, Policy Network Map, and Transitions Assessment: priorities for organizations or individuals, based on various units of analysis of the sample checklist of specific problems** (Appendix C)

(based on M. Reich's "Political Mapping of Health Policy", Jun. 1994)

STAKEHOLDER ANALYSIS:

3.1 What are the main objectives or interests of your of your organization in the proposed policy decision? (Each organization or individuals (units of analysis) within their own system rank themselves (high, medium, low) in relation to their present positions to the HIV/AIDS district response policy)

3.2 How important to the organization are those interests in the proposed decision: high, medium, or low priority? (Each organization or individual prioritize by order (1, 2, 3) the three most important questions/ issues of the checklist of its own system: specify which are the main constraining factors, and which main enabling factors would help to overcome the problem(s))

3.3 What would the organization be willing to accept at a minimum from the proposed decision?

3.4 What are the main interests in the decision of another involved organization? (and Each organization or individuals (units of analysis) rank (high, medium, low) the other systems as a whole)

3.5 Each organization or individual prioritize by order the three most important actors (units of analysis) of the checklists of the other systems: specify for each the main enabling and constraining factors

POLICY NETWORK MAP:

3.6 Which organizations affect your organization on the proposed decision? How strong is the influence and what are the main forms of influence (finances, information, people)?

3.7 Which other organizations does your organization influence on the proposed decision? How strong is the influence? What are the main forms onf influence (finances, information, people)?

TRANSITIONS ASSESSMENT:

3.8 What current transitions are occurring in the group or project responsible for implementation of the proposed decision?

3.9 What current transitions are occurring in the major organizations likely to be affected by the proposed decision?

3.10 What current transitions are occurring the broader political and economic and health (sector reform) environment that could affect the proposed decision?

4. Categorizing the types of organizations running each system
based on "Mintzberg on Management Inside our Strange World of Organizations," 1989)

4.1 External final assessment and classification of the type of organizations running each system (entrepreneurial, machine, diversified, professional, innovative / adhocracy, ideology and missionary, politics and political)
4.2 Consequences in terms of management and organizational set-up

5. Assessment of the community managed response

(specific, for the "Communities Organization System" based on WHO/ TDR "Qualitative research Methods", Resource Paper No. 3, and for 5.4 based on the new approach to community participation assessment Bjaras, Haglund, Rifkin, Health Promotion International 1991)

5.1 Assessment of the communities' roles in response to HIV/AIDS (ref 1.1, 1.2, 1.3)
5.2 Which systems could help you most in the future in improving the response to HIV/AIDS and why?
5.3 What are the three major positive aspects, your community has accomplished to improve the response to HIV/AIDS and what are the three major obstacles?
5.4 Assessment of the degree of present community participation based on the ranking of the following process indicators
    - needs assessment

- leadership

- organization

- resource mobilization

- management

5.5 Optional (for countries with an advanced reporting system in place already, i.e. Uganda ...): setting up of a sensitive surveillance system for monitoring the diffusion of new norms of behavior, and attitudes in relation to utilization and quality of HIV/ AIDS services in the health but other systems as well, using semi-structured interviews at the village level.

MATRIX TO DESCRIBE VULNERABLE POPULATIONS
RESULTATS DES TRAVAUX DU GROUPE TECHNIQUE: MATRICE POUR DECRIRE LES POPULATIONS CIBLES

Cibles	Taille	Comportement à risque	Facteurs influençan les risques d'infection		Possibilité que la population s'infecte ou infecte les autres (E,M, F)	Importance relative	Intervention présentes		Intervention futures
1. Les jeunes	30 % de la population	Précocité des rapports sexuels non protégés	Harcellement sexuel	funérailles et autres fête	Elevé	primaire	Formation des volontaires communautaires	prise en charge des patients (MST)	Apprécier l'importance relative des interventions présentes
		partenaires multiples	Lévirat	Alcool			jeu radiophonique	EMP dans les école (secondaire)	impliquer de nouveaux partenaires
			Migrations	Marchés de nuit			Magasins radio-diffusés	fourniture des condoms	s'informer sur ce qui se fait avec les service agricoles(Ver de guinée VIH/SIDA
			l'excision	tolérance des			theatres dans les village	lutte contre la pratique	

				rappor ts sexuel s hors maria ge				de l'excisio n	
			consom mation d'euphor isants	Haute préval ence de la malad ie au sein des jeunes			Distributi on de boites à images au FS et aux associatio n Causeries et projection de film	Confére nces dans les établisse ments scolaires	
2.Les femme s en âge de procré er	22,8 % de la popul ation	Idem aux comport ement des jeunes	Idem aux facteurs des jeunes		Elevé e primai re	Idem aux interve ntion pour les jeunes			Idem aux actions futures pour les jeunes
			Accouch ement septique s						
			Mariage s précoces						
			la polygam ie						
3.Patie nts MST									
4. Migrant s									
5. Orpheli ns									
6.Milita ires									
7. Routier									

s								
8.Priso nniers								
9. Personn es ayant le VIH								
10.Pros titués								

SYNTHESIS TABLE

TABLEAU DE SYNTHESE (PLANIFICATION ET CONSENSUS) DES 5 OBJECTIFS PRIORITAIRES DE LA REPONSE ELARGIE AU VIH/ SIDA1998-2000/ 2003:

DISTRICT DE GAOUA, BURKINA FASO

Chaque représentant d'une institution ou organisation, devait pour chaque objectif prioritaire, stratégie et intervention définir son apport en terme de:

1 - Apport d'expériences
2 - Apport de compétences (ressources humaines qualifiées et disponibles)
3 - Apport de moyens didactiques
4 - Apport de moyens matériels
5 - Apport de moyens financiers
6 - Mise en oeuvre d'une stratégie ou intervention déjà planifiée.
7 - Appui dans la mobilisation des populations

Tableau de synthèse de l'objectif prioritaire 1

OBJECTIF PRIORITAIRE 1	Intervenants (objectifs1)			
La prevention de l'infection VIH dans les groupes cibles est assurée	ONUSIDA 5 PROMACO 1,2,3,4, 6		GTZ 1,2 CNLS 2,3,4,6	
Stratégies Objectifs 1	Intervenants (Stratégies Objectifs 1)			
Promouvoir l'adoption de comportement sexuel Sûrs chez les jeunes de moins de 35 et les femmes en âge de procéer Promouvoir les comportements sexuels sûrs au sein des jeunes et des migrants	CNLS 4,2		GTZ 1,2,3,6	
Rendre disponibles les préservatifs dans la communauté Impliquer les personnes vivant avec le VIH dans les activités IEC et conseils (témoignage)	GTZ/PPF 6	ECD/FS 6	<u>PROMACO</u> 6	PIB 6
Education des jeunes par des jeunes	Croix rouge 1,2,7 <u>Jeunesse sport</u> 7	PIB 4-6	Coeur vaillants 7 Scouts 1,7,2	
Education des femmes par des femmes (groupements association	Scouts 7	ABBEF 1,2,7	<u>APFG</u> 1,2,7	

NB: Les mots ou sigles soulignés désignent le chef de file de la stratégie ou de l'intervention.

Les chiffres au bas ou à côté des mots ou sigles indiquent le domaine dans lequel le partenaire peut s'engager. Par exemple l'ONU/SIDA se propose d'intervenir pour le financement (5) de l'objectif prioritaire 1.

Par contre pour le même objectif prioritaire la GTZ apportera de l'expérience (1) et des compétences (2).

Tableau de synthèse de l'objectif prioritaire 1 (suite et fin)

Interventions sur l'objectif prioritaire 1	Intervenants Objectifs

Poursuivre la sensibilisation sur les moyens de protection contre l'infection du VIH/SIDA	Agri Resp. Sect3 Commun.,Cath. Scouts
	7 7 Mobilisation 2-7
	                                                        7
	
	Pénitencier APFG RG Enseig. Sécon.
	7 1 7 2
	
	PIB APASP APHPG APFG
	1,3,5,6,2 7,6 7 6
	
	+ rouge Prefet ECD enseig. Prim.
	7 7 (Stand Santé) 2
	                                                    6
	
	<u>CRESA/DRS</u> ATEFO FILPAH
	Jeu. Sport
	     1,2 6,7,2 2
	7
	
	PROMACO Resp musul. ABBEF
	Action social
	     6 7 2,7
	6

Informer les populations sur les voies de transmission du VIH dans leur milieu	PIB <u>R.G</u> GTZ/PPF 2,1,6,5 4,7+1 3 Assoc.pr Epanuis- ECD/PF APFG sement enfance au 1,3,4 2 Poni 7 Scouts trpe théat. + rouge 1,7 7 2,1
Encourager la population à faire le test	CHR SCOUT APASP Trpe Théat. 2,6 2 7 2 Club Unesco R.G Action sociale 7 2 6
Les jeunes et les migrants sont informés sur les voies de transmission du VIH/SIDA en leur milieu	Préfet R.G 7 4+7-1 Jeunesse et sport PIB 7 3,5,6

Tableau de synthèse de l'objectif prioritaire 2

Objectif prioritaire 2	Intervenant Objectifs (priorité) 2			
La participation multi sectorielle et communautaire est assurée	CNLS 1		GTZ 1,2,4,5,6	
	processus de reponse élargie		Accompagnement du	
	ONUSIDA 5		PSD 2	
Stratégies sur l'objectif prioritaire 2	Intervenants strategies/objectif 2			
Les ONG et les agents techniques travaillent en collaboration avec la communauté				
Impliquer l'ensemble des secteurs de développement à la lutte contre le SIDA	ECD 6			
Intervention sur l'objectif prioritaire 2	Intervenants			
Améliorer la communication entre les secteurs en vue de la lutte contre le VIH/SIDA	PIB 2-6			
Evaluer le niveau des interventions dans la lutte contre le VIH/SIDA	CRESA/DRS Appui 1-6	PSD 2		
Impliquer les responsables politico-administratifs dans l'encadrement des intervenants				
Mettre en place dans le District un organe efficace multisectoriel et communautaire de coordination des interventions de lutte contre le VIH/SIDA				

Tableau de synthèse de l'objectif prioritaire 3

Objectif prioritaire 3	Intervenant Objectifs 3			
Les soins et les conseils en matière de MST/SIDA sont assurés (FS et communauté)	GTZ 1,2,3,6	ECD 2,3		
	ONUSIDA 5	CNLS 1;5		
Stratégies sur l'objectif prioritaire 3	Interveants			
Responsabiliser la médecine traditionnelle	Préfet 2;7	mairie 4,7		
Former le personnel de santé sur la prise en charge des patients MST/SIDA	P I B 5	ECD 2;3		
Former les agents d'animation aux techniques de counselling pour la prise en charge	P I B 5	Action sociale 2	ECD 2;3	
Former le personnel de santé en counselling pour la prise en charge	P I B 6	ECD 2;3		
Assurer une surveillance chez les enfants nés de mères seropositives	Action Sociale 2	CHR 1,2		

Interventions sur objectif prioritaire 3	Intervenants
Améliorer les compétences des agents de santé sur la prise en charge des MST/SIDA Rendre disponible le test VIH	N E A N T

Tableau de synthèse de l'objectif prioritaire 4

Objectif prioritaire 4	Intervenants objectif 4		
Le SIDA est ressenti comme priorité par les groupes cibles (importance, gravité, comportements à risque)	GTZ 1,2,4	PROMACO 6	CNLS 2,3
	ONUSIDA 5	ECD/CHR 6	
Stratégies sur objectif prioritaire 4	Intervenants stratégie/objectif		
Informations des personnes ressources sur le VIH			
Mise à jour et diffusion régulières sur l'évolution de la prévalence VIH/SIDA et de ses conséquences	ABBEF 1-7	Mairie 4 7	Scouts 7-1	Préfet 7
renforcement des capacités de l'IEC d'exposer le problème du VIH/SIDA	Trpe théat. 1	APASP 7	Action sociale 2
Interventions sur objectif 4	Intervenants		
Mettre en place un mécanisme de coordination entre ECD et secteur Privé pour un plaidoyer VIH/SIDA			

Tableau de synthèse de l'objectif prioritaire 5

Objectif prioritaire 5	Intervenants sur objectifs 5		
L'impact socio-économique du SIDA et des MST est réduit dans le District	ONUSIDA 5	CNLS 2	GTZ 1,2,3,6
Stratégies sur objectif 5	Intervenants		
Développer des stratégies pour favoriser un comportement social qui démystifie le SIDA Promouvoir des activités pour reduire les conséquences socio-economiques du VIH/SIDA Mettre en place une stratégie de suivi et de prise en charge des enfants orphelins du SIDA	NEANT		
Interventions sur objectif prioritaire 5	Intervenants		
Apporter un soutien social aux personnes atteintes, leurs familles IEC sur la séropositivité	Act. sociale 2	APASP 7	Eglise ECD catholi. (Ajout santé) 4 6
IEC MST pour population	PROMACO 1,2,6		
Appuyer les activités génératrices de revenus pour les familles affectées par le VIH			

APPENDIX 5C

EXPLANATORY FACT SHEET OF THE FRAMEWORK
FOR THE TOOLS USED FOR THE IMPLEMENTATION OF THE HEALTH
REFORM
AND HIV AGENDA IN VARIOUS NATIONAL SETTINGS (version of
19.2.99)

Update of: day/ mo./year

1. Tool Category: (select one)
1. to conduct a situation analysis (sectorial, community…)
2. to assess the institutions' and sectors' roles and capacities
3. to assess the existing policies vs. needs and realities
4. to calculate intervention costs
5. to mobilise resources
6. to monitor and evaluate the program

2. Tool Name: Self-explanatory

3. Purpose and Objectives of the Tool: Self-explanatory

4. Level(s) of Application: National, Regional/ Provincial, District/ Local,
Communities

5. Description of Methods: Brief type of methodology used

6. Contribution to Programme Planning, Monitoring and Evaluation:
How is the tool contributing to the determination of planning and/ or monitoring
and/ or evaluation? How are results fedback to the informants (individuals,
communities, institutions…)?

7. Role in the Determination of Strategies and Interventions:
How is the tool contributing to the determination of strategies and interventions?

8. Advantages: of using this tool

9. Limitations: of using this tool

10. Primary Users: of this tool

11. Preferred or Suggested Technical Background and Training for Users of Tool:
Expertise or technical background preferred to use the tool
Time requested for training the user(s) (if accomplished)

12. Resources Needed to Apply the Tools: Time, human resources, cars, computers …

13. Used by and Location:
Institutional: Ministry, Agency…
Geographical: Country, District…

14. Original References:
Original document/ report etc. full reference. (number of pages)
Sources for availability (ref. ordering through Agency or Web-site address below)

15. Source of Technical Advice:
Name and e-mail or other contacts for technical purposes
NOTA: The tool may be obtained from the following web address: UNAIDS.ORG/PSR
pointing to "Reform HIV"

16. Tool Summary Description:
1-2 pages max. (Content and others, including Additional References related to the Tool)

APPENDIX 5D

SUMMARY TABLES OF SIX CATEGORIES OF KEY TOOLS FOR THE IMPLEMENTATION OF THE HEALTH REFORM AND HIV AGENDA IN VARIOUS NATIONAL SETTINGS

(vers. Update 19.2.1999)

CATEGORIES OF TOOLS:	TOOLS REFERENCES:
1. Situation Analysis see attached detailed outline	1.1. Guide to the Strategic Planning Process for a National Response to HIV/ AIDS: Situation Analysis. UNAIDS, Module 1 1.2. Guide to the Strategic Planning Process for a National Response to HIV/ AIDS: Strategic Plan Formulation. UNAIDS, Module 3 1.3. Strengthening health management in districts and provinces (AIDS technical function), A. Cassels and K. Janowsky (Additional specific situation analysis are documented in Categories 2 to 6 as well)
Reference List of additional tools either existing or in development	"Situation analysis for a district HIV/ AIDS programme" Ties Boerma and Marc Urassa, in HIV prevention and AIDS care in Africa. A district level approach. Japhet Ng'weshemi et al. Ed. Royal Tropical Institute-The Netherlands 1997
	Rapport Initiative ONUSIDA/ OMS/ GTZ de Riposte Elargie au niveau du District. Etude de Cas du Burkina Faso (District de Gaoua). C. Pervilhac. Mai/ Juin 1997
	Report on the District Expanded Response Initiative (DRI) UNAIDS/ WHO/ GTZ, Case-Study of Kabarole District, the Republic of Uganda, Vol. 1 Report, Vol. 2 Detailed Documentation of Study Findings and Questionnaires, C. Pervilhac et al., Dec. 1997
	"Patterns of HIV Spread in the Four Districts" (Participatory Rural Appraisal (PRA) methods), The Zambian HIV/ AIDS District Response Initiative. An Assessment of Four Districts in Zambia. James K. Sulwe. March 1998
	"Guidelines for conducting a review of a National Tuberculosis Programme" WHO/TB/98.240. WHO. 1998 (AIDS Programme identified as a potential site for field visit)

"Young people and HIV/ AIDS: Background discussion paper on the elements of a global strategy" Programme Coordinating Board (UNAIDS/PCB(7)98.3. 21 October 1998) with a detailed list of 7 sets of action (policies, participation, peer and youth groups, parents and policy-makers and media and religious organisations mobilisation, school programmes, youth-friendly health services, orphans and young people living with HIV/ AIDS)

Rapid Assessment of the Continuum of Care of PLHA and Chronically Ill Patients in Botswana, AIDS/ STD Unit in collaboration with WHO, July 1998, E. Van Praag et al.

Tools and Methods for Health System Assessment: Inventory and Review. WHO Div. of Analysis, Research and Assessment. WHO/ ARA/ 98.4. 1998. Phyllida Travis and David Weakliam.

Vulnerable Groups, UNAIDS (in development, to be published in 1999)

Mainstreaming Gender into National Strategic Plans, UNAIDS (in development, to be published in 1999)

Key Questions to issues relating to Human Rights UNAIDS (in development)

Rapid Assessment of Community Initiatives at local levels (in development, Best Practice on Community Mobilization to be published in 1999)

417

CATEGORIES OF TOOLS:	TOOLS REFERENCES:
2. Institutions' and Sector's Capacity Assessment see attached detailed outline	2.1. Guide to the Strategic Planning Process for a National Response to HIV/ AIDS: Response Analysis. UNAIDS, Module 2
	2.2. Rapid Organisational Review (ROR), Burkina Faso, Uganda, 1997, C. Pervilhac
	2.3. "Mapping of Institutional Relationships and Decision-Making (Power Relationships Flows) in Public Sector" in Progress Report on Tanzania District Response Initiative Study, Hamisi I. Mahigi and Damas S. Muna, March 1998
	2.4. Rapid Assessment of Access to Care and HIV/ AIDS-Related Drugs in Communities and the Health System, Malawi, UNAIDS and WHO, January 1999
Reference List of additional tools either existing or in development	"Coordinated care in different settings" in TB/ HIV A Clinical Manual WHO/TB/96.200, WHO, 1996, pp.119-122
	"Integration and Sustainability" Gijs Walraven and Japheth Ng'weshemi, in HIV prevention and AIDS care in Africa. A district level approach. Japhet Ng'weshemi et al. Ed. Royal Tropical Institute-The Netherlands 1997
	"Human Rights and HIV/ AIDS: Effective Community Responses" International Human Rights Documentation Network, May 1998 (case-studies related to Law Reform, Developing HIV/ AIDS Charters, Advocacy Work, Networking, Education Information-Gathering and Documentation, and Services for People Living with HIV/ AIDS
	"Organising the integration of voluntary counselling and testing for HIV infection in antenatal care. A practical guide " (with 10 key elements) Richard Baggaley and Eric van Praag, WHO (draft 15/12/98)
	Guidelines on Human Rights for Parliamentarians, UNAIDS, to be published 1st trim. 1999.
	"Country Health System Profiles" data bank (at least 55 from AFRO, PAHO, EMRO, EURO, SEARO, WPRO Regions) to be available (at least 55 countries planned for 1999) from WHO/ EIP including national data related to organisation and management, health care finance and expenditure, service delivery, financial resource allocation, and health care reforms

CATEGORIES OF TOOLS:	TOOLS REFERENCES:
3. Assessment of Existing Policies vs. needs and realities see attached detailed outline	3.1. "Decentralisation and Health Systems Change: A Framework for Analysis" Revised Working Document, WHO/ SHS/NHP/95.2 3.2. "Health Financing Reform A Framework for Evaluation" Revised Working Document, WHO/SHS/NHP/96.2 3.3. "HIV/ AIDS and Human Rights International Guidelines" United Nations, 1998
Reference List of additional tools either existing or in development	Guidelines on Human Rights for Policy-Makers, to be published in 1st trim. 1999 M. Maluwa. Guidelines on Human Rights for Parliamentarians, to be published in 1st trim. 1999 M. Maluwa. Guidelines on Human Rights for NGOs, to be published in 1st trim. 1999 M. Maluwa. planned for 1999: Key questions and issues relating to Human Rights. M. Maluwa. United Nations and National Response in Countries towards HIV/ AIDS: Qualitative Assessment Guidelines, Nefise Bazoglu, to be published in 1999

419

CATEGORIES OF TOOLS:	TOOLS REFERENCES:
4. Calculation of intervention costs see attached detailed outline	4.1. "Costs of district AIDS programmes" Ties Boerma and Japheth Ng'weshemi, in HIV prevention and AIDS care in Africa. A district level approach. Japhet Ng'weshemi et al. Ed. Royal Tropical Institute-The Netherlands 1997 4.2. Costing Guidelines for HIV/ AIDS Prevention Strategies. A companion volume to Cost Analysis in Primary Health Care. A Training Manual for Programme Managers. World Health Organisation. Lilani Kumaranayake, Jane Pepperall, Hilary Goodman, Anne Mills, 1998 4.3. "Distribution of Intervention Costs (Proportions)" in "HIV and Health Care Reform in Phayao From Crisis to Opportunity" (Draft Apr. 8. 1998) UNAIDS, PAAC, Health Care Reform Project, HIV/ AIDS, A. Tanbanjong, Piyanat, J.L. Lamboray
Reference List of additional tools either existing or in development	none reported

CATEGORIES OF TOOLS:	TOOLS REFERENCES:
5. Resource mobilisation see attached detailed outline	5.1. "Resource Mobilisation and Allocation" in District Response Initiative on HIV/ AIDS. Ghana Case-Study, J. Amnan et al., Nov. 1997 5.2. Calculation of Origins of Project Funding. UNAIDS, PAAC, Health Care Reform Project, HIV/ AIDS epidemiological and behavioural monitoring and evaluation in "HIV and Health Care Reform in Phayao From Crisis to Opportunity" (Draft Apr. 8. 1998) A. Tanbanjong, Piyanat, J.L. Lamboray
Reference List of additional tools either existing or in development	Guide to the Strategic Planning Process for a National Response to HIV/ AIDS: Resource Mobilisation. UNAIDS, Module 4, for publication in 1999

420

CATEGORIES OF TOOLS:	TOOLS REFERENCES:
6. Programme monitoring and evaluation see attached detailed outline	6.1. "Monitoring and evaluation (a district level approach)" Awene Gavyole, Ties Boerma and Dick Schapink, in HIV prevention and AIDS care in Africa. A district level approach. Japhet Ng'weshemi et al. Ed. Royal Tropical Institute-The Netherlands 1997 6.2. Using a Simplified Tool: A Monitoring Tool for Assessing, Analysing and Improving the Health Sector Response to HIV/ AIDS, in HIV and Health Care Reform: Making Health Care Systems Respond Effectively to HIV and AIDS. A Tool for Local Assessment, Analysis and Action by and for Peripheral Managers and Communities, March 1 1998 Agnès Soucat with inputs of J.L. Lamboray, P. Jongudomsuk, P. Daveloose, R. Msiska, W. Sittitri, A. Tanbanjong. Office of Health Care Reform-AIDS Division and Ministry of Public Health Thailand, UNAIDS 6.3. HIV/ AIDS epidemiological and behavioural monitoring and evaluation (Phayao District, Thailand) in "HIV and Health Care Reform in Phayao From Crisis to Opportunity" (draft Apr. 8. 1998), UNAIDS, PAAC, Health Care Reform Project 6.4. Protocol for Setting and Monitoring Locally Acceptable Standards of Counselling in relation to HIV Diagnosis, UNAIDS, July 1994 draft, for publication in 1999 6.5. Care Programs for People Living with HIV/ AIDS"(chap. 7) in Operational Approaches to the Evaluation of Major Programme Components, by E. Van Praag and D. Tarantola, for publication in 1999
Reference List of additional tools either existing or in development	Relationships of HIV and STD declines in Thailand to behavioural change A synthesis of existing studies. Key Material. UNAIDS Best Practice Collection. UNAIDS/ 98.2. Looking deeper into the HIV epidemic: A questionnaire for tracing sexual networks. Key Materials. Best Practice Collection. UNAIDS/ 98.7.

APPENDIX 5E
Sample of Seven Tools Reviewed
Update of: 11/ 02/1999

1. Tool Category:
Category 1: to conduct a situation analysis (sectorial, community…)

2. Tool Name:
1.1. Guide to the Strategic Planning Process for a National Response to HIV/ AIDS: Situation Analysis. UNAIDS, Module 1

3. Purpose and Objectives of the Tool:
For UNAIDS country programs, donor agencies, NGOs to conduct a situation analysis of HIV/ AIDS at a national or decentralized level

4. Level(s) of Application:
National, Regional/ Provincial, District/ Local

5. Description of Methods:
Document review, field visits with qualitative methods (interviews, group discussion etc.).

6. Contribution to Programme Planning, Monitoring and Evaluation:
Preliminary step of the planning stages comprising next the Response Analysis (Module 2, ref. Cat. 2), followed by the Strategic Plan Formulation (Module 3, ref. Cat. 1). Maximum openness in the dissemination of the report recommended to general population and vulnerable groups and communities: public presentations, simple publications, media releases, posting information on the Internet.

7. Role in the Determination of Strategies and Interventions:
Preliminary stage to the determination of strategies and interventions.

8. Advantages:
Step approach to planning concentrating on the situation analysis only.

9. Limitations:
The situation analysis covers a broad spectrum of areas for enquiries which can overwhelm the team into details, and can at the end make prioritization difficult.

10. Primary Users:
The situation analysis team, followed by the group who analyses the response, and then by the people who formulate the strategic plan, or in a nutshell, ultimately the national or local planners and managers.

11. Preferred or Suggested Technical Background and Training for Users of Tool:
Multi-disciplinary team, e.g. economist, civil servant, community organizer, anthropologist, private sector market specialist, sociologist... and person(s) living with HIV.
2 weeks to 8 months (longer for first situation than subsequent analysis and pending upon depth of analysis).

12. Resources Needed to Apply the Tools:
Time and human resources as per above. Cars depending of data collection needs. Word processing facilities necessary.

13. Used by and Location:
Presently a dozen Ministries in West Africa, and several in the East Africa, Asia, Latin America Regions.

14. Original References:
Guide to the Strategic Planning Process for a National Response to HIV/ AIDS: Situation Analysis. UNAIDS, Module 1. UNAIDS/98.19. 32 pages. Sections: Introduction, Responsibilities, The Situation Analysis Process (a steps approach), Next Steps: towards the response analysis, Bibliography.

15. Source of Technical Advice:
Clément Chan Kam, Department of Country Planning and Programme Development, UNAIDS. E-mail: ?
Pierre M'Pele, Strategic Planning for Gaoua District, Burkina Faso, 1998. E-mail: ?

NOTA: The tool may be obtained from the following web address: UNAIDS.ORG/PSR
pointing to "Reform HIV", or available at UNAIDS Information Center, Geneva

16. Tool Summary Description:
Guide to the Strategic Planning Process for a National Response to HIV/ AIDS: Situation Analysis. UNAIDS/98.19, Module 1

The rationale to conduct a complete situation analysis points to the necessity to identify:
- who is vulnerable to HIV/ AIDS and why;
- the most serious obstacles to expanding the response;
- the most promising opportunities for expanding the response.

The overall responsibility in-country to own and carry out the process is described, as well as the ideal composition of the team.

The main phases to conduct the situation analysis's main work are broken down into:
1. Preparatory Work
2. Team Briefing
3. Information Gathering. This key section is well designed and contains the main questions to be asked and answered: guiding principles, main factors determining the spread of HIV and its impact (underlying factors, risk behaviours, epidemiological considerations) and identification of determinants, obstacles, opportunities for priority areas. Topic areas to enquire into are detailed as well: population issues, health issues, social issues, political/ legal/ economic issues, social services, partnerships.
4. Analysis: identified as the most important step in the analysis with the team analysing the response using next the results of this analysis
5. Production of the Report. The section gives a suggested format under the form of Tables which can be used to layout findings (needs, obstacles and opportunities), and a Report Outline
6. Circulation of the Report for Comments and Finalization

Bibliographical References: list of 14 references
M.S., DRS Gaoua, D.S. Gaoua. Plan de Lutte contre le VIH/SIDA et les MST dans le District Sanitaire de Gaoua. (Pierre M'Pele, 1999)

Update of: 11/ 02/1999

1. Tool Category:

Category 1. to conduct a situation analysis (sectorial, community…)

2. Tool Name:

1.2. Guide to the Strategic Planning Process for a National Response to HIV/ AIDS: Response Strategic Plan Formulation. UNAIDS, Module 3

3. **Purpose and Objectives of the Tool:** for UNAIDS country programs, donor agencies, NGOs to conceive a strategic plan or general framework to implement the response, and detailed strategies necessary to change the current situation, and the successive intermediate steps needed to reach stated objectives.

4. Level(s) of Application:

National, Regional/ Provincial, District/ Local

5. Description of Methods:

Document review, field visits with qualitative methods (interviews, group discussion etc.)

6. Contribution to Programme Planning, Monitoring and Evaluation:

Third step of the planning stages, preceding the Resource mobilization (Module 4, Cat. 5, in development), following the Situation Analysis (Module 1, ref. Cat. 1) and Response Analysis (Module 2, ref. Cat. 2). Dissemination of the final strategic plan to all those who have participated in the process, and to everyone interested in the Response or whose partnership is sought.

7. Role in the Determination of Strategies and Interventions:

End-stage of planning with the determination of strategies and interventions, before the Resource Mobilization (Module 4, Cat. 5, in development).

8. Advantages:

Step approach to planning concentrating on the strategic planning process only. Clarifies what is a strategy, and detailed explanation of all the steps necessary to set objectives in priority areas in order in turn to determine the most effective strategies

9. Limitations:

The Strategic Plan Formulation does not address how to develop targets and indicators, workplans with time tables and budgets to operationalize the strategies, or the very last stage of the planning process (ref. may be necessary to other documents such as Logical Framework Planning exercises, or Objectives-Oriented Project Planning…)

10. Primary Users:

The programme managers who implement activities that seek to diminish the spread of HIV and its impact. Reference to everyone seeking to contribute to the Response.

11. Preferred or Suggested Technical Background and Training for Users of Tool:

Strategic Plan Formulation team: solid Government representation, all key stakeholders, if necessary appropriate expertise, team(s) who conducted the situation and response analyses

12. Resources Needed to Apply the Tools:

Time and human resources as per above. Word processing facilities necessary. Meeting space.

13. Used by and Location:

Presently a dozen Ministries in West Africa, and several in the East Africa, Asia, Latin America Regions.

14. Original References:

Guide to the Strategic Planning Process for a National Response to HIV/ AIDS: Strategic Plan Formulation. UNAIDS, Module 3. UNAIDS/98.21. 28 pages. Sections: Responsibilities, Formulation of a Strategic Plan, Producing a Strategic Plan Document, Next Steps: resource mobilization, operational plans, implementation. Bibliography: 7 references.

15. Source of Technical Advice:

Clément Chan Kam, Department of Country Planning and Programme Development, UNAIDS. E-mail: ?
Pierre M'Pele, Strategic Planning for Gaoua District, Burkina Faso, 1998. E-mail: ?

NOTA: The tool may be obtained from the following web address: UNAIDS.ORG/PSR

pointing to "Reform HIV", or available at UNAIDS Information Center, Geneva

16. Tool Summary Description:

Guide to the Strategic Planning Process for a National Response to HIV/ AIDS: Strategic Plan Formulation. UNAIDS/ 98.21, Module 3

The rationale for strategic plan clarifies how the planning process is based on situations which are different according to the population group addressed, and to the changes over time. Strategies are tailored to be flexible enough to adapt to situation changes, based on realistic limited resources, or taking advantage of initiatives developing with built-in resources.

Three possibilities to design the Strategic Plan Formulation, among the multitude existing based on each country administrative structures, are illustrated: national level planning, national priorities with local strategies, and province setting the agenda.

The key section of the Module consists of the Formulation of a Strategic Plan explaining in details the main steps in strategic plan formulation:

1. Re-examine the guiding principles (ref. Policies outlined in the Situation Analysis)
2. Confirm priority areas for a response
3. Set objectives in priority areas
4. Develop strategies to reach objectives in priority areas
5. Develop a strategic framework for the response
6. Examine the strengths and weaknesses of proposed strategies
7. Revise objectives and strategies when necessary
8. Plan flexible management and funding to ensure support for emerging strategies

The steps are illustrated using as an example a "Strategy formulation for one priority area: Reducing HIV transmission among young people." 4 specific objectives and their strategies to achieve those are outlined.

Finally the Module documents how to produce a strategic plan document.

Bibliographical References: list of 7 references

M.S., DRS Gaoua, D.S. Gaoua. Plan de Lutte contre le VIH/SIDA et les MST dans le District Sanitaire de Gaoua. (Pierre M'Pele, 1999)

Update of: 11/ 02/1999

1. Tool Category:

Category 2. Institution's and Sector's Capacity Assessment

2. Tool Name:

2.1. Guide to the Strategic Planning Process for a National Response to HIV/ AIDS: Response Analysis. UNAIDS, Module 2

3. Purpose and Objectives of the Tool: for UNAIDS country programs, donor agencies, NGOs to assess how various Institutions and Sectors are responding to HIV/ AIDS at a national or decentralized level

4. Level(s) of Application:

National, Regional/ Provincial, District/ Local

5. Description of Methods:

Document review, field visits with qualitative methods (interviews, group discussion etc.)

6. Contribution to Programme Planning, Monitoring and Evaluation:

Second step of the planning stages following the Situation Analysis (Module 1, ref. Cat. 1), and followed by the Strategic Plan Formulation (Module 3, ref. Cat. 1). Maximum openness in the dissemination of the report recommended to general population and vulnerable groups and communities: public presentations, simple publications, media releases, posting information on the Internet.

7. Role in the Determination of Strategies and Interventions:

Mid-stage to the determination of strategies and interventions.

8. Advantages:
Step approach to planning concentrating on the response analysis only. Gives good illustrations on how to analyze data to understand better and improve the present response in specific areas.

9. Limitations:
The response analysis is limited to few focus areas only in comparison to the broad spectrum of interventions available for program managers: one on care, one on mitigating the impact, six on prevention, and one on human rights.

10. Primary Users:
The response analysis team supported by a governing (or local) committee, followed by the group who formulates the strategic plan, or in a nutshell, ultimately the national or local planners and managers.

11. Preferred or Suggested Technical Background and Training for Users of Tool:
Multi-disciplinary team, e.g. economist, civil servant, community organizer, anthropologist, private sector market specialist, sociologist... and person(s) living with HIV, preferably same team as the one used for the situation analysis. A one-off exercise of 1 to a few weeks pending upon depth of analysis.

12. Resources Needed to Apply the Tools:
Time and human resources as per above. Cars depending of data collection needs. Word processing facilities necessary.

13. Used by and Location:
Presently a dozen Ministries in West Africa, and several in the East Africa, Asia, Latin America Regions.

14. Original References:
Guide to the Strategic Planning Process for a National Response to HIV/ AIDS: Response Analysis. UNAIDS, Module 2. UNAIDS/98.20. 28 pages. Sections: Responsibilities, Steps for the Response Analysis (from preparatory work to circulating the report for comment and finalize), Next Step towards the strategic plan formulation.
Bibliography: 8 references.

15. Source of Technical Advice:

Clément Chan Kam, Department of Country Planning and Programme Development, UNAIDS. E-mail: ?

Pierre M'Pele, Strategic Planning for Gaoua District, Burkina Faso, 1998. E-mail: ?

NOTA: The tool may be obtained from the following web address: UNAIDS.ORG/PSR

pointing to "Reform HIV", or available at UNAIDS Information Center, Geneva

16. Tool Summary Description:

Guide to the Strategic Planning Process for a National Response to HIV/ AIDS: Response Analysis. UNAIDS/ 98.20, Module 2

Clarification of the difference between a response analysis and a programme review with emphasis in the changing situation, and considering the broader social and economic sectors' contribution.

Identification of the overall responsibility, the response analysis team, and the response analysis governing committee.

Suggested process steps of the response analysis process are outlined:
1. Preparatory work
2. Brief the response analysis team
3. Gather information from documents, interviews and field research
4. Analyse (2 examples: "Expanding the syndromic treatment of STDs in Zimbabwe" and "Reducing HIV transmission among young people")
5. Produce the Report
6. Circulate for comments, finalize

The main questions to be answered (section 3) constitute the main section of the Guide:
a) What is the situation?
b) What is being done to respond to HIV?
c) Is the national response relevant to the current situation?
d) Is the response working in priority areas?
e) Why is a response working or not working?

Bibliographical References: list of 14 references

M.S., DRS Gaoua, D.S. Gaoua. Plan de Lutte contre le VIH/SIDA et les MST dans le District Sanitaire de Gaoua. (Pierre M'Pele, 1999)

Update of: 12/02/1999

1. Tool Category:
Category 3: to assess the existing policies vs. needs and realities

2. Tool Name:
3.1. Decentralization and Health Systems Change: A Framework for Analysis

3. Purpose and Objectives of the Tool:
A framework to systematically review the development and implementation of decentralization policies, and to examine concurrent changes in the health system that may, at least in part, be ascribed to decentralization.

4. Level(s) of Application:
National, Regional/ Provincial, District/ Local through "streams of decentralization," i.e. local governments, different levels and institutions within the Ministry of Health and other relevant Ministries in the context of democratization, social insurance funds, and various provider institutions in the public and private sectors.

5. Description of Methods:
Qualitative and impressionistic rather than quantitative and factual. Rapid rather than exhaustive assessment. Literature review, routine health information system and/ or special existing studies, semi-structured questionnaires of key informants and focus group discussions with various representatives (national, district, sub-district and health units).

6. Contribution to Programme Planning, Monitoring and Evaluation:
The tool can be applied for programme planning, or monitoring, or evaluation:
- for planning: to focus in the "Situation Analysis" (UNAIDS, Guide to the Strategic Planning Process for a National Response to HIV/ AIDS, Module 1) in the political and legal and partnership issues and identify needs, obstacles, and opportunities
- for monitoring: to consider variables to be monitored for prospective study of the effects of decentralization
- for evaluation: for a retrospective analysis to study the effects of decentralization on equity, efficiency and quality

Dissemination recommended as per Strategic Planning Process (UNAIDS) to all those who have participated in the process, and to everyone interested in the

Response or whose partnership is sought. 2-3 days Workshop suggested for feedback.

7. Role in the Determination of Strategies and Interventions:

The tool allows to understand the environment in which the strategies and interventions for a response to HIV/ AIDS takes place, and be able too understand better the policy needs, or to take advantage of the opportunities, or to overcome the obstacles.

8. Advantages:

The tool is structured in a "Framework for Analysis" which is a stepwise approach that can be used based on the different stages of decentralization the country has reached: 1) Countries in which decentralization has been in place for some time: analysis of structure and functions, 2) Countries at mid-stage of decentralization: analysis of organsational structures and processes, 3) Countries with mature stage of decentralization: analysis of equity, efficiency, and quality.

9. Limitations:

Long term processes with important contextual enabling or disabling factors over which HIV/ AIDS response has little or no control. Difficulty in the case of countries in the mature stage to choose among the 27 facettes of the framework which ones to use.

10. Primary Users: the national or local authorities to take action or catalyze some of the processes.

11. Preferred or Suggested Technical Background and Training for Users of Tool:

Policy implementers, Consultants or Academicians or Social Scientists (e.g. Economists, Sociologists…) from University setting

The tool is not planned to be disseminated and replicated through training exercises but national or local policy-makers involved in the use of the tool will definitely learn and benefit from the process as well as feel more committed to the long-term processes.

12. Resources Needed to Apply the Tools

Team of 2 to 4 people. Other resources (time, vehicles …): unknown

13. Used by and Location:

27 countries in the mid-nineties from Africa, Latin America, Asia and Europe in a global comparative project aiming to establish generalizable links between decentralization and changes in health systems in different countries.

14. Original References:

"Decentralization and Health Systems Change: A Framework for Analysis" Revised Working Document WHO/SHS/NHP/95.2, March 1995 (26 pages) Sources for availability: ref. Web site or WHO/ SHS

15. Source of Technical Advice:

Name and e-mail or other contacts for technical purposes:

Katja Janovsky, WHO: email:

Andrew Creese, WHO: email

Phyllida Travis, WHO: email

NOTA: The tool may be obtained from the following web address: UNAIDS.ORG/PSR

pointing to "Reform HIV"

16. Tool Summary Description:

5 Components of the following Table

Decentralization and Health Systems Change

Framework for Analysis: Overview

(to insert Table p. 3)

Bibliography:

WHO/ARA/CC/97.3. Barbara McPake and Joseph Kutzin. "Methods for Evaluating Effects of Health Reforms" Div. of Analysis, Research and Assessment. Current Concerns ARA Paper number 13

WHO/ARA/CC/97.6. Sara Bennett, Ellias Ngalande-Banda, with annotated bibliography by Ole Teglgaard. "Public and Private Roles in Health. A Review and Analysis of Experience in sub-Saharan Africa." Current Concerns ARA Paper number 6

WHO. Health System Decentralization in Africa: An Overview of Experiences in Eight Countries" (Botswana, Burkina Faso, Ghana, Kenya, Mali, South Africa, Uganda, Zambia) Background Document Prepared for the Regional Meeting on Decentralization in the Context of Health Sector Reform in Africa, no date

Update of: 16/02/1999

1. Tool Category:

Category 4. to calculate intervention costs

6.

2. Tool Name:

4.1. Costs of district AIDS programmes

3. Purpose and Objectives of the Tool: To compare the costs and benefits of different interventions and their relative costs in relation to their effectiveness, in order to set priorities based on the resources available

4. Level(s) of Application:

Regional/ Provincial, District/ Local, Communities

5. Description of Methods:

Costs estimation per year of HIV prevention and AIDS care

6. Contribution to Programme Planning, Monitoring and Evaluation:

The tool allows to determine priorities to plan which interventions to prioritize in relation to funding levels, and assess the necessary additional efforts to be made to attract additional funding (ref. category 5 Resource Mobilization). Information can be shared and discussed with the participants of the strategic planning workshop.

7. Role in the Determination of Strategies and Interventions:

The tool allows to prioritize which interventions are the most cost-effective, and give tips on how to reduce costs under limited resources (focus on high transmission areas, including vulnerable populations, STD management services etc.)

8. Advantages:

Comparative costs and benefits with assessment of effectiveness for 8 preventive, 2 both preventive and curative, and 2 curative interventions.

9. Limitations:

Costs estimated for a population of 300,000, including 125,000 adults/ adolescents and an estimated 100,000 sexually active individuals with an HIV prevalence of 5% to 10%: needs to be adapted to the local situation

10. Primary Users:
Program planners and managers at the local level

11. Preferred or Suggested Technical Background and Training for Users of Tool:
Economic or accounting background. No time assessed to train the users in the application of the tool.

12. Resources Needed to Apply the Tools:
No resources estimated.

13. Used by and Location:
Institutional: TANESA Project, Mwanza Region, Tanzania

14. Original References:
"Costs of district AIDS programmes" Ties Boerma and Japheth Ng'weshemi, in HIV prevention and AIDS care in Africa. A district level approach. Japhet Ng'weshemi et al. Ed. Royal Tropical Institute-The Netherlands 1997, pp. 353-370

15. Source of Technical Advice:
Ties Boerma e-mail:
John Bennett e-mail:
NOTA: The tool may be obtained from the following web address: UNAIDS.ORG/PSR
pointing to "Reform HIV"

16. Tool Summary Description:
The tool estimates the costs of HIV prevention and AIDS care for:
1) Preventive interventions:
- promotion of safer sexual behaviours: general population
- promotion of safer sexual behaviours: youth
- promotion of safer sexual behaviours: high-transmission areas
- STD control: general population
- STD control: core groups
- condom promotion and distribution
- reduction of HIV transmission through blood transfusions
- reduction of HIV transmission through injections
2) Preventive and curative interventions:

- AIDS care: training of health workers
- counseling

3) Curative interventions:
- care for AIDS patients
- survivor assistance

Comparing interventions for a comprehensive HIV intervention programme covering the whole district with 300,000 people (5-10% HIV prevalence) with STD control, intensive health education, youth activities, condom promotion and distribution, training of health workers, and a safe blood supply, amounts to US$ 350,000 or US$ 1.16 per person ($3.50 per sexually active adult), excluding capital costs or most government or other staff salaries.

An estimated US$ 200,000-300,000 per year may be needed for basic care of AIDS patients, including a home-based care programme and a fund for survivor assistance, or US$ 1 per capita per year, or US$ 3 per adult.

Based on 5 different categories of resources available from very limited (US$ 25,000) to high (US$ 300,000), a Table illustrates in a useful manner for program managers the different options available for district AIDS programmes at different funding levels for the example of that district.

Bibliographical References:
WHO. The costs of HIV/ AIDS prevention strategies in developing countries. WHO/GPA/DIR/93.2. Geneva, 1993.
WHO. Provision of HIV/ AIDS care in resource constrained settings. Geneva. n.d.
The hidden cost of AIDS: the challenge of HIV to development. The Panos Institute. London. 1992
Soderlund N. et al. The costs of HIV prevention strategies in developing countries. Bulletin of the WHO 1993, 71: 595-604.

Update of: 19/ 02/1999

1. Tool Category:

Category 5. to mobilise resources

2. Tool Name:

5.1. "Resource Mobilization and Allocation" in the District Response Initiative on HIV/ AIDS Ghana Case-Study

3. Purpose and Objectives of the Tool:

To broader the spectrum of HIV/ AIDS activities from a vertical health sector focused approach towards an integrated multisectoral and development-oriented approach with the following objectives:

a) Review the policy and organisational environment within participating countries and their districts

b) Review responses to HIV/ AIDS and relevant social sector experiences

c) Advice on districts' responses to HIV/ AIDS

d) Development assessment tools to assist districts and communities to determine options for social and developmental challenges including HIV/ AIDS

e) Develop a framework that will take districts through a capacity-building process, to ensure greater intersectoral problem identification and problem-solving.

4. Level(s) of Application:

Three-tier nature of the system in Ghana surveyed: National, Regional/ Provincial, District/ Local

5. Description of Methods:

Documents and Reports review, interviews

6. Contribution to Programme Planning, Monitoring and Evaluation:

The main conclusions and recommendations of the Study address planning issues to improve not only resource allocation, but also other important areas such as how to influence policy-making, to strengthen intersectoral collaboration, to address district capacity issues, and to promote opportunities for the District Response Initiative.

Feedback through debriefing sessions with the central administration of the district assemblies and group discussions at area council or community levels. Discussion at the national level, debriefing meeting with the national Multisectoral Taskforce.

7. Role in the Determination of Strategies and Interventions:
The tool gives general orientations to determine strategies useful at the national level (Ministries, Donors/ NGOs), and key Regional and District partners. Identified more attention to be paid to interventions for the promotion of attitude and behaviour changes.

8. Advantages:
Allows to capture quickly and comprehensively the national, regional, and district levels for some of the key issues to expand the response to HIV/ AIDS

9. Limitations:
Tool does not include the interviews schedules. No thorough review of the community needs.

10. Primary Users:
Decision-makers at the different levels of the system

11. Preferred or Suggested Technical Background and Training for Users of Tool:
5 consultants with the following overlapping expertise: public health physician, health economist, development planner, HIV/ AIDS specialist, demographers, home-based care specialist, social anthropologist, health systems analyst, manpower planner
Users: not trained (consultants)

12. Resources Needed to Apply the Tools:
Time, human resources, cars, computers: not specified

13. Used by and Location:
Institutional: Ministry of Health in Ghana and UNAIDS
National and Regional levels, including Wenchi, Adansi West, and Fanteakwa Districts

14. Original References:

"Resource Mobilization and Allocation" in the District Response Initiative on HIV/ AIDS Ghana Case-Study, November 1997 (43 pages)

Sources for availability (ref. ordering through UNAIDS or JSA Consultants Ltd., P.O.Box A408, La-Accra, Ghana, or Web-site address below)

15. Source of Technical Advice:

Joe Annan, e-mail:

NOTA: The tool may be obtained from the following web address: UNAIDS.ORG/PSR

pointing to "Reform HIV"

16. Tool Summary Description:

Broad review of the key institutional reform and decentralisation

Findings:

- national policies and strategies
- donor/ NGO findings
- regional level assessment
- mapping of institutional authority and resource allocation

Three District Case-Studies and comparative analysis of district findings

Discussion of the Expanded Response by national, regional and district levels, with additional aspects related to interventions and participation

Conclusions and Recommendations for: resource allocation, policy-making, intersectoral collaboration, district capacity issues, and opportunities to promote the District Response Initiative.

Update of: **18/ 02/1999**

1. Tool Category:

Category 6. to monitor and evaluate the program

7.

2. Tool Name:

6.2.Using a Simplified Tool: A Monitoring Tool for Assessing, Analyzing and Improving the Health Sector Response to HIV/ AIDS

3. Purpose and Objectives of the Tool:
The tool aims to assess, analyze, and consequently design and take actions both for management (local level) and reform (local and national) purposes.

4. Level(s) of Application:
Regional/ Provincial, including District/ Local and Communities, with a total of about 500,000 population

5. Description of Methods:
Rapid assessment methods with focus groups, interviews, reviews of local data

6. Contribution to Programme Planning, Monitoring and Evaluation:
The tool is used for planning and monitoring the implementation of the District Response to HIV/ AIDS. Results are fedback to the informants of community organization, associations, and representatives of staff from health center, and district level by including them in the local analysis of data and problems, and the elaboration of actions to solve problems identified, and the synthesis of experiences, and elaboration of recommendations for Reform.

7. Role in the Determination of Strategies and Interventions:
The tool is geared to identify the necessary interventions/ actions that are relevant at different levels: individual and household, community organizations and associations, health system and services, and policy.

8. Advantages:
The tool provides a number of grids and examples of problem-solving frameworks, and indicators for planning and monitoring for key preventive and curative and sustainable interventions which can be adapted to a local situation.
Detailed background information on the Health Care Reform and HIV provided (original ref. pp. 1-34), including two examples form Thailand and Côte d'Ivoire of "packages of interventions" offered at community, sub-district, and district levels.

9. Limitations:
The process of adapting the tool to the local situation may be difficult for local managers if not assisted by a multi-disciplinary skilled team (e.g. economists, policy analysts, community specialists with experience in qualitative methods etc.)

10. Primary Users:
Regional and District health managers

11. Preferred or Suggested Technical Background and Training for Users of Tool:
Program managers (taking into consideration the limitations identified in sect. 9)
Time requested for training the user(s): twice, three days

12. Resources Needed to Apply the Tools:
2 months plus a preliminary step of 1 week or 2 to adapt the tool.
Human resources, cars, computers: no indication

13. Used by and Location:
In Phayao District, Thailand by the Office of Health Care Reform-AIDS Division and Ministry of Public Health Thailand and UNAIDS

14. Original References:
"Using a Simplified Tool: A Monitoring Tool for Assessing, Analyzing and Improving the Health Sector Response to HIV/ AIDS," in HIV and Health Care Reform: Making Health Care Systems Respond Effectively to HIV and AIDS. A Tool for Local Assessment, Analysis and Action by and for Peripheral Managers and Communities, March 1 1998 Agnès Soucat with inputs of J.L. Lamboray, P. Jongudomsuk, P. Daveloose, R. Msiska, W. Sittitri, A. Tanbanjong. Office of Health Care Reform-AIDS Division and Ministry of Public Health Thailand, UNAIDS (pp. 1-34: background information, pp. 35 to 55: tool)

Sources for availability (ref. ordering through UNAIDS or Web-site address below …)

15. Source of Technical Advice:
Agnès Soucat, UNAIDS, Thailand, e-mail:
Jean-Louis Lamboray, UNAIDS, Geneva, e-mail:
NOTA: The tool may be obtained from the following web address: UNAIDS.ORG/PSR
pointing to "Reform HIV"

16. Tool Summary Description:
1) Analysis of Response for community-based monitoring and planning at individual and household level:

Knowledge, skills, attitude and behavioral change by General population and Specific groups, General population and Families of HIV+people, and pregnant women

Problem-Solving Framework for Behavioral Change: Example of IEC for Safe Sexual Behavior

2) Analysis of Response for community organizations and associations or interface level:

Life Skills Training and Condom Distribution, Psychological and Social Support, Home-Caring Support, Co-management of health services, Community-Based Problem-Solving and Planning looking at various stages or determinants (equity, autonomy, quality, continuity, utilization, access, availability of resources, target population).

Problem-Solving Framework for Analyzing the Response at the interface level: example of life-skills training and condom distribution

3) Analysis of Response for health system and services:

Conceptual Framework for Monitoring the Production of Sustained Health Outcomes

Conceptual Framework for the Production of Sustained Response

Indicators for Planning and Monitoring the Implementation of the Process of Production of Sustained Outcomes to address the HIV Epidemic in the Health Care System. Example of Effectiveness Indicators.

Example of necessary conditions to be fulfilled to ensure final effective coverage with prevention of vertical transmission, monitoring and the three phases of the intervention: screen, treat, care.

Indicators for Planning and Monitoring the Implementation of the Process of Production of Sustained Outcomes to address the HIV Epidemic in the Health Care System. Example of Effectiveness Indicators for Curative Interventions.

Indicators for Planning and Monitoring the Implementation of the Process of Production of Sustained Outcomes to address the HIV Epidemic in the Health Care System: Coverage, Cost, and Funding

4) Analysis of Response for policy:

Policy Monitoring Framework

Problem-Solving Framework for Analysis of Management and Policy Factors affecting Effectiveness, Efficiency, and Financial Viability at Health Center level, Management Factors: Policy Factors

Example of Corrective Management Actions to improve Effective Coverage, Efficiency, and Financial Viability of the Health Sector Response to HIV/ AIDS Matrix for Monitoring the Cost and Funding Issues on the Policy Response to HIV/ AIDS

Additional information:
- 2 months schedule of the activities, duration and actors to be involved in the Assessment, Analysis and Feedback of the Health Sector Response to HIV/ AIDS.
- Methods of data collection and list of informants, and list of questionnaires to be developed.

Fourteen References on the subject, including:
Lamboray J.L., "Can we develop a common framework for analysis and action?" South East Asian J. Trop. Med. Public Health. Vol. 27, no. 2, Jun. 1996
Mills A., "Current Policy Issues in Health Care Reform from an international perspective: the battle between bureaucrats and marketers in Health Care Reform: at the frontier of Research and Policy Decisions"

APPENDIX 5F: A Tool for Partnerships and Consensus Building at the Local Level

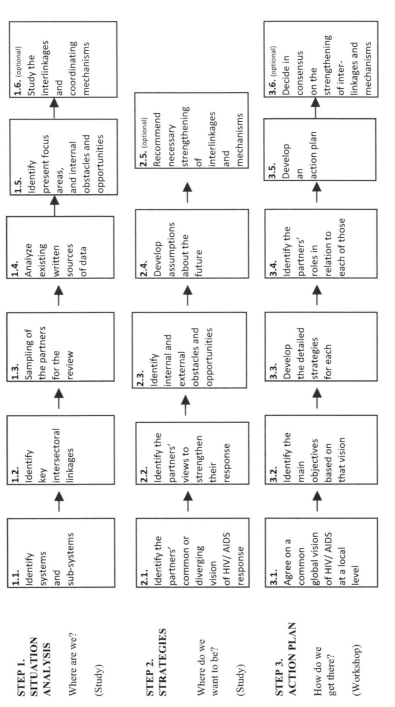

**STEP 1.
SITUATION
ANALYSIS**

Where are we?

(Study)

| 1.1. Identify systems and sub-systems | → | 1.2. Identify key intersectoral linkages | → | 1.3. Sampling of the partners for the review | → | 1.4. Analyze existing written sources of data | → | 1.5. Identify present focus areas, and internal obstacles and opportunities | → | 1.6. (optional) Study the interlinkages and coordinating mechanisms |

**STEP 2.
STRATEGIES**

Where do we want to be?

(Study)

| 2.1. Identify the partners' common or diverging vision of HIV/ AIDS response | → | 2.2. Identify the partners' views to strengthen their response | → | 2.3. Identify internal and external obstacles and opportunities | → | 2.4. Develop assumptions about the future | → | 2.5. (optional) Recommend necessary strengthening of interlinkages and mechanisms |

**STEP 3.
ACTION PLAN**

How do we get there?

(Workshop)

| 3.1. Agree on a common global vision of HIV/ AIDS at a local level | → | 3.2. Identify the main objectives based on that vision | → | 3.3. Develop the detailed strategies for each | → | 3.4. Identify the partners' roles in relation to each of those | → | 3.5. Develop an action plan | → | 3.6. (optional) Decide in consensus on the strengthening of inter-linkages and mechanisms |

445

APPENDIX 5G

Introduction Sheet to the Rapid Organizational Review (ROR) tool

for the HIV/ AIDS District expanded Response Initiative (DRI)

(\RORDRITOOL.doc)

Purpose:

The Rapid Organizational Review (ROR) tool to be used during –but not limited to-- the planning stages of a program aims to contribute to a situation analysis of the effectiveness and efficiency of organizations functioning at the local level as partners for the HIV/ AIDS District expanded Response Initiative (DRI), and on the long term to improve their inputs and to monitor and evaluate their progresses.

Description:

The Rapid Organizational Review (ROR) tool assists the District or local level managers to review rapidly in one particular aspect --the organizational one-- of the situation analysis some of the key organizations from the public and the private sectors, including communities, which are present or can be future potential partners in HIV/ AIDS activities by:

- first, carrying an inventory,
- second, mapping these organizations into active or not, and for those active (if possible) estimate how much,
- third, appraising their present capacities and limitations,
- finally, defining better their roles in relation to the information collected and the future needs for planning purposes.

Developed by:

Cyril Pervilhac

Users:

- District Health Management Team

- District Project Planning Teams

- District Monitoring and/ or Evaluation Teams

Application:

Ministry of Health-German Technical Cooperation (GTZ) Projects in the UNAIDS-WHO-GTZ collaborative efforts in the planning stage of the DRI:

- Gaoua District, Burkina Faso

- Kabarole District, Uganda

Advantages:

- Rapid Assessment Procedures (RAP) approach with existing qualitative methods

- Focus possible on the public, or private (NGOs), or communities (CBOs), or a mix of those as needed

- Option to understand in more details the intersectoral linkages and multisectoral approaches

- Looking more at why and how much the response (process oriented) is occurring and sustained rather than considering only outputs and outcome

- Collection of data feasible with a team of 2-4 maximum in 5-10 days

- Data analysis feasible in 2-3 weeks maximum

- Use as organizational/ institutional baseline possible

- No particular software or special skills needed

- Method to look at "Partnerships" as one of the "Topic areas for enquiry" (UNAIDS, "Guide to the strategic planning process for a national response to HIV/ AIDS Situation Analysis", 98.19), with the "Response Analysis" (UNAIDS, 98.20) at the district level

Limitations:

- Difficulties to collect data related to finances at a local level (sensitive)

- Answers are soft data, difficult to verify or cross-check,

- Difficulties to distinguish in the answers between present and future, real activities and planned one

- Users need minimum interest and curiosity in social sciences and the methods used

- Policy analysis not included in this tool (ref. to other tools, e.g. *"PolicyMaker"* by Michael R. Reich, Harvard SPH, or Joe Annan, Ghana DRI Case-Study Report, 1997, JSA Consultants Ltd.), but possible through the district level data collection

- Community participation not included in this tool (ref. to other tool, G. Bjaras et al., 1991), the survey at the community level can combine these data collection as well

- No magic bullet approach or solution, but part of a planning process with emphasis on organizations and institutions, or the local partners

Recommendations for Users:

- Should be familiar with qualitative methods and techniques (group discussion, focus groups, key informants…)

- Adapt the tool and matrices, develop questions and pre-test for first time use in a country, preferably with the expertise of a social scientist (sociologist…)

- Accompany the review team for the first rounds to make sure questions are consistent

- Use if possible a team which collect data as impartially and objectively as possible (i.e. not the DMO, or an influential person), for example a retired instructor or nurse etc.

- Analyze the data immediately following the survey, and if possible on the spot

- Use a brief (2-3 days) planning/ consensus workshop at the local level for feedback and applications of findings

- The ROR exercise can be a useful local preparation or preliminary step to a broader Objectives Oriented Project Planning (ZOPP)

Report Attached:

- Roger Salla et al., "Handout Supplement" of the "District Response Initiative (DRI): Fostering Partnership in HIV/ AIDS Control. Situation Analysis in Burkina Faso." Poster Presentation. 12th World AIDS Conference, Geneva.

Reports and Publications:

- C. Pervilhac, Rapport Initiative ONUSIDA/ OMS/ GTZ de Riposte Elargie au Niveau du District. Etude de Cas du Burkina Faso. 1997. GTZ: Eschborn.

- C. Pervilhac, W. Kipp, and D. Babikwa, Report on the UNAIDS/ WHO/ GTZ Initiative of the expanded District Response Initiative. Case-Study from Uganda. 1997. GTZ. Eschborn.

- C. Pervilhac, "Rapport de Synthèse de l'Atelier sur l'Initiative de la Réponse Elargie au VIH/ SIDA: District de Gaoua, Burkina Faso." GTZ. Eschborn.1998.

- Joe Annan, DRI Tools ?, Accra. 1998.

- C. Pervilhac et al., "Handout Supplement" of the "District Response Initiative (DRI): Missing Link in HIV/ AIDS Control. A Situation Analysis in Uganda. Poster Presentation. 12th World AIDS Conference, Geneva.

Background Publications:

- UNAIDS Best Practice Collection, "Expanding the global response to HIV/ AIDS through focused action" UNAIDS/ 98.1

- Soucat Agnès, "HIV and Health Care Reform: Making Health Care Systems Respond Effectively to HIV and AIDS. A tool for local assessment, analysis and action by and for peripheral managers and communities. Office of Health Care Reform-AIDS Division, Ministry of Public Health Thailand-UNAIDS. March 1, 1998.

- Bjaras G., B. Haglund, S. Rifkin, "A new approach to community participation assessment", Health Promotion International, 6, 3, 1991, pp. 199-206.

- Reich M., "*PolicyMaker*" Political Mapping of Health Policy. A Guide for Managing the Political Dimensions of Health Policy," Harvards SPH, 1994, at web site: //www.polimap.com/pmintro.html

Languages:

English

Instrument:

The three steps of the Rapid Organizational Review (ROR)

ROR guides you through three steps of applied organizational analysis for strengthening and building partnerships at a district/ local level to generate strategies and plans tailored to the local needs and possibilities. The present illustrations are coming from the Case-Study of Gaoua District, Burkina-Faso. (ref. Report Attached)

The three steps correspond to, the normal stages of any planning strategy, and therefore complement those. It is designed to improve the understanding and functions of the various partners, e.g. organizations, with a sequential analysis, and accompanying visualization (illustrations) through three steps:

- Step 1: Situation Analysis
Where are we: who is doing what at the present time?

- Step 2: Strategies
Where do we want to be: who is willing to contribute to what, and how in the

future?

- Step 3: Action Plan
How do we get there: what is the consensus and what is the plan?

Each step and their detailed sequences can be illustrated under the form of a path analysis as per attached "***Rapid Organizational Review (ROR): Building the Organizational Plan***" scheme, and summarized with an overview as follow. Each step and their detailed sequences are explained in the last section, **Users' Guide**. (Appendix 6H)

APPENDIX 5H

Users' Guide to the Rapid Organizational Review (ROR) Tool

(\RORUSERSGUIDE.doc)

A full detailed guide of the various steps and sequences of each sub-category follows.

STEP 1: SITUATION ANALYSIS

Where are we: who is doing what at the present time?

Illustration: *Model of the District and Communities Systems*

1.1. Identify and define the various systems and sub-systems (inputs and processes) in the program cycle (inputs, process, outputs, and outcome), as well as the main strategies existing presently.

Rationale: Inventory taking and categorization. Moving the thinking early on in the planning stages from individual focus to broader groups, e.g. communities and organizations, and visualizing the process. Distinguishing and categorizing 3 key systems at the local level, and their actors (sub-systems): the public sector (including projects contracted with a Ministerial bi-lateral Government agreement), the private sector, and the communities placing the latter at the center of the overall system.

1.2. Identify the key intersectoral linkages, and illustrate the main ones: first, within or between the public sector partners (with health, or between other Departments), second, between the partners of the public and private sectors, third, between the Communities and the partners of either sector. Identify the key intra-sectoral linkages within the Ministry of Health (between Departments or sections).

Rationale: Identification of relationships, and/ or of coordinating mechanisms existing or needed.

1.3. Sampling of the partners for the review: an equal sample of approximate a dozen partners from the public and a dozen from the private, including at the community level, sectors.

Rationale: This sample size allows to have a full picture of the public sector (i.e. to sample all or the large majority of the public sectors which work or can work in HIV/ AIDS activities), and sufficient numbers of different types of organizations from the private sector, including at the community level (4 communities). As aggregate data, the reviewers can understand as a whole the activities in the public, in the private sectors, including at the community level.

1.4. Analyze existing written sources of data from the various partners.

1.5. Identify the present focus areas (strategies, interventions) for each partner. Identify internal issues (population, health, social political and legal and economic and social and partnerships in "Situation Analysis" UNAIDS 1998, pp. 15-25), and some of the main factors which are predisposing to the risk and vulnerability of infections (epidemiologic and demographic factors, support services factors, political and cultural factors, social and economic factors) (GPA 1995, p. 25 and UNAIDS, A Guide for Strategic Planning Process, Working Vers. Draft 3, 16 Apr. 1997, p. 5-7) and hence identify as a consequence the opportunities for the present activities.

1.6. Study of the interlinkages and coordinating mechanisms (optional): finally, as an option, in addition to the individual interlinkages, the global coordinating mechanisms between the three systems necessary to strengthen the partnerships, are reviewed.

Rationale: for more mature programs where decentralization is already advanced down to the communities' level (e.g. Uganda)

STEP 2: STRATEGIES

Where do we want to be: who is willing to contribute to what, and how in the future?

Illustration: *Institutional Landscape of the Partners from the Public and Private Sectors (present situation or organizational baseline)*

2.1. Identify the partners' common or diverging global vision of HIV/ AIDS response at a local level

2.2. Identify how the partners envision to strengthen their response in the focus area(s) they are presently involved in, and how much? The same, in another new area of need?

2.3. Identify internal obstacles or organizational factors of contstraints (experiences, competencies, didactic and other materials, financial means, specific present activities, population mobilization…) and external obstacles ("super-structural factors" or background and environmental factors which neither individuals nor governments can change in the short or medium term, ref. UNAIDS A Guide for Strategic Planning Process, Working Vers. Draft 3, 16 Apr. 1997, p. 5-7), and opportunities for the future activities

2.4. Develop assumptions about the future

2.5. Recommend necessary strengthening of interlinkages and mechanisms to facilitate those (optional)

STEP 3: ACTION PLAN

How do we get there: what is the consensus and what is the plan?

Illustrations:

Institutional Landscape of the Partners from the Public and Private Sectors (future situation)

Planning and Consensus Synthesis Matrix by Objectives and Inputs

(temporary version in French, to be translated)

3.1. Agree on a common global vision of HIV/ AIDS at a local level

3.2. Identify the main objectives based on that vision

3.3. Develop the detailed strategies for each

3.4. Identify the partners' roles in relation to each of those (ref. Strategies 2.2)

3.5. Develop an action plan (priorities and calendar of implementation)

3.6. Decide in consensus on the strengthening of interlinkages and mechanisms to facilitate those (optional)

APPENDIX 6A

SYNTHESIS TABLE

TABLEAU DE SYNTHESE (PLANIFICATION ET CONSENSUS) DES 5 OBJECTIFS PRIORITAIRES DE LA REPONSE ELARGIE AU VIH/ SIDA1998-2000/ 2003:

DISTRICT DE GAOUA, BURKINA FASO

Chaque représentant d'une institution ou organisation, devait pour chaque objectif prioritaire, stratégie et intervention définir son apport en terme de:

1 - Apport d'expériences

2 - Apport de compétences (ressources humaines qualifiées et disponibles)

3 - Apport de moyens didactiques

4 - Apport de moyens matériels

5 - Apport de moyens financiers

6 - Mise en oeuvre d'une stratégie ou intervention déjà planifiée.

7 - Appui dans la mobilisation des populations

Tableau de synthèse de l'objectif prioritaire 1

OBJECTIF PRIORITAIRE 1	Intervenants (objectifs1)			
La prevention de l'infection VIH dans les groupes cibles est assurée	ONUSIDA 5 PROMACO 1,2,3,4, 6		GTZ 1,2 CNLS 2,3,4,6	
Stratégies Objectifs 1	Intervenants (Stratégies Objectifs 1)			
Promouvoir l'adoption de comportement sexuel Sûrs chez les jeunes de moins de 35 et les femmes en âge de procéer Promouvoir les comportements sexuels sûrs au sein des jeunes et des migrants	CNLS 4,2		GTZ 1,2,3,6	
Rendre disponibles les préservatifs dans la communauté Impliquer les personnes vivant avec le VIH dans les activités IEC et conseils (témoignage)	GTZ/PPF 6	ECD/FS 6	PROMACO 6	PIB 6
Education des jeunes par des jeunes	Croix rouge 1,2,7 Jeunesse sport 7	PIB 4-6	Coeur vaillants 7 Scouts 1,7,2	
Education des femmes par des femmes (groupements association	Scouts 7	ABBEF 1,2,7	APFG 1,2,7	

NB: Les mots ou sigles soulignés désignent le chef de file de la stratégie ou de l'intervention.

Les chiffres au bas ou à côté des mots ou sigles indiquent le domaine dans lequel le partenaire peut s'engager. Par exemple l'ONU/SIDA se propose d'intervenir pour le financement (5) de l'objectif prioritaire 1.

Par contre pour le même objectif prioritaire la GTZ apportera de l'expérience (1) et des compétences (2).

Tableau de synthèse de l'objectif prioritaire 1 (suite et fin)

Interventions sur l'objectif prioritaire 1	Intervenants / Objectifs

Poursuivre la sensibilisation sur les moyens de protection contre l'infection du VIH/SIDA	Agri Resp. Sect3 Commun.,Cath. Scouts
	7 7 Mobilisation 2-7
	                7
	
	Pénitencier APFG RG Enseig. Sécon.
	7 1 7 2
	
	PIB APASP APHPG APFG
	1,3,5,6,2 7,6 7 6
	
	+ rouge Prefet ECD enseig.
	Prim.
	7 7 (Stand Santé) 2
	                    6
	
	<u>CRESA/DRS</u> ATEFO FILPAH
	Jeu. Sport
	   1,2 6,7,2 2
	7
	
	PROMACO Resp musul. ABBEF
	Action social
	   6 7 2,7
	6

Informer les populations sur les voies de transmission du VIH dans leur milieu	PIB <u>R.G</u> GTZ/PPF 2,1,6,5 4,7+1 3 Assoc.pr Epanuis- ECD/PF APFG sement enfance au 1,3,4 2 Poni 7 Scouts trpe théat. + rouge

	1,7	7	2,1

Encourager la population à faire le test	CHR SCOUT APASP Trpe Théat. 2,6 2 7 2 Club Unesco R.G Action sociale 7 2 6
Les jeunes et les migrants sont informés sur les voies de transmission du VIH/SIDA en leur milieu	Préfet R.G 7 4+7-1 Jeunesse et sport PIB 7 3,5,6

Tableau de synthèse de l'objectif prioritaire 2

Objectif prioritaire 2	Intervenant Objectifs (priorité) 2		
La participation multi sectorielle et communautaire est assurée	CNLS 1		GTZ 1,2,4,5,6
	processus de reponse élargie		Accompagnement du
	ONUSIDA 5		PSD 2
Stratégies sur l'objectif prioritaire 2	Intervenants strategies/objectif 2		
Les ONG et les agents techniques travaillent en collaboration avec la communauté			
Impliquer l'ensemble des secteurs de développement à la lutte contre le SIDA	ECD 6		
Intervention sur l'objectif prioritaire 2	Intervenants		
Améliorer la communication entre les secteurs en vue de la lutte contre le VIH/SIDA	PIB 2-6		
Evaluer le niveau des interventions dans la lutte contre le VIH/SIDA	CRESA/DRS Appui 1-6	PSD 2	
Impliquer les responsables politico-administratifs dans l'encadrement des intervenants			
Mettre en place dans le District un organe efficace multisectoriel et communautaire de coordination des interventions de lutte contre le VIH/SIDA			

Tableau de synthèse de l'objectif prioritaire 3

Objectif prioritaire 3	Intervenant Objectifs 3			
Les soins et les conseils en matière de MST/SIDA sont assurés (FS et communauté)	GTZ 1,2,3,6	ECD 2,3		
	ONUSIDA 5	CNLS 1;5		
Stratégies sur l'objectif prioritaire 3	Interveants			
Responsabiliser la médecine traditionnelle	Préfet 2;7	mairie 4,7		
Former le personnel de santé sur la prise en charge des patients MST/SIDA	P I B 5	ECD 2;3		
Former les agents d'animation aux techniques de counselling pour la prise en charge	P I B 5	Action sociale 2	ECD 2;3	
Former le personnel de santé en counselling pour la prise en charge	P I B 6	ECD 2;3		
Assurer une surveillance chez les enfants nés de mères seropositives	Action Sociale 2	CHR 1,2		

Interventions sur objectif prioritaire 3	**Intervenants**
Améliorer les compétences des agents de santé sur la prise en charge des MST/SIDA Rendre disponible le test VIH	N E A N T

Tableau de synthèse de l'objectif prioritaire 4

Objectif prioritaire 4	Intervenants objectif 4			
Le SIDA est ressenti comme priorité par les groupes cibles (importance, gravité, comportements à risque)	GTZ 1,2,4	PROMACO 6	CNLS 2,3	
	ONUSIDA 5	ECD/CHR 6		
Stratégies sur objectif prioritaire 4	Intervenants stratégie/objectif			
Informations des personnes ressources sur le VIH				
Mise à jour et diffusion régulières sur l'évolution de la prévalence VIH/SIDA et de ses conséquences	ABBEF 1-7	Mairie 4 7	Scouts 7-1	Préfet 7
renforcement des capacités de l'IEC d'exposer le problème du VIH/SIDA	Trpe théat. 1	APASP 7	Action sociale 2	
Interventions sur objectif 4	Intervenants			
Mettre en place un mécanisme de coordination entre ECD et secteur Privé pour un plaidoyer VIH/SIDA				

Tableau de synthèse de l'objectif prioritaire 5

Objectif prioritaire 5	Intervenants sur objectifs 5		
L'impact socio-économique du SIDA et des MST est réduit dans le District	ONUSIDA 5	CNLS 2	GTZ 1,2,3,6
Stratégies sur objectif 5	Intervenants		
Développer des stratégies pour favoriser un comportement social qui démystifie le SIDA			
Promouvoir des activités pour reduire les conséquences socio-economiques du VIH/SIDA	NEANT		
Mettre en place une stratégie de suivi et de prise en charge des enfants orphelins du SIDA			
Interventions sur objectif prioritaire 5	Intervenants		
Apporter un soutien social aux personnes atteintes, leurs familles	Act. sociale 2	APASP 7	Eglise catholi. 4
IEC sur la séropositivité			ECD (Ajout santé) 6
IEC MST pour population	PROMACO 1,2,6		
Appuyer les activités génératrices de revenus pour les familles affectées par le VIH			

HIV Prevention in Europe.

A review of Policy and Practice in Europe.

Caren Weilandt (WIAD)
Cyril Pervilhac (WIAD)
Wolfgang Heckmann (SPI)
Michael Kraus (SPI)

Acknowledgements

The authors of this report would like to express gratitude to all those who contributed information and advice in the compilation of country reports and this summary report, particularly the country collaborators, listed below. In addition we would like to thank the European Commission, DG V, for their support for this project.

Country Collaborators

Austria	Frank M. Amort
Belgium	Douchan Beghin
Bulgaria	Tonka Varleva
Czech Republic	Jaroslav Jedlicka
Denmark	Sigrid Paulsen & Else Smith
Estonia	Nelli Kalikova
Finland	Silja Hormia
France	Geneviève Paicheler
Greece	Demosthenes Agrafiotis
Iceland	Sigurdur B. Thorsteinsson
Ireland	Deirdre Seery
Italy	Felice Grieco
Latvia	Melita Sauka
Lithuania	Marija Caplinskiene
Netherlands	Theo Sandfort
Norway	Siri P. Hole
Poland	Arkadiusz Nowak
Portugal	Maria Odette Santos Ferreira
Romania	Galina Musat
Slovakia	Daniel Stancek
Slovenia	Irena Klavs
Spain	Jordi Baroja
Sweden	Gunila Rådö
United Kingdom	Wendy Macdowall

Executive Summary

The purpose of the project "HIV Prevention in Europe: Review of Policy and Practice" was the carrying out of an exhaustive inventory and comparative analysis of the various aspects of national HIV and AIDS policies in all the Member States of the European Community (Austria, Belgium, Denmark, Finland, France, Germany, Greece, Ireland, Italy, Luxembourg, Portugal, Spain, Sweden, the Netherlands, United Kingdom) those EFTA countries which are signatories to the Agreement on the European Economic Area (Iceland, Liechtenstein, Norway), and the associated countries of Central and Eastern Europe (Bulgaria, Estonia Poland, Hungary, Lithuania, Latvia, Romania, the Czech Republic, Slovakia and Slovenia).

The objectives were:

- To have a better common understanding of national HIV/AIDS prevention policies and measures in Europe
- To identify the current and future developments in the field of HIV prevention
- To identify the common features as well as the differences among the national policies
- To develop the necessary knowledge base for the adaptation of future action at community level.

The methodology used was the analysis of primary and secondary sources (reports, documents at national and international level), the collection of standardised data and information in the individual countries in close co-operation with national HIV/AIDS experts (country reports). A further step was an analysis through consultations with experts and interviews with key persons from international organisations and finally standardises interviews with a wide range of key players within the field of HIV in each country about the perception of the system, current debates and likely policy changes.

This analysis focused on the following general goals of HIV prevention:

- Minimising the HIV incidence
- Preventing the discrimination of vulnerable groups
- Providing an adequate patent care including the possibility to die with dignity.

For each country involved, an exhaustive description and inventory of the various aspects of HIV/AIDS policy and prevention practices has been carried out. It describes the current situation as well as significant developments with respect to the general population and specific vulnerable subgroups. This covers the following aspects:

- Short history/chronology in the respective country
- General policy on HIV/AIDS
- Institutional structures of policy implementation
- Summarising the main legal framework
- The surveillance and monitoring system of HIV and AIDS in the respective country
- Epidemiological data on HIV/AIDS
- Primary HIV prevention
- Social and economic measures of support for HIV positive persons
- HIV/AIDS treatment and care
- 1 to 2 examples of the best model projects in HIV prevention and/or care for HIV positive persons
- Estimation of the overall costs of the HIV/AIDS epidemic in the respective country
- Perception of the system

For each of the above-mentioned aspects, the country reports are also providing quantitative information as far as available and appropriate. The development of policy since the emergence of the HIV epidemic was analysed, with the identification of relevant influences contributing to evident changes.

The comparison of the country reports showed a great variety of developments in the different countries for each topic. The outcome of the comparative analysis of the country reports and of the results of the exhaustive discussions with the country collaborators during the two meetings in Berlin is a set of conclusions and recommendations for action and future research concerning the following topics:

The comparison of the chapter "History and Chronology" highlighted the following topics as essential for prevention policy:

- Creating a favourable and permissive environment

- Large campaigns for the general population combined with solidarity information
- Integration of HIV prevention and care activities, with other existing structures

For the "Institutional Structures of Policy Implementation" the following recommendations were found to be important:

- Involvement of vulnerable groups in the various formal structures of the making of policies at different levels
- Decentralisation of HIV activities to the local levels
- National Government commitment, with HIV/AIDS activities high in the agenda of public priorities
- Central co-ordination of activities

Concerning "Legal Aspects" important recommendations are:

- Updating and developing laws adapted to the new emerging vulnerable groups
- Close examination of laws and regulations can reveal the loopholes
- The introduction and adaptation of existing laws within a reasonable time period is an indicator of governmental commitment

Further research is recommended to answer the following questions:

- What are the mechanisms which can accelerate the introduction or updating of laws facilitating HIV prevention policies in Europe?
- What is the influence of larger EU treaties, and is there room for more guidance of the EU in relation to legal developments?
- How are laws introduced to combat the underlying factors increasing the vulnerability to HIV?

Recommendations concerning "Epidemiology/Surveillance System":

- Epidemiological data can offer persuasive evidence for instituting measures aimed at the more vulnerable groups
- AIDS epidemiological data need to be complemented with HIV data
- The analysis of risk behaviours to complement the present epidemiological data is needed to tailor improved intervention strategies

Recommendations for future research:

- How to improve the use of the surveillance systems for decision-making at the local level?
- How to combine HIV/AIDS epidemiological monitoring with behavioural surveillance data collection at minimum costs?

Recommendations concerning the "System of Primary HIV Prevention":

- Find ways to adjust to the marginalisation: empowering instead of victimising vulnerable groups
- Action research and documentation of best practices
- The known gaps to address the vulnerable groups' needs must be urgently addressed in each country
- The power and dynamism of the voluntary sector and NGOs can have more impact on the formulation of HIV prevention policies at local and national levels
- Integration of HIV activities with STDs and HEP activities
- Ensure equal access to services (migrants and prisoners)
- Continue to address the prevention related to gay men

Recommendations for future research

- What is the best mix of strategies to continue to inform the general population, and at the same time to reach the vulnerable groups, with scarcer resources?
- How to promote and use best practices experiences?
- How to build-in action research in existing strategies, particularly for pioneer work with the emerging vulnerable groups?
- What are the best prevention messages and strategies to reach the young female group in each country?
- What is the best mix of national and local structures to support the development of HIV prevention policies?

Recommendations concerning "Treatment and Care":

- Guidelines or continuing education through experts provide a favourable environment to adapt and promote quality HIV treatment in a rapidly changing field of intervention
- Best practices in each country can offer persuasive evidence for instituting and programme change
- Adapt to continuous medical advances, especially in the field of care

Recommendations for future research:

- How to measure the effectiveness of treatment and care identify the bottlenecks and recommend solutions?
- How to facilitate compliance to treatments?

Recommendations concerning "General Policy on HIV and AIDS":

- Refining through the EU the HIV prevention policies "golden" standards may stimulate and encourage countries to follow those with more exchange between policy-makers at an international level
- Barriers faced presently in Europe due to the normalisation of the disease, its medicalisation, the decreasing budgets, the medical advancements which are still unsatisfactory, need to be overcome
- National plans are essential guidance tools to translate HIV prevention policies into reality
- Inter-sectoral and multi-disciplinary inputs are essential
- Involvement of the voluntary sector at all levels of the system
- More attention needed to the increasing drug scene with the early introduction of harm reduction

The following gaps in HIV prevention and support for PWLA need to be overcome:

- Insufficient response to new vulnerable groups (prisoners, migrants, young women, young MSM)
- Quality and specificity of the messages for vulnerable groups
- Issues related to the lack of political commitment in prevention policy and decreasing resources
- Unequal accessibility to treatments for rural populations and specific target groups

To summarise the following future challenges for Prevention Policies in Europe are presented:

- To keep HIV/AIDS as an important and relevant theme
- To make or keep funds available for prevention
- Integration of the response at different levels of the system

- Quick adaptation of strategies to new vulnerable groups (i.e. migrants, prisoners, young women, young MSM)

The different situation in the countries of Central and Eastern Europe requires additional challenges:

- Allocation of financial support for prevention (false feeling of security due to low incidences)
- Monitoring of behavioural change in specific at risk populations and early intervention
- Training for medical staff and counsellors
- Increase of acceptance of marginalised groups
- Control the increasing numbers of IDUs and STDs (e.g. harm reduction measures)
- Increase public awareness and media coverage
- Apply good practise examples particularly for IDUs

1. Introduction

1.1 Background

"The spread of HIV can be curtailed and the impact of AIDS alleviated. Countries everywhere need to base their response on policies known to be effective against AIDS – and setting these policies can take political courage. Countries also need financial resources to confront AIDS" (UNAIDS Report 1999).

The HIV/AIDS epidemic in Europe is a patchwork of different complex epidemics accompanied by various social and economic factors and disparate behaviour patterns. " HIV travels along the fault-lines of society. Vulnerability to HIV is aggravated by many factors – such as migration, economic disparities, inequalities between men and women, and industrial development policies that attract workers to jobs far from their families. Directly and indirectly, these factors deprive individuals of their control over HIV exposure. In many contexts, AIDS prevention involves tackling the epidemic at its social, cultural and economic roots." (UNAIDS Report, 1999). This assessment which refers above all to Third World countries, also goes for Europe, especially for its central and eastern regions. In Europe, the HIV/AIDS epidemic still primarily affects homosexual men and intravenous drug users, but heterosexual infection rates are steadily rising. The increase of human trafficking requires particular attention. Violence against girls and women increases their HIV risk considerably. In western Europe alone as many as half a million women are affected by human trafficking. Targeted prevention strategies are necessary to protect these diverse groups. Hence, the United Nations Drug Control Programme (UNDCP) defines restrictions on demand and supply, particularly for young people, as a central strategy. But additional strategies are necessary to protect those who already use drugs against HIV infection or prevent transmission of the virus to their partners (NIH 1997). These prevention strategies normally comprise education measures for drug users and their partners [e.g. travel tips for mobile drug users in Europe (Broering & van Duifhuizen, 1996)], drug therapy programmes, free access to condoms, "bleach" or sterile needles and syringes. It has been shown for England (Stimson, 1995) that such prevention programmes have a major impact on the behaviour of drug addicts, although their impact is less clear in the Euregio Maas-Rhine (Franken & Kaplan 1997).

In addition, the European regions differ in their social mentalities (Danzinger, 1998). In some countries of eastern Europe and the former USSR compulsory HIV tests used to be the rule. In these countries it was particularly important to show that the protection of human rights can also be a major contribution of HIV prevention. Discrimination and stigmatisation impede effective HIV prevention by helping to push the problems under the rug and restricting access to urgently needed institutions of medical and psycho-social care.

The diversity of these factors with an impact on the emergence and spread of the epidemic in individual European countries requires a comprehensive analysis in order to find adequate prevention strategies that can be effectively used against the background of ever scarcer resources in Europe. First of all, this calls for an exact description of the HIV/AIDS situation in the European countries. This includes:

a) Identification of the focus areas of local epidemics,
b) Identification of factors that contribute to spreading the epidemic, such as opinions on sexual behaviour and drug use and
c) Documentation of access to and acceptance of prevention aids such as condoms and sterile needles.

The second major issue is the analysis of strong and weak points of individual national prevention policies with all their measures. This also includes the identification of particularly effective strategies such as approaches based on "social marketing" (Lamptey & Price, 1998) or on the concept of "community empowerment" (Becker et al., 1998).

Based on these analyses highly effective prevention strategies can be recommended for diverse needs. "To succeed in preventing HIV transmission, countries need to work simultaneously on many fronts – for example, through schools and health facilities, in the workplace, through media campaigns, and through outreach to sex workers. Drawing on practical experience from countries around the world, they must use effective approaches – the policies, strategies and technologies that UNAIDS calls 'best practice' ". (UNAIDS Report 1999)

Against this background, the Wissenschaftliches Institut der Ärzte Deutschlands (WIAD) - Scientific Institute of the German Medical Association - and the Sozialpädagogisches Institut (SPI) - Social Education Institute - jointly implemented the project Inventory and Comparative Analysis of National HIV/AIDS Prevention Policies in Europe on behalf of the European Commission.

1.2   Focus of the project

The purpose of the project was the carrying out of an exhaustive inventory and comparative analysis of the various aspects of national HIV and AIDS policies in all the Member States of the European Community (Austria, Belgium, Denmark, Finland, France, Germany, Greece, Ireland, Italy, Luxembourg, Portugal, Spain, Sweden, the Netherlands, United Kingdom) those EFTA countries which are signatories to the Agreement on the European Economic Area (Iceland, Liechtenstein, Norway), and the associated countries of central and eastern Europe (Bulgaria, Estonia Poland, Hungary, Lithuania, Latvia, Romania, the Czech Republic, Slovakia and Slovenia).

The aims of the programme were the following:

- To have a better common/mutual understanding of national HIV/AIDS prevention policies and measures in Europe;
- To identify the current and future developments in the field of HIV prevention;
- To identify the common features as well as the differences among the national policies;
- To develop the necessary knowledge base for the adaptation of future action at Community level.

The work carried out is related to the following fields:

a) *Exhaustive inventory by country*

For each country involved, an exhaustive description and inventory of the various aspects of HIV/AIDS policy and prevention practices has been carried out. It describes the current situation as well as significant developments with respect to the general population and specific vulnerable subgroups. This covers the following aspects:

- Overall national policy on HIV/AIDS, including links with policies concerning other communicable diseases (STD's, viral Hepatitis etc.)

- Institutional structure of policy implementation: Public institutions, Role of NGOs, National/regional co-ordination of HIV prevention policies
- Legal aspects: HIV testing, Prisons, Drug abuse, Rights of homosexuals, Prostitution
- Surveillance and monitoring of HIV and AIDS
  (particular attention is paid to the current development of the epidemic in central and eastern European countries – with special regard to intravenous drug use and illegal prostitution – and the consequences for the HIV policies in these countries)
- Primary prevention (information/education): Policy priorities, Who does what (public sector, NGOs), Prevention for special target groups (vulnerable subgroups)
- Social and economic support for HIV positive persons: Policy priorities and actors
- Treatment and care: National policy, services providing treatment and care, Access to treatment
- Estimation of the overall cost of the HIV/AIDS epidemic at governmental and non govern mental level

For each of the above-mentioned aspects, the country reports are also providing quantitative information as far as available and appropriate. The development of policy since the emergence of the HIV epidemic is analysed, with the identification of relevant influences contributing to evident changes.

b) *Comparative analysis at the European level*

The descriptive inventory for each country is supplemented by a comparative analysis at the European level. This was carried out for each of the subjects dealt with by the inventory.

In particular, this analysis shows:

- The main characteristics (objectives, means, methods, costs, results) of HIV/AIDS prevention policies at the European level;
- Common (or dominant) aspects and approaches among the various national policies and practices;
- The main recent or anticipated developments at national and European level;

- Significant divergence's between the various national policies and practices;
State of co-operation and coherence among national policies and practices.

2.   Materials and methods

2.1   Research questions and analytical framework

A recent review of health target and priority setting in 18 European Countries "Health Policies on Target?" (van de Water, van Herten, 1998) presented a useful framework for policy analysis. Since the 1970s, there has been a shift from structure-oriented health policy towards population health as the starting point. The Minister of Health of Canada, Marc Lalonde, presented this innovative perspective in "A New Perspective on the Health of Canadians: A Working Document".

It has since inspired many institutions, including the World Health Organisation in the process of formulating its "Health for All strategy". According to this concept for a new health policy model, better health depends on influencing the determinants of health which were grouped into five categories:

• the biological factors (e.g. hereditary properties of individuals),
• the physical environment (e.g. air, water, soil and temperature, sound, radiation and micro-organisms),
• the social environment (e.g. the influence of family and society on the (mental) health of the individual),
• the lifestyle factors (e.g. smoking, nutrition, physical exercise, use of alcohol and drugs), and
• the health care services.

For the purpose of the present research focusing on HIV Prevention Policies in Europe, we developed, based on the previous mentioned model, an Analytical Framework which encompassed key questions (ref. Appendix A) to understand the various components of HIV/AIDS policies.

The analytical framework of the HIV prevention policy is not a causal model but attempts merely to describe the various components of HIV/AIDS policies.

Illustration 1: *Analytical Framework of the HIV Prevention Policy in Europe*

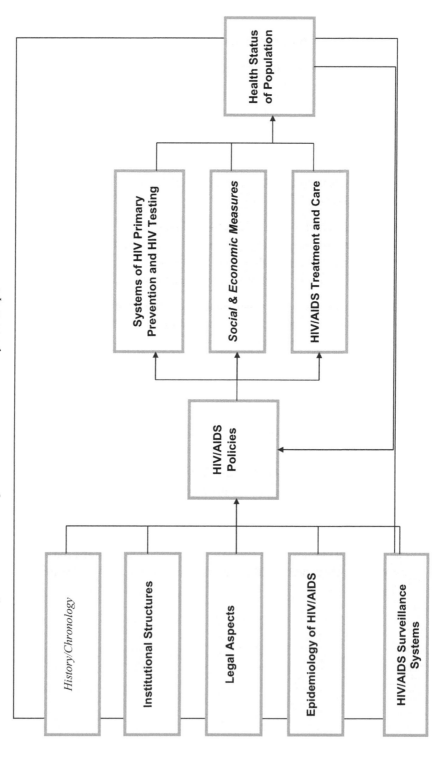

Source: WIAD adapted from Ministry of Welfare, Health and Cultural Affairs, Canada, 1987

The analysis focuses on the more recent 1996 onwards period, and the components are documented in the various sections (mentioned as paragraph, "Para.") of the present study.

The questions are:

- How has the history and chronology of the HIV epidemic developed in the country and influenced the early making of HIV prevention policy (Para. 3.1)?
- How have the institutional structures facilitated the policy implementation (Para. 3.3)?
- What are the legal aspects specific to policies for more vulnerable groups, and other groups (e.g. PLWAs, health care professionals) (Para. 3.4)?
- How has the epidemiology of HIV/AIDS (Para. 3.5), and the surveillance systems (Para. 3.6) been instrumental in guiding policies?

These various factors influence the development of HIV/AIDS Policies (Para. 3.2). In complement, the making of HIV/AIDS policies are reflected through three HIV/AIDS Services, or intervention policies, which we used as proxy measures for HIV/AIDS policies as well:

- the Systems of HIV prevention (Para. 3.7), and HIV testing (Para. 3.13) as a primary prevention measure,
- the social and economic measures of support for HIV positive persons (Para. 3.8),
- and the HIV/AIDS treatment and care (Para. 3.9), and HIV testing as a secondary prevention measure.

The health status of the population is the ultimate outcome which can be measured through the epidemiological data (Para. 3.5), and the surveillance data (Para 3.6), and finally, influence in turn the HIV/AIDS policies (Para. 3.2).

Some of the main partners' opinions of the perception of the different components of the system, and the current debates and likely policy changes, are summarised separately as an overall recent update of the situation in each country (Para. 12).

2.2 Methodological considerations for the country reviews

HIV/AIDS prevention policies depend on many complex factors in each individual country. If such policies are examined in different countries, the complexity and diversity of these factors increases significantly. This goes in particular for the countries of Europe, which have developed differently in disparate social systems over the past 50 years, for example, if we compare western Europe with eastern and central Europe. But even within the countries of western or eastern Europe cultural and social idiosyncrasies generate distinct developments which can have a major impact on prevention policies. Other factors include geographic features, demographic trends and, not least, the country's economic situation. In order to understand the specific prevention policy of a country, we should consider all these factors, but such an approach would go far beyond the scope of this project. Still, it is important to find explanations in such factors, when reviewing the seemingly chance diversity of prevention policies.

In order to assess and compare prevention policies, we must record the differences between a country's professed prevention policy and what measures it actually puts into practice. This requires a targeted and systematic approach. Kronemann & van der Zee (1997) provide a good overview of the advantages and disadvantages of possible analytical methods:

Tab. 1: Analytical approaches and their potential advantages and disadvantages

Method	Advantages	Disadvantages
Analysis of primary sources	- reveals initial intention of policy - exact norms and rules can be found	- possible high translation costs - uncertainty about actual implementation
Analysis of secondary sources	- gives an overview of reform - reveals inconsistencies lack of clarity, which prompt further investigations	- sometimes too global, to give real insight - global nature of the information may lead to apparent contradictions
Analysis through consultations with experts	- reveals the actual course of the implementations and subsequent problems - indicates unintended effects	- experts may give biased information - no exact information about implementation dates (because of retrospective nature)

Our method in this project is to combine these approaches in order to investigate the most valid information and rule out the mentioned disadvantages as far as possible. The analysis of primary and secondary sources was performed by experts in the individual countries, who consulted further experts and key contacts in the country to gain further information. To ensure standardised surveys of the examined European countries, this was co-ordinated, following the project management's specifications, between all project experts at the first preparatory meeting. The result of this co-ordination meeting is the questionnaire and structure plan for the country reviews in annex A. Still, an "expert bias" cannot be completely ruled out for the individual country reports. However, this bias has been minimised, as the statements of the country reports were revised by national experts from other institutions.

2.3 Material for the country reviews

The 25 country reviews were created by the experts of each country. In content and structure, these reviews meet the standardised specifications of the questionnaires (see annex A). To answer the questionnaires, the experts assessed the available written primary and secondary sources in each country and interviewed further experts both verbally and in writing.

The following primary and secondary sources were consulted:

HIV/AIDS-related legislation texts, political agreements, official national reports, published and unpublished articles, prevention material, progress reports and available written material, where accessible for literature analyses and Internet research, as well as all information available from health ministries, national AIDS committees, AIDS co-ordinators, public health authorities, NGOs and other prevention-related institutions. Each country review is available in the country's official language and in English.

Experts were either interviewed directly or in written form, with a focus on question 12 (Perception of the Systems of HIV/AIDS Prevention) of the questionnaire. The interviewed experts include representatives of ministries of health and other public institutions as well as representatives of NGOs, to enable a comparison of both viewpoints.

HIV testing, an important part of prevention policy, was not covered by this study, as its was examined by another EU-funded project implemented in 1998 ("HIV Testing in Europe: A Review of Policy and Practice", London School of Hygiene and Tropical Medicine, 1999).

The comparative analysis of AIDS prevention policies in Europe by the project co-ordinators is based primarily on the available information of the country reviews and the results of the two work meetings with involved country experts in Berlin. And we integrated information from higher-ranking European organisations such as the European Union, the WHO regional office for Europe in Copenhagen, UNAIDS in Geneva and the European Centre for the Epidemiological Monitoring of AIDS, Saint-Maurice in Paris. These sources, which generally cover country-specific information on all European states, were analysed to complement the country reviews. The results of the comparative analyses were sent to the experts for revision and corrected on receipt of the corresponding feedback.

3. Policy and practice of HIV prevention: comparative analysis

3.1 History and chronology of the response to HIV/AIDS

In its analyses of HIV/AIDS prevention policies in Europe, this report mainly focuses on the period from 1995. However, a historical-chronological account of how the HIV/AIDS issue was handled in different countries is of major importance for the development of prevention policies. "The problem-solving cycle of health policy development is the background for setting health targets" (Water & Herten, 1998, p. 31). This cycle, which leads from perception of the problem, here HIV/AIDS, through the analysis of the problem, suggestions on how to solve the problem, implementation of attempts to solve the problem to the evaluation and, based on this, re-analysis, generating different approaches in each European country, can only be understood in a historical context.

In the country reviews, opinions were voiced in reply to the following eight questions on historical development:

- When and how was the HIV epidemic first perceived by the public?
- When was the first HIV infection diagnosed? Did this happen before or after the problem of the HIV epidemic had been publicly perceived? When was the first case of AIDS identified?
- When was the first information campaign developed for the mass media? For which target groups? When was it first used?
- When and in what order were the first HIV/AIDS-related laws, official decrees or legal skeleton laws enacted?
- When was the first AIDS-specific NGO founded, or when did existing NGOs take on HIV/AIDS-related tasks? What were the original reasons for the commitment of NGOs in this field?
- When did treatment methods for HIV/AIDS patients become available and when were they first used? What antiretroviral therapies were available and who had access to such treatment?
- When were the first needle exchange programmes or corresponding other low-threshold prevention measures introduced for IDUs?
- Was there a significant change within HIV/AIDS prevention policies from a special top-priority status to a more normalised status among other diseases, e.g. as a subarea of infectious diseases?

Regarding these questions we can expect similar chronologies in many European countries. Still, the eastern European countries, for example, will differ clearly in some points from western European states. Rosenbrock et al. (1999) observed that in western European countries with different national development patterns the predominant phase of 'AIDS-exceptionalism' at the start of the epidemic was followed by a "normalisation" phase in 1996. The following summary of country reviews shows to what extent central and eastern European countries correspond to this pattern.

3.1.1 Western and Southern Europe

Western and Southern European countries report the first AIDS cases detected in the early 1980s. The media largely influenced the general perception of the public that the disease came from abroad, with the threat was often followed by panic and fear related to the virus. A major impact on public awareness occurred in a few countries from Southern Europe only later, with the HIV infection and death in 1985 of the American actor Rock Hudson.

The countries report in common vigorous original measures which covered usually the following spectrum of activities:

- the gay community was involved from the origins in almost all countries, and the haemophiliacs as well in some, who both contributed to mounting public awareness and get other structures to move on the issue,
- compulsory ELISA testing of blood donors for the presence of antibodies and opening of anonymous and free screening centres, and setting up of HIV and AIDS epidemiological surveillance,
- first general population campaigns (between 1985 and 1987 in general) through information leaflets, radio, cinemas, television, bill boards, and in some countries directed to groups considered to be at increased risk for contracting the infection, particularly homosexual males, on the virus transmission and prevention (e.g. to increase the use of condoms), and solidarity with HIV patients (e.g. the "compassion" campaign in the Netherlands in 1990), and set-up of information telephone services,
- the often illegality of homosexuality and injecting drug use (IDU) in some countries, and responses for those have delayed the targeting of information to these groups,
- specific information campaigns were directed to the health services and hospitals,
- original legislation addressing the regulation of blood transfusions, legalisation of unrestricted sales of syringes in pharmacies (in Western Europe in general), and legislation on diagnosis and treatment free of charge,
- relaxation of restrictions to the sale or to the advertising of condoms,
- mobilisation or creation of Non-Governmental Organisations (NGOs), e.g. Deutsche AIDS-Hilfe, and the Church, (sometimes compensating the absence of response from the public sector, to organise training for social and medical care-givers and to encourage prevention among various vulnerable groups, particularly homosexuals and bisexuals, but as well among intravenous drug

users (IDUs), prostitutes of both sexes, and, to a lesser extent, migrants, and accommodation for homeless and/or socially disadvantaged AIDS patients,

- a response to targeting the "at risk",
- creation and public financing of pilot or experimental projects,
- implementation of risk reduction programmes among drug users, e.g. needle exchange programmes and/or methadone programmes and/or outreach programme distributing free kits containing sterilised needles and condoms (late eighties to early nineties) with some countries having pioneered those earlier (e.g. the Netherlands),
- original introduction of the anti-retroviral treatment AZT (around 1987),
- the set up of co-ordinating public ad-hoc structures (advisory, fund-raising, policy-making and regulation) which sometimes were introduced already in the mid-eighties whereas in some countries in the late-eighties or early nineties only, with accompanying commitments of AIDS being a public health priority, with sometimes a "wartime response" (e.g. in England).

In the mid nineties the standard double, or triple combination therapies are being considered standard treatment methods in AIDS therapy.

In the late nineties, countries have adapted their responses to the evolution of the endemic and emerging vulnerable groups, the development of preventive measures and the introduction of the new multi-drug therapies, the public knowledge and prevailing attitudes and practices among the population. Consequently, countries have more recently moved into:

- alarmism has dropped progressively,
- legality of homosexuality and injecting drug use in the early nineties has facilitated the targeting of campaigns and interventions in the late nineties,
- introduction of the multi-drug therapies combining anti-viral and anti-protease molecules (around 1996) with a shift of interest from prevention to the patients' care,
- large campaigns integrating HIV and STD in the public safe sex campaigns (e.g. the Netherlands),
- specific public campaigns addressing target specific groups (e.g. homo- and bisexuals; IDUs with low-threshold institutions and/or needle exchange programmes and/or mobile offerings) have started in general mid- or late-nineties only,
- a response to targeting the "new" vulnerable groups, and involvement of prisons in harm reduction programmes,

- regrouping of organisations specialising in HIV due to the beneficial effects of new treatments but also due to scarcer resources and to less involvement of the original groups,
- anchoring HIV/AIDS activities within the scope of a broader health promotion is the general move,
- policy change towards a focus on a combined approach of prevention, care and treatment,
- decentralisation of HIV prevention and care activities into the regions and departments,
- preparation of updated strategy for the new millennium.

Each country has had its own degree of response to the above mentioned measures depending of different components: such as (but not limited to) the dimension of the epidemic, the different types of victims (homosexuals or haemophiliacs, or IDUs), the organisational structures, the tradition of the medical and social sciences field, the existing movements (e.g. gay), and mobilisation of citizens.

Some delays of a few years have occurred in the introduction of timely measures for some countries which may explain in the nineties some of the epidemiological impact: e.g. in France, a noticeable exception signalled which has been well covered by the media is the delay in introducing testing with the consequent haemophiliac scandal; or, the risk-reducing campaigns to drug users introduced late (1995) in comparison to other countries.

Late starters may nevertheless become full supporters of new programmes, through public support and political commitment, e.g. in France, in 1995 the establishment of substitution programmes and legalisation of the free distribution of syringes to drug users by HIV and Hepatitis prevention organisations, and in 1996, a decree permitting the State to grant financial assistance to market materials for prevention of HIV and Hepatitis, and to reduce the prices of these materials when sold to users or to organisations involved in prevention programmes.

The public health and social scientists have concentrated on different areas of interests over that twenty years period (Aggleton, 1995): early on, in the social perception of the phenomenon, then at the end of the eighties and beginning of the nineties on the sexual behaviour and its social dynamic, and in the late nineties on the study of groups and situations, multi-disciplinary research, and the factors of vulnerability.

3.1.2 Northern, Central and Eastern Europe

For the northern European states of Denmark, Finland and Sweden - just like in western and southern Europe - the early 1980s marked the start of public interest in the HIV/AIDS problem. This rather fast response, despite the lack of diagnosed cases in some countries, was due, among other things, to existing ties between national gay associations, e. g. in Denmark and Sweden.

In Norway things developed more slowly, hence there was no public discussion of the topic until the mid-, and especially last third of the 1980s, triggered by information campaigns of the health authorities.

In contrast, the eastern European countries show a different development pattern. In most of these countries the media first covered the issue in the mid-1980s. State control and influence conveyed an image of AIDS as a "disease of the western world", caused by promiscuity and moral decay, which was just a further symptom of the decline of the collapsing capitalist system. Taken to extremes (Romania), this led to the denial of diagnosed cases of HIV and AIDS in one's own country to the public at large. The decline of the socialist system led to more objective media coverage.

The first NGOs were already founded in the Scandinavian countries in the early 1980s – a process that only started in central and eastern Europe after the collapse of communism. Slovenia is an exception. Just like in Scandinavia, gay associations in Slovenia took instant action, by integrating the topic immediately in their work. In contrast, the foundation of western-style AIDS help organisations was the rule in other central and eastern European countries, albeit mostly with a delay of approx. five years.

In northern Europe widespread information campaigns were implemented in the mid-1980s, mostly organised by the ministries in charge. In 1985, for example, Denmark saw the first information campaigns, which reached all households in the form of direct mailings. Its first mass-media campaign was in 1987. The only countries to implement such early measures in central and eastern Europe were Bulgaria and Slovenia. The other states only started to provide targeted information to the general public and select risk groups in the late 1980s and early 1990s. These campaigns comprised the following measures, to name a few:

• Production and broadcast of video clips on television, and their distribution in night-clubs, subculture venues, schools etc.,

- Publication of brochures informing about modes of transmission, protection measures, contacts for counselling and advice, and treatment options,
- Performances of popular bands and artists at charity and info events,
- Thematic training courses for teachers,
- Events to boost condom acceptance,
- Annual campaigns on 1 December - World AIDS Day,
- Articles and reports in media used by the public at large,
- Campaigns to dissipate prejudices against those affected and increase their general acceptance.

These measures were mostly organised by the relevant ministries of social affairs, health or education, and in some cases NGOs, the Red Cross and - in central and eastern European countries - often the WHO. In this context, one should point out that the member states of the former Soviet Union all date the start of their central AIDS prevention campaigns to after they reached independence. Only Romania has reported of no central measures so far. To date, only NGOs have initiated sporadic campaigns.

The first legislative state measures - mostly decrees on blood product testing or STD control - are dated by most reports to the mid-1980s.

Right after the approval of zidovudine (AZT) in the USA, corresponding treatment started in Denmark, Finland, Norway and Sweden. Slovenia, Czechoslovakia, Finland, Poland, Romania, Lithuania and Latvia rapidly followed suit over the following three years. In Bulgaria and Estonia the drug wasn't available until 1995 and 1997 respectively, at a time when the application of dual and tri-therapy was already the norm elsewhere.

Needle exchange - programmes as a low-threshold measure are now established in virtually all countries, but again with delays in central and eastern European countries. Most of them only introduced methadone programmes in 1996 (e.g. Latvia), but much earlier in Scandinavia, where targeted Methadon treatment was already used as an HIV prevention measure in 1985, as in Denmark for example.
In their chronology of events and historical development of HIV policies, the Scandinavian countries hardly differ from the western European countries described in 3.1.1. But the development differs considerably from that in central and eastern European countries. Although these countries were aware of the HIV/AIDS epidemic at the same early date, none of them - apart from Slovenia - started prevention policies similar to those practised in western Europe until

1990, after the collapse of communism. At this time none of them - again apart from Slovenia - had NGOs, and prevention policies were solely determined by state authorities, in most cases with the WHO's support and in line with its goals. Western-style NGOs only emerged in the context of increasing liberalisation and took on major prevention tasks from 1992, as for example in Lithuania. The WHO's goals were generally accepted on paper, but their implementation often turned out to be difficult, since, despite reforms, its liberal approaches often collided with moral values, rules and laws that partly date back to the Soviet regime but still influence attitudes in parts of the population and in public institutions. Still, the phase of 'AIDS Exceptionalism' is already in transition to the normalisation phase in central and eastern Europe, for example in Lithuania HIV/AIDS is ranked as a health problem equal to many others.

3.2   The present status of the HIV/AIDS prevention policies

"Policy deficits are the most important factor contributing to the ongoing spread, and associated dynamics of the HIV/AIDS pandemic and its numerous sub-epidemics around the world." (Rosenbrock, 1994)"

A recent review of the "The AIDS Policy in Western Europe" noticed that there is "no universal or unilinear path" in governmental policies and public reactions towards AIDS in the different European countries but a "generally shared trajectory" with "specific configuration" to each country (Rosenbrock et al., 1999).

The normalisation of AIDS since 1996 approximately in Western Europe, which is the period of more interest to the present research, presents the following characteristics: successful prevention measures to HIV infections and AIDS have lead most countries of Western Europe to endemic equilibriums far below the levels feared, and have even declined. The alliance between health care professionals and social movements dealing with AIDS which has spearheaded an effective response is showing signs of fatigue. Broader health systems changes such as health sector reform in market-oriented cost-containment policies are gaining acceptance and changing the traditional health care delivery. New antiretroviral therapies extend survival times dramatically changing and challenging the traditional health care delivery as well (ambulatory patients).

Some of the innovations in prevention and care achieved with exceptionalism are placed in question, including as a consequence cut back, and a change towards integration into normal course of politics, administration, prevention and health care.

AIDS-related task forces and specific government agencies are being cut back or re-integrated in normal hierarchic/ bureaucratic organisations. (Cattacin, 1998) Some of the resources for prevention and research are being drastically reduced due to different sound reasons: first, to "overestimated pressures," second, to AIDS-related innovations which have gained acceptance and have become institutionalised-normalisation as the stabilisation of exceptionalism, and third, to new development that have stood the test in respect to AIDS and have become generalised. On the other hand, the cuts are often to "the expense of prevention efficacy and the quality of care."

Rosenbrock (1993) claimed already in the early nineties that the key elements to successful AIDS policies are:

- priority to primary prevention and timely risk perception and assessment (early intervention),
- policies for special and general populations including addressing new social norms (consistency),
- the formulation of a coherent policy which is integrated into the more general public health programmes (integration).

First, three general goals of HIV prevention are outlined which are international common sense:

(1) Minimising the HIV incidence.
(2) Preventing the discrimination of risk groups and infected or ill persons.
(3) Providing an adequate patient care including the possibility to die with dignity.

The social framework conditions vary strongly from region to region. The main differences can be seen in the risk structures. But there are also different disposable public resources that determine the provisions of the specific public health systems, patient care and social movements.

Some general rules for anti HIV and AIDS strategies outlined by Rosenbrock still valid today are:

- A decentralised organisation of the prevention strategies has to be embedded into the specific cultural and local contexts. Universal and culturally unbound approaches, following the top-down-principles are proven not to be very effective.
- In that sense strategies have to take into account the different social frameworks and material resources in given specific risk structures.
- Because of the long latency period between HIV and AIDS, prevention strategies must be designed with long term perspectives to facilitate the development of a time table facilitating the social and individual self-control in potential risk situations.

Furthermore, experiences from all over the world make it possible to derive three dogma of a successful HIV/AIDS prevention policy. Because of their intercultural characters, these can be generalised to:

a) Early interventions

The earlier an intervention starts the more successful the corresponding prevention policy will be. Consequently there must be given priority to primary prevention. This is a historical public health experience resulting from the fight against various infectious diseases.

However, early intervention mostly is hindered by different social and political obstacles. In the case of HIV/AIDS the difficulty to start a public discussion about issues like sex or drug abuse has to be overcome first. Normally the affected risk groups are not accepted because they are discriminated against, and public scandals and small resistance are the usual consequences which hamper a timely early intervention supported by appropriate policies.

The best proven means to put pressure on the political actors are the mobilisation of the affected persons and the issue of HIV/AIDS as a common and not only a minority problem.

b) Consistent interventions

A consistent strategy has to fulfil three preconditions:

- its instruments have to focus on all relevant aspects;
- it must be supported by all relevant actors;
- the sub-strategies must not be contradictory.

Particularly referring to the last point, two distinct approaches are regarded to be incompatible and therefore should not be mixed. The aim of the so-called control and containment strategy is to find and control all individuals and groups that are infected with or endangered by the virus. The activities based on repression and force are not adequate to create a climate of confidence and consultation.

In contrast, the co-operation strategy tries to initiate a social learning process which enforces a time stable and voluntary self-control. Its instruments are: first, the widespread central information and messages; second, socially, regionally and culturally bound campaigns for specific target groups; and finally, emphatic consultation for single persons. The co-operation strategy aims to establish new and commonly accepted social norms for all and not just for risk groups. Beyond pure medical care this modern form of an epidemic policy enforces a co-operative action circle of medicine, public health, science, police, social movements, mass media and private economy that must be guided by political actors.

c) Integrated intervention

An HIV/AIDS prevention strategy must be integrated in two aspects:

- The responsibilities must be divided under the premise of the greatest competence. The social movements of the affected groups need a framework of policy making that allows them to create their own group specific strategies. The competencies of the medical system must not be overestimated. Particularly in primary and secondary HIV/AIDS prevention, the efficiency of the medical system is very limited (e.g. to preventive HIV-testing or preventive medication).
- To avoid either underestimation or overestimation, HIV and AIDS policy should be integrated in the complete set of the societal and political efforts of the health sector. In most countries HIV and AIDS are neither the only nor the biggest health related problem. In that sense the social distribution of risk behaviour and information has to be evaluated in the same way as the epidemiological parameters used such as incidence or prevalence. Diseases that are related to HIV/AIDS, like STDs and TB, should be more and more

integrated in epidemiological investigation and surveillance. The statistical parameters of health reports should allow a comparative perspective of related health phenomena. In that way the common ground of different infectious diseases can be explored more accurately (e.g. conditions as poverty, political injustice, or the destruction of social structures), concurring with the recent findings in "HIV/AIDS prevention and 'class' and socio-economic related factors of risk of HIV infection. (Luger, 1998).

The following analysis is largely based on Steffen (1996) in an international public policy comparison between four European countries (France, Great Britain, Germany, and Italy), unless stated otherwise.

AIDS policies development have been hampered by two factors:

- first, an epidemic in the first stage which appeared as a disease of a minority striking an elite and particular groups, and which later surfaced as a mass epidemic that affects the misfits of society and different vulnerable groups;
- second, AIDS has been a trans-sectoral public health problem (health policy, various social policies, scientific research) dependent to be acted upon successfully of the collaboration and good will of different actors, be it government or private agencies, institutions, and interest groups.

The diversification and nature of AIDS policies in Europe have varied based on the fracture points and debates which were different in each country.

The original only model of prevention imported from the USA explains the influence on the way the private association initiatives and public interventions were balanced in Europe. All countries quickly put AIDS on their political agenda. Despite the fact European homosexuals did not make up an acknowledged pressure group in the political systems, in comparison to the USA, they were able to organise themselves and influence policies in different manners (e.g. Deutsche AIDS Hilfe). The presence of homosexuals in the nascent AIDS policy networks contrasted with the embarrassing silence of haemophiliacs, and the voiceless population of drug users and the prison community. Homosexuals have had direct access to the political system, and political integration has prevailed in the eighties in comparison to earlier radical currents. They have followed the example set by young Social-Democrats, left wing doctors and other militant minorities of the seventies who work in the normal structures of public life to have their particular cases heard in political parties, trade unions, professional organisations.

As observed in the eighties and nineties, AIDS has acted as an innovative force to operate readjustments in fields considered before as taboo, or reputed for their conservatism, for example the penal health systems in all countries, the surveillance of the pharmaceutics industry (e.g. Germany and France), sexual education (e.g. Italy), anti-drug policy (e.g. France). Shortcomings in socio-sanitary policies, and long resisted structural changes have finally been addressed due to the crises provoked by AIDS.

Comparing the institutionalisation processes in AIDS policies clarifies the general mechanisms of public policies which in turn determine national policies. Differences portray how actors are inserted institutionally which in turn vary according to context. In Europe, the alarm initially sounded by outsiders from the public system, with positions on the fringes of decision-making, hampered them from initiating a social policy. The help of the Health Administrations was required, hence the central state authority intervened to legitimise the problem carried by a minority when the national interest seemed threatened. Policy processes were influenced in each country by the strength or weakness of the respective public health administration, the efficiency of the inter-government co-ordination bodies, and by the Associations.

Cattacin et al. (1997) remind us that politics and policies are determined not only by the existing traditions of the "State-providence", but also the politico-institutional or social structures (decision-making process and actors' participation) which strongly influence public politics, more so than the individual epidemiological profiles. These structures may also explain the different choices in European politics. Beyond Steffen's position (1996) that HIV/AIDS policies can be explained by national traditions, the authors notice how HIV/AIDS have changed fundamentally these traditions.

The comparative study (Steffen, 1996) does not confirm the hypothesis that the pressure of the HIV epidemics fuelled quicker policy responses. Both Germany and Great Britain, the least affected were those that mobilised institutional resources the quickest, in comparison to France and Italy.

The fears of social stigmatisation combined with the desire to preserve the general population from the onslaught rather than epidemiological data explains changes in targeting more affected regions and groups. This distortion illustrates the autonomy of the political sphere for which public policies did not follow the reality of the epidemic. Besides France, all countries have been continually using the condom for contraception and extra-marital sex (making it an intervention both feasible and well-accepted).

The institutional contexts of Great Britain, Italy and Germany have supported the adaptation of the health sector and social policies for AIDS, in contrast to France. A more decentralised organisation of the public health apparatus, that left more autonomy to actors in the infra-national strata to private organisations, facilitated the introduction of new actors in the debates.

The direct and increased role of politicians in AIDS prevention can be explained by the necessity over time that the State has faced to intervene in the safety of blood transfusions and medicine products, or "social misfit" groups (IDU), in comparison to prevention based on the availability of condoms and their promotion and use (homosexual organisations and public information campaigns).

Efficiency in AIDS policies depends upon 2 factors:

- the extent to which policies are receptive to the specific needs of threatened groups,
- the capacity for co-ordination between all the health and social policies concerned by AIDS.

In the nineties, Cattacin et al. (1997) point how the disease has become a normal disease among others, with a broader spectrum of institutions contributing, from specialised to more general ones. Decentralised institutional support has followed (from urban to rural or regions). The content of the combat against HIV/AIDS has also normalised through education in schools, public health for general population, IDUs with messages to reduce risk. Finally, normalisation has occurred due to the availability of treatments which allow to control the negative physical effects, even it cannot yet be cured.

Based on our review, and collection of data, we concur with Cattacin et al. (1997) that the changing "macro-constellation" of the response to HIV/AIDS operates first, in an enabling positive environment of the "integration process of Europe" which facilitates in turn the adaptation of national policies, the "normalisation" of AIDS. Second, the information exchange through conferences etc. and the scientific community are also promoting new ideas.

Societies have had to face and invent new approaches to manage this new social risk.

Based on the positive experience of HIV/AIDS, lessons could be learnt and applied to other preventive programmes. Experiments to evaluate and implement other programmes could be based on what has been learnt from HIV/AIDS (distribution of syringes), or from the reinforcement of the collaboration of State and private actors.

Just like the variety of the epidemic of HIV/AIDS in Europe, consequently, individual countries have responded with a variety of policies. The European Union has launched in the context of the new public health policy within the Community (Decision No 647/96/EC of 29 March 1996 of the European Parliament and the Council), several policies through the Second Community Programme for the Prevention of AIDS (1996-2000) which fall into four areas and are supported through a number of various activities financed by the EU: surveillance and monitoring of HIV/AIDS and communicable diseases, combating transmission, information education and training, and the support for persons with HIV/AIDS and combating of discrimination.

A recent survey in the Spring of 1999 of the state of the public opinion towards the European Union revealed that the "Fight against cancer and AIDS" does not appear on the top priority list of the European Parliament attention. It ranked seventh (20%) among a number of areas identified for priority action, preceded first by employment (55%), the fight against drug trafficking and organised crime (36%), environmental and consumer protection, and foreign policy and security (both 25%). The fight against cancer and AIDS made the top four priorities in Portugal (28%) and Denmark (23%). People in Finland (13%), Germany (14%), and Sweden (15%) were the least likely to consider it a priority for the European Parliament (EU Eurobarometer 51, Jly 1999, pp. 85-86).

This situation can explain why the EU has more support and leverage as an institution to refine policies and actions in relation to some of the top areas of other priorities than HIV prevention policies.

3.2.1 Western and Southern Europe

In general countries have adopted the WHO, and more recently UNAIDS, recommendations for prevention activities, and formulated those in strategic plans (e.g. 1998-2002 five-year plan in Belgium, or 1995-1999 in France) or a more flexible "Evolving Strategy" plan (UK). Austria has been strongly influenced by the WHO concepts of health promotion (Alma-Ata, Ottawa, Jakarta) but does not have any national documents, agendas or regulations on prevention work. The policies are grounded on three main goals, as reflected in the example of The Netherlands: first, the prevention of further spread of HIV (primary prevention) with the promotion of safer sexual behaviour, especially for youth; second, the prevention of the development of AIDS in people with HIV (secondary prevention); the improvement of the quality of life of people with HIV/AIDS (tertiary prevention), and the improvement of the quality of AIDS control in a general sense.

The National Committees on AIDS are the implementing bodies for the plans, and address and advise on policy issues. The national Government or the Ministries of (Public) Health play a co-ordinating role. These plans are generally based on fundamental principles which where laid out at the onset of the epidemic, such in France for example, the solidarity, and non-discrimination and respect for the rights of HIV patients and of the most vulnerable groups. Within the plans each country defines its own sets of objectives, and within those new strategies can evolve on a yearly basis, through different documents (e.g. Guidelines, Sexual Health Strategy). In general countries have developed over the past decade a co-operative strategy in contrast to control and containment strategy. The governments have drawn in their advisory committees, or sub-committees (e.g. Education and Prevention, Care and Management, Surveillance) for HIV/AIDS policies multi-disciplinary teams of experts from the political arena and/or senior civil servants, and medical and social sciences field, and/or inter-ministerial (Health, Education, Justice, Defence, Home Office and Employment, Social Affairs, Scientific Research, Foundations) committees. Policies are often made and evolve through those. The committees include sometimes People Living with HIV. In complement, informal channels have plaid an important role too in the making of policies, for example, the tradition of organisations for homosexuals in particular involved in legal and political activities against AIDS. Some countries, such as Ireland, signal a community development, socially inclusive and partnership approach to the making of HIV/AIDS national policies. The voluntary sector can represent in common a powerful voice to the statutory or more formal sector, for example in the UK (National AIDS Trust, the Terrence Higgins Trust, the UK Coalition of PLWAs and Stonewall). Some countries have been more successful (e.g. The Netherlands, Germany) than others (Southern European countries) to have their politicians not to politicise AIDS, and to avoid unnecessary debates around sexual politics. The States have generally plaid a fundamental role in both the delivering of health and welfare services, and the funding.

These plans allow to bring some consistency in the implementation of HIV prevention policies, and hence political changes have in general not hampered in a major way policies. National plans are sometimes translated into specific programmes (the "Know, make accountable, inform, act" CRIA Programme in Portugal) which are relayed at the local level into local programmes, through newly created District Committees for the Combat against AIDS (CDLCS). The implementation of the policies outlined in the plans vary according to the local authorities and the degree of the decentralisation and autonomy of those in each country. A number of countries have been over this past decade embarking into efforts of "regionalisation", or the improved partnership of social organisations and local authorities. Advisory councils to co-ordinate the work between public administration and the NGOs can be found down to the local structures. As an example, in The Netherlands, the "AIDS-platforms" are a formalised process of structures representing the territories of the regional public health authorities in which local and regional organisations participate to the formulation and content of local policies.

Active (formulation, evaluation, commissioning) national, and/or regional Parliaments can catalyse and facilitate the implementation of innovative HIV/AIDS prevention policies through political and public mobilisation, or more liberal views. As a corollary, the arbitrating, accompanying, legitimating roles of the Law and Justice (example of the Asylum and Immigration Act in the UK) can also influence positively the policy-making. Forming a national consensus to adopt a liberal policy against AIDS through smooth processes facilitate the positive making of HIV prevention policies.

Prevention policies appear to be constantly evolving due to different developments: for example, improved attention towards and consciousness of the socially and economically disadvantaged, the discovery of new treatments against HIV infection leading to AIDS as a chronic illness and a need for long-term prevention. In The Netherlands, the effectiveness of combination treatments has recently changed the Health Council's position to a more pro-active test policy, particularly for pregnant women. Policies develop along the needs of sections most affected by HIV in each country, and are stimulated by independent working groups or tasks forces, by changes in laws, and special studies. For example, in Ireland, following the 1992 national formulation of strategy, public policy towards the gay community related for HIV prevention among gay men made considerable progress, and was accelerated by the decriminalisation of homosexuality in the 1993 Criminal Law Sexual Offences Act, and a special study on "Poverty, Lesbians and Gay Men: The Economic and Social Effects of Discrimination in 1995"; in 1993, an amendment to the Health Family Planning Act allowing condoms to become widely available; for drug users, the current policy was set later, in 1996, by the First Report of the Ministerial Task Force on Measures to Reduce the Demand for Drugs; in 1994, the ministry of justice ceased the segregation of prisoners with HIV; in 1998/99, an initiative by the Department of Education and Science enabling schools to develop policies on sex education.

The countries have at least a common denominator in attempting to tailor targeted HIV prevention policies to their different vulnerable populations. In Austria, a number of in depth studies in the nineties have been benchmarks influencing policy changes (effectiveness of sex education in schools in 1993, adolescent sexuality and AIDS in 1994, adult sexuality and AIDS in 1996, doctor-patient study related to gynaecology in 1999 etc.).

Although the countries do not mention being directly influenced by other countries in the making of HIV/AIDS policies, we found remarkable similarities and patterns in terms of development of specific programmes and using the positive experiences from some countries which have had positive experiments for some strategies and approaches (e.g. some of the IDUs strategies of the Netherlands). Countries do mention to use some exchange networks to strengthen HIV prevention, e.g. the co-operation between Nordic countries. The countries rarely mention any specific influence of the EU in the making of policies, with the exception of the EU Health Education Programmes influencing the Greek policy, or Iceland and Italy for HIV policy in general. Country national policy-makers are members of the EU Management Committee on AIDS and Other Communicable Diseases. As such, they participate in a multiplicity of EU and other international networks which update them of the latest policies in other countries. This process in turn influences national policy-making. Finally, countries signal that epidemiology may become increasingly important in informing policy, while the media may be losing ground in comparison to the past. Summits or Conferences contribute to influence national policies, e.g. the Paris AIDS Summit Declaration of 1994 "*to involve fully non-governmental and community-based organisations as well as people living with HIV/AIDS in the formulation and implementation of public policies*" to draw up the national UK plan "An Evolving Strategy".

HIV/AIDS is not anymore, in comparison to the eighties, an everyday topic, while topics like migration, and drug trafficking are now more frequently taken up. This can be reflected in the rather low profile "World AIDS Day" campaigns mobilised on 1st December 1999, in comparison to previous years.

In some cases, the civil society and local organisations have been drawn into the Government's attention due to local circumstances, e.g. the HIV-contaminated blood affair in France. Bottom-up approaches to planning vary depending of several factors: the tradition of implementing bottom-up approaches, the influence of socially vulnerable groups, the centralisation of Government structures, to mention a few. In other cases, pressure can be made on a temporary basis for the development of policies by and for some vulnerable and well-organised, sometimes politically powerful, groups, but if the country is small, e.g. Greece, the accumulated experience and power may not be sufficient to self-sustain itself, in comparison to France or Germany for example. Some Governments have legitimised early on one partner as the main interlocutor (e.g. "Deutsche-AIDS Hilfe" in Germany) instead of a multitude of smaller or less formal local associations.

Generally speaking, political, religious and legal organisations have concurred with the AIDS policies established by Government authorities, with some local national cultural specificity, such as the restrictive interpretations of the application of HIV/AIDS policies to prevent HIV/AIDS with respect to sex education in schools, the use of condoms, programmes for IDUs and people involved in prostitution both by the Italian Government in the early nineties, and the Catholic church still up to now. Sometimes the lack of involvement of the Church (e.g. Lutheran church in Iceland) is perceived as a deterrent to the development of HIV/AIDS policies, and in parallel, the moral legitimisation of sexual behaviour and faith and morality for the prevention of AIDS (e.g. the Protestant Church in Germany) can contribute to its success.

HIV/AIDS prevention policies are in general set within the broader context of other preventive and health promotion activities, such as, in Belgium, the combats against smoking and against accidents, the detection of breast cancer and promotion of low-fat nutrition. Although there is a general tendency towards the integration and horizontal approaches, and as a consequence an overlap of policies and personnel involved in interventions of HIV/AIDS, for example working with other programmes such the prevention of Hepatitis C, or STDs, Tuberculosis, or other infectious diseases, and towards decentralisation (to the Regions in Spain or France, Federal States in Germany, Districts in Portugal), those vary based on country-specific health systems and political structures (ref. Section 7). Evolving national safer sex campaigns have started to integrate HIV with STD prevention, and the prevention of unwanted pregnancies. In Austria, the approach is increasingly moving towards a comprehensive HIV-related health promotion, with a focus on sexual health.

Governments have made contractual agreements with implementing organisations which are non-profit bodies of a private, public or semi-public nature. In general, a degree of professionalisation and innovation have occurred within all organisations working on care and prevention over the past few years. The people HIV-infected have grown stronger through the support of special organisations of gay men and women, drug users and haemophiliacs. In some countries, or sub-communities (e.g. French-speaking community in Belgium), the recent dissolution of the prevention agencies and/or their integration into other departments or sections accompanied by reduction in budgets (France, Germany) are sometimes perceived by the general population or public sector agencies as a set back or a disinterest by the Government.

Public campaigns are well categorised. Some countries have successfully used grassroots organisations and their advice and concepts to reduce the misconceptions and prejudice against HIV/AIDS. They are evaluated by independent organisations and priority groups clearly circumscribed. Policy reviews fall into the national evaluations which are also carried out by independent bodies (National Evaluation Council, independent experts). The national bodies, e.g. National Commission, or the MOH, usually identify and design the evaluation indicators. A few countries (e.g. Greece, Iceland) have not yet had any national evaluations of their prevention policies or interventions.

In general countries do not use any theoretical frameworks to formulate the general policies, although those can be grounded on theories. Research or interventions can draw upon some theories (social network theory on HIV diffusion in Iceland, or cognitive behavioural theory in the Gay Men Fighting AIDS groups in the UK).

3.2.2 Northern, Central and Eastern Europe

In general, the WHO and UNAIDS recommendations had a major impact on the development of HIV/AIDS prevention policies in these countries, with central and eastern European countries rating this impact as particularly significant.

The main goals of the respective national AIDS prevention strategies in northern, central and eastern European countries are:

- To minimise the number of new infections: Bulgaria and Romania play a special role here, as they focus on HIV transmission via blood transfusion and perinatal transmission.
- To provide optimum treatment to HIV positive persons or PLWAs: While Finland, Norway, Poland and the Czech Republic aim to provide the best possible treatment and care to those already infected, Romania is still fighting for better access to diagnostic facilities and the creation of modern day clinics.
- To improve the quality of life of people living with HIV or AIDS: to ensure respect for and dignity of those affected in all spheres of life and encourage solidarity with infected persons in society (Poland, Finland, Sweden, Slovakia, Slovenia).

Some Eastern European countries are still fighting for a rationalisation of the existing HIV/AIDS prevention system and for a more effective allocation of available funds (Poland, Romania).

Both in Scandinavia and eastern Europe health promotion and health education of the public at large and risk groups are explicitly proclaimed goals, with information on modes of transmission and protection measures taking priority for these target groups. Moreover, Norway and Slovakia consider it important to improve the expertise of health and social workers.

In virtually all countries participating in the study it was the ministries of health and social affairs who were responsible for formulating national AIDS strategies and to whom the involved institutions were accountable. The fact that none of the decision-makers in the Estonian government are health experts has an accordingly adverse impact on the development of effective strategies.

For the co-ordination of activities most countries founded committees composed of - depending on country - health experts, the relevant minister, representatives of youth organisations, the Red Cross, the churches, NGOs or even relevant foundations. In Romania the formation of such a committee is still at the planning stage.

In Sweden and Estonia the influence of NGOs on national AIDS strategies is rated as particularly large, while it is rather small in other central and eastern European states, in stark contrast to western Europe. This is mostly due to their recent inception, as they didn't exist before the collapse of communism and were later only set up gradually according to the western model, partly even by government institutions. In the public awareness of these countries NGOs still play an minor role.

Of course, the political reforms of 1989 had a decisive impact on all major HIV/AIDS-related aspects in eastern Europe. The responses to questions on the effects of later changes of government differed considerably. For example, in Norway there have been no fundamental changes to AIDS prevention policy since the mid-80s despite some political changes. In Lithuania, in contrast, four changes of government over the last ten years have generated the same number of HIV/AIDS prevention concepts. A debate on the legalisation of prostitution came to an abrupt halt in Estonia after the elections. In the Czech Republic the rise to power of a more liberal party improved tolerance towards homosexuals, even if the introduced bill on registered partnerships still hasn't been ratified to date. Political instability from 1997 to 98 was the reason why Romania has so far been unable to realise plans to found a co-ordination committee.

Like in western European countries the theoretical foundations of prevention policy are rarely mentioned or explicitly denied, for example in the Estonian, Danish, Norwegian and Czech reports. In Bulgaria certain projects may be based on theories that are not specified here. In Lithuania the Health Belief model serves as a basis for safer sex education measures. The Theory of Reasoned Action is the foundation of HIV/AIDS programmes at schools. According to the Romanian report, its primary prevention elements are based on the Health Belief model, because it seems to be a suitable approach for information, education and communication. In general, there is no theoretical foundation for most prevention policies in the countries of northern, central and eastern Europe.

International organisations like the WHO, UNAIDS, EU, UNFPA, UNICEF and World Bank are ascribed a major influence on the respective AIDS strategies of central and eastern European countries. The former Global Programme on AIDS (GPA) contributed considerably to the first planned AIDS prevention strategies.

In all countries involved in the study HIV/AIDS prevention policies are based on national programmes or strategies. These plans often have a defined timeframe (e.g. 1997 to 2000 in Estonia and Slovakia or 1999 to 2004 in Poland). They vary in term from two to five years. Many of them were preceded by other short or medium-term programmes.

In general, organisations that backed and looked after the interests of certain risk groups had quite an appreciable impact on the development of national prevention strategies. This goes above all for gay associations that have a strong lobby in Sweden, the Czech Republic and Slovakia and whose representatives partly work in decision-making forums. The Bulgarian report mentions PLWA self-help groups. The Roma, who are supported in Slovakia by PHARE and UNICEF, for example, play a special role. The rising number of HIV-infected IDUs made the Estonian planning committee modify parts of the programme. In Latvia public institutions try to delegate tasks to NGOs, without giving them the necessary funds.

The influence of international organisations has already been quoted as decisive. In this vein, the WHO recommendations were essential for the development of national strategies (Denmark, Finland, Lithuania, Slovenia) and the instructions were incorporated directly in legislation (Bulgaria, Finland). Estonia mentions UNAIDS, which upgraded the role of NGOs in a 1996 study. In the Czech Republic the UNAIDS "Best International Practice" documents were very helpful. In Norway, however, it is apparently difficult to measure the degree of influence, despite the large number of EU, WHO or UNAIDS programmes Norway was or is involved in. Romania has received similar recommendations and instructions but has not yet put them into practice.

Hardly any of these reports mentions a specific country as a model of its own AIDS policy. Only Lithuania mentions that it took example of the Swiss policy for developing its national AIDS prevention programme. Latvia asked the National Institute for Public Health in Stockholm for support as of 1993, but without taking direct example of the Swedish model. Romania's National AIDS Commission is modelled on its Canadian counterpart. NGOs orientated themselves on programmes from France, the UK, the Netherlands and the USA. Lithuania consulted experts from different western European countries. There was a regular exchange of information and ideas between Norway, Denmark and Sweden, co-operation between the Scandinavian countries is strong in general. Despite the foundation of two sovereign states in 1993, the Czech Republic and Slovakia still co-operate closely in the field of AIDS prevention, among others, and are still using previously established structures and connections. And we can speak or orientation in the opposite sense, as well, when we see Bulgaria using its observations of epidemiological developments in Ukraine, Russia and Moldavia as a warning.

Partly, the countries use specific programmes for orientation. For example, Hungary's needle exchange programmes, Lithuania's methadone programmes, Norway's youth work and Finland's and Sweden's work with PLWAs are role models for Estonia. The Czech Republic adopted the ABC programmes for young people performed by the Centres for Disease Control (CDC Atlanta) in the USA.

The transition from secondary to primary prevention (1992), the introduction of voluntary and anonymous AIDS-Tests (1994), and the fact that intervention programmes now rather target risk groups than the general population, are rated as recent key trends by Bulgaria, among others.

Until the collapse of communism the former socialist states had no frank discussion of topics like homosexuality, drug abuse or prostitution, for which the social conditions were allegedly not given. Making these topics subjects of public debate, was one of the first little steps towards a change in policy (e.g. Lithuania).

Over the last three years (this was also the term of the first National Programme of Prevention) Poland has seen a particularly dynamic development, marked by the establishment of certain organisational structures at the public level, by successful fund raising, support of NGOs and assignment of responsibility for drug and AIDS prevention to the health minister. Information and education measures no longer simply comprise general information on modes of transmission and protection, but should serve to improve the attitude towards PLWAs. Political reshuffles between 1990 and 1994 slowed down the installation of corresponding structures. Only since 1994 has there been some progress. While from 1985 to 1992 district and municipal governments took the main responsibility in Sweden, it has now been transferred to the National Institute for Health Promotion.

Virtually everywhere in northern, central and eastern Europe we find a close connection with measures for the prevention of other communicable diseases. In most countries many of the structures already in place for hepatitis or STD prevention, now benefit HIV/AIDS prevention, as well. In the Czech Republic, for example, the concept used since the 1950s for STD surveillance, also served for AIDS monitoring until around 1992. In Lithuania and Norway the national AIDS prevention programme is integrated in concepts for the prevention of other communicable diseases, of drug abuse and in family planning measures. Existing networks and financial and staff resources are used jointly. Other countries implement measures that serve both to prevent AIDS and STDs (Estonia). In Bulgaria it is recommended that certain tests (HIV, TBC) should follow certain diagnoses (STD; HIV). In Slovenia some STD clinics also offer AIDS tests and corresponding counselling. AIDS prevention measures, especially those targeted at young people, are often intended for STD prevention, as well (Poland).

And there are other fields of health promotion that are closely linked with HIV/AIDS prevention. This goes especially for family planning and sex education measures (Bulgaria, Estonia, Norway). In the Czech Republic the "National Anti AIDS Fight Programme" in co-operation with the ministry of education promoted a training programme for teachers that served to integrate health education in the school curriculum. Ten Slovak schools are members of the European, another six hundred members of the national Health in Schools network. Sex education and the prevention of STDs are part of the curriculum

Studies for the evaluation of measures performed so far have mostly been commissioned and financed (Estonia, Finland) by international organisations or the relevant national ministries. For example, in 1995 WHO experts evaluated the medium-term strategy plans of Bulgaria and Latvia. Financed by UNAIDS and under the guidance of a former GPA staff member, an independent study was performed on the effectiveness of the Czech Republic's National Anti AIDS Fight Programme in 1996. In the same year a corresponding UNAIDS study upgraded the role of NGOs in Estonia. Every year the co-ordination committee of the National Prevention Programme submits a report on the programme's realisation to the Latvian ministry of health. The situation is much the same in Slovakia. The HIV/AIDS prevention measures of the Norwegian Board of Health up to 1994 have been evaluated by various research institutes, likewise its individual projects. And an evaluation study on the effectiveness of the Plan of Action for Combating the HIV/AIDS Epidemic 1996-2000 has already been commissioned. NGOs have commissioned evaluations for subareas of their activities, many of which are financed by public funds. In Sweden the executive institutions are responsible for evaluating certain measures. In 1995, for example, there was a corresponding evaluation of the allocation of the government budget. In 1999, for example, the National Institute for Public Health reported to the government about the status of HIV prevention work in big city areas. No evaluation measures have been conducted or commissioned in Romania, with the exception of NGOs, whose international sponsors demand a corresponding assessment of their programmes. Neither are official evaluation results available from Slovenia. There were plans to conduct a study on sex behaviour in the general population in 1999/2000.

In summary, the Scandinavian countries are comparable with western Europe in every respect regarding their HIV/AIDS prevention strategies. Only the influence of the church plays a rather minor role in these countries. In their intentions, the countries of central and eastern Europe follow the same policies but have not been able to complete their implementation yet. Apart from a few exceptions, they lack the driving force of NGOs, which are only gradually developing according to the western model and have only little influence on policies so far. The work of NGOs and state prevention strategies are often restricted by a lack of financial resources and additionally impeded by still prevailing attitudes left from the socialist regime, for example in medical associations. Despite the communist past, the church has regained considerable influence in these countries and should be considered in prevention policy measures.

3.3 Institutional structures of policy implementation

A recent study on sexual behaviours and HIV prevention carried out in Western Europe (Sandfort et al., 1998) concludes with the observation that the political climate is changing and is paying less attention to AIDS, and that a solution to efficient HIV programme may be to integrate it into a more global health programme, following the example of a few countries. In addition with the influence of people within and beyond borders, and less visible frontiers, an international sexual health policy may be even more beneficial.

Kenis et al. (1997) describe the results of the "Managing AIDS project" which started in 1989 as a WHO Collaborative Study with a design developed in close collaboration with the WHO and the European Council of AIDS Service Organisations (EURO CASO). The data collected between 1992 and 1995 refer to six countries: Switzerland, Netherlands, Sweden, Belgium (Flanders), Austria, and Italy. The study design focuses attention on the meso-level of organisations, or the intermediate level i.e. the level on which organisations are located, instead of the traditional studies referring to the micro-level of individual behaviour or the macro or national level. The study is less to be seen as a public policy analysis of national HIV/AIDS policies, but rather more as a study of the response of a wide variety of sources of collective action, such as public organisations, private organisations, non-profit organisations, community-based organisations etc. Those in turn provide a wide variety of activities (e.g. prevention, care, policy co-ordination, interest mediation, fund-raising etc.). The degree of the organisational response (being the dependent variable in the study) is defined as the degree to which an organisation or group of organisations responds to HIV/AIDS, i.e. where they develop specific activities to deal with the problems of HIV transmissions and/or to reduce the negative personal and social consequences of HIV/AIDS. Any organisation having at least one activity in the area of HIV/AIDS in the study is considered as having an organisational response. The degree of the response can be analysed on different levels.

Some of the key findings of the study are:

- The organisational response can neither be explained by the case-load (i.e. epidemiological size), nor by the size of the country. No society applied the existing epidemic laws to deal with this problem, but rather mobilised (to a larger or lesser extent) societal actors to deal with the problem.

- The organisational response is neither equally distributed across social groups nor across geographical areas within any one country.
- Questions regarding the degree of responsiveness with the three essential dimensions (types of activities, types of organisations and forms of distribution) have been found to constitute a useful minimal framework to explain the organisational response and to be measurable.

In the last few years a number of organisations were created to respond to European issues related either specifically to HIV and AIDS, or to European Health Policy. For example, the European Public Policy Network (EPPNA) has evolved from the Standing Conference of European Parliamentarians on HIV/AIDS held in Barcelona in 1995 where ways were explored to have the problem of HIV and AIDS in Europe remain a political, social and economic priority. This priority has become EPPNA original mandate which appears in the "EPPNA Review" (Journal of the European Public Policy Network on HIV and AIDS). The network is a forum and co-ordinating body for politicians, experts, business and community leaders, academics and organisations and aims to promote good public policy-making on HIV and AIDS issues within both national and local governments across the European Union and non-EU countries of the WHO European Region including Eastern Europe, and to share information and ideas. EPPNA has organised meetings on some current issues of HIV/AIDS in Europe, e.g. Social and Economic Consequences of New Treatments", and Mobility and HIV/AIDS: The Problem of Cross-Border Infection (1997).

Another example can be found in the "Public health policy in a European context" of the recent European Health Forum held in October 1999 in Gastein, Austria. In Europe, nowadays, the fact is known that health policy decisions can no longer be taken according to purely national concerns. Issues for the European level such as "newly emerging communicable diseases, including HIV/AIDS... are being paid more and more attention" (Rumpf, 1999: Issues in European Health Policy).

3.3.1 Western and Southern Europe

A mix of involvement of different institutional structures are to be found at the national level, often under the leadership of the ministry of public health, or other equivalent denomination.

In general, the public sector has dominated prevention for the public at large, research and medical care, and often the ministry of public health has been responsible for specific tasks, such as epidemiological surveillance. Within ministries of health, the tendency has been that special units for AIDS to become integrated into or with other units, e.g. communicable diseases, directorate of health. Some ministries, such as the ministry of social affairs in Belgium, are playing an increasingly important role because of the new emphasis in care and support structures (hospitals and first-level structures, insurances) with the introduction of the multi-drug therapies. The voluntary sector, on the other hand, has by large worked more in the field of prevention, psycho-social support, and education, and in some cases (universities, private institutes) research.

National AIDS Committees function through a set of structures, for example in Portugal, the Executive Board of Directors, the Advisory Board, and the Clinical Work Party. Despite the fact the National AIDS Committees may formulate policies and recommendations, the final responsibility to implement those or not lie in many countries, ultimately, either on the various responsible Ministries or on the local administrations' agreements with the national policies, or both. Some ministries are slower to accept changes in roles and functions (e.g. ministry of justice, ministry of the interior, ministry of employment) than others (e.g. ministry of social affairs, ministry of education). Rare are the national committees which cover the full spectrum of responsibilities such as, in Portugal, the elaboration of the programme, the co-ordination of its execution, the enforcement of its principles, and the assessment of the results.

Although committees have attempted to have some of the more vulnerable groups to participate, those are not always well represented. For example in Greece, the national steering committee has no representatives from the directly interested parties, e.g. homosexuals.

In some countries, special committees or tasks forces relay national policies to different structures, e.g. "National Advisory Committee" coupled with an "Inter-ministerial Working Group" in Germany, "AIDS task force" in France to organise hospital and medical care, "Commission for AIDS Policy (CAB) and Advisory Board for AIDS Research (WAR) in the Netherlands.

Public structures, either national or regional, have been providing the main financial resources both to the public and the voluntary sectors. Yet, private donations and fund-raising have plaid a non-negligible role as well, through national Foundations and NGOs initiatives. UK has set up a system obliging its district health authorities (HAs) to spend 50% of their prevention allocation to work within the vulnerable groups identified in their national plan.

Federal structures have found usually sound working relations by delegating the education or information activities to national agencies, parastatal or semi-private, for example the Flemish Institute for the Promotion of Health (VIG) in Belgium, or the Federal Centre for Health, Education, AIDS Programme (BZgA) in Germany. Twenty years into HIV prevention activities, the integration of special agencies, e.g. AIDS prevention Agency in the French-speaking community of Belgium, into larger existing structures, e.g. into health promotion departments, can be seen as a positive step to sustaining and normalising the response. Such transition is smoother, though, once the decentralisation at the local level is already fully functional and well-experienced. On the negative side, it can lead to a reduction of specifically earmarked funds for prevention, including for media campaigns, and to a loss of visibility and credibility among the public at large.

The co-ordination, execution, and implementation of activities are often delegated to a special unit, or independent body, either integrated into the ministry of health, or sometimes outside the ministry, e.g. the Flemish AIDS Co-ordination (IPAC), in Greece the Centre for the Control of Infectious Diseases (KEEL), in The Netherlands the AIDS Foundation complemented in this country with two additional important structures, the STD Foundation and the SAD-Schorer Foundation. These structures can in turn be in charge of special activities (e.g. information centre, library, documentation centre, counselling).

Despite the mechanisms just described, weaknesses in co-ordination do exist as illustrated with the following examples. In Belgium, the lack of structured co-ordination between the two Ministries for the Flemish- and the French-speaking communities involved in the efforts to stem the endemic. In Spain, due to the decentralisation of the National Health Care System, the redundancy in tasks between Agencies due to inadequate co-ordination, despite the Inter-territorial Council of the National Health Care System for the communication between the regional health authorities, and despite the commissions. In The Netherlands, the myriad of institutions provoking sometimes a barrier to co-ordination, although there are examples of successful well co-ordinated projects too.

National structures, through the various above mentioned structures, play an important role in policy implementation at the national level, and in supporting local or regional levels policies through projects carried out locally by local health authorities or by the voluntary sector.

Countries have had some success in decentralising activities, often driven by a local action plan, through local networks, e.g. co-ordination centres or health promotion centres in Belgium, the creation of District Committees Against AIDS in Portugal, the use of the existing district health authorities (HAs) in the UK, the "Regional Health Boards" in Ireland, the national information campaign branch of the AIDS Operating Centre (COA) in Italy. Yet, in Italy, decentralising may also mean ironing out and overcoming "regional divisions" with a common policy of action for the whole country. The activities can also be specific to vulnerable groups, e.g. the national network of Services for Drug Addicts (SerT) in Italy. The structures mentioned are in turn delegating activities and programmes (for example the army in Greece), or projects, to local authorities (health care centres, infectious diseases departments, gynaecology and obstetric departments etc.), schools (ministry of education), and Associations or local networks (of family counsellors in northern Italy). Local co-ordination can be facilitated through formal structures, e.g. the boards for health and social affairs of the various departments, or regions in France, in charge of implementing ministerial policies at the local levels, and with the collaboration of local partner groups, or the regional or county health councils in Italy. Decentralisation entails often local financing and accountability.

Decentralisation may also be a constraint to the implementation of sound HIV prevention policies as illustrated next. In France, decentralisation has not been a smooth process and can lead to tensions. Conflicts arise between the role of public structures and NGOs, with the latter complaining that their original objectives and activities are being re-appropriated by the State. It therefore needs special nurturing and preparatory steps. In Germany, and in other countries (Rosenbrock, 1999), primary prevention has not been institutionalised in a homogenous way. This is due to the fact responsible institutions differ by policy types (behavioural prevention, structural prevention, health enforcement, mixed forms), and fields of intervention (work, community, social groups, environment). Decentralised organisational structures are an adequate form to divide responsibilities. On the other hand, there is no responsibility for the complex as whole. The problems resulting from this lie either in dual responsibilities, or in responsibilities gaps, or both. An example is the lack of adequate response presently stated by the countries in addressing HIV/AIDS prevention issues related to migrants. In the example of Germany, on one hand, migrants fall as a particular vulnerable group under the large NGO (Deutsche-AIDS Hilfe), on the other hand it can be seen as particular segment of the general population falling under the public services. In Ireland, co-ordination of services vary from region to region, depends upon individuals, upon ill-defined roles, and the structures can, as a consequence, be erratic. In The Netherlands, the decentralisation was accelerated in 1990 through a law whereby the local/regional authorities play a key role in the allocation of resources for prevention activities which makes AIDS prevention dependent of local policies, leading in turn to "less optimal situations".

The various countries underline the essential roles plaid at the grass-root level by NGOs which have been instrumental in carrying out the functions the public sector cannot fulfil. Austria signals a close co-operation between the ministry of health and the AIDS NGOs characterising the country situation. NGOs have been able to complement the national campaigns and reach the more vulnerable communities or specific target groups, and able to meet the challenge of the needed diversification of responses. They are characterised by specialisation in different areas, such as telephone counselling, psychological care and social support, legal assistance, lobbying and being a voice for some of the more discriminated groups, to mention a few.

AIDS Reference Centres, subsidised by Governments, have different roles in different countries: HIV screening tests and counselling, training of health care professionals, collection of data, publications, information and publication centres.

Despite these structures, "institutional inertia to new responses", as stated by Ireland but implicit among other countries as well, may result in some organisations or individuals blocking initiatives which are relevant to progress in an area, and need innovation.

3.3.2 Northern, Central and Eastern Europe

As in western Europe, chief responsibility for the co-ordination and supervision of HIV/AIDS prevention measures lies with the national ministries of health and social affairs in virtually all northern, central and eastern European countries.

These ministries delegate relevant tasks and allocate available funds. In general, the relevant minister is also a member of the National AIDS Committee. Normally the ministry has a subordinate department of public health as an executive organ.

In many cases, the ministry of health is the initiator of the National AIDS Prevention Committee, whose members are recruited from a diversity of institutions. The committee co-ordinates the work of various sectors and institutions, supervises the observation of a time plan and is responsible for financial planning. Often the AIDS Committee is accountable to the ministry and has to report regularly on the progress or situation of the commissioned implementation of measures, programmes etc. (Estonia, Latvia Lithuania, Slovakia, the Czech Republic). In Sweden those responsible are grouped in two different committees that work together, the National AIDS Council and a working group composed of the National Agency for Education, the National Prisons and Probation Administration, the Board for Occupational Safety and the Health and Immigration Board. In Slovenia committee members are directly appointed by the minister of health.

Individual central institutions or organisations are assigned various tasks - in line with their other responsibilities - in the field of HIV/AIDS prevention. Therefore, responsibilities can differ between individual states:

Recording and documentation of epidemiological data, corresponding research and information falls under the scope of the Centres for Communicable Disease Control (Bulgaria, Slovakia, Sweden) or, like in Norway, the National Institute of Public Health.

The ministries of education integrate sex and health education in the national public curriculum (Bulgaria, Norway, Poland, Slovenia).

International networking and participation in co-operation programmes can be the responsibility of the foreign ministry (Finland).

The work of National Centres for the Prevention of Drug Addiction (Bulgaria, Slovakia) with IDUs naturally includes AIDS prevention measures.

The prevention of communicable diseases in prison and the establishment of needle exchange programmes falls under the scope of the ministries of the interior or justice. AIDS prevention is also part of the police training curriculum in some states (Bulgaria, Finland, Norway, Poland, Slovenia).

The Institutes for Occupational Safety develop guidelines for workplace safety, e.g. for staff of medical institutions (Finland, Sweden).

In Finland and Poland, for example the ministry of defence is in charge of organising preventive measures for conscripts.

At the regional and local level municipal authorities - school, social and health authorities - are the executive organs.

In most cases the work of all these institutions is co-ordinated and supervised by the National AIDS Committees. In Lithuania the UNAIDS Theme Group provides support by co-ordinating the prevention activities of 20 co-operating partners.

The organisation of NGO activities and their co-operation among each other and with public institutions differs greatly between individual countries. In Slovenia, for example, there is no co-ordination of NGO activities. The Czech government delegates the implementation of virtually all prevention measures for the chief risk groups to NGOs. In return, the state provides a large part of their funds. NGOs in Denmark are responsible for providing information to their target groups themselves. Simultaneously, public institutions make corresponding funds available. Co-operation takes place through the national AIDS programme. In Estonia the AIDS Prevention Centre co-ordinates the co-operation between the government level and the NGOs. In Slovakia state institutions and NGOs only very rarely work together.

Church organisations are mentioned separately only in the Slovenian report. Here the Catholic church organises campaigns of its own, for example for World AIDS Day, and Caritas has its own rehabilitation centre for IDUs.

Depending on the form of government, the distribution of responsibilities differs between the central and decentralised level and the degree of influence that public organisations have on regional and local decision-makers. For example, every government district in Denmark has a network of "Key Persons" involved in local prevention measures. As cities and municipalities are largely autonomous, guidelines developed by a ministry may not be put into practice at the local level. In Sweden the county councils bear the chief responsibility at the local level for measures addressed to individuals. They are independent and can organise their work according to the respective circumstances. In some councils there are separate departments for HIV/AIDS prevention work, in others this aspect is integrated in the general scope of public health work. All county councils work on the basis of specific plans of action. Contacts are part of a well-functioning network. In the Czech Republic eight district epidemiologists (also for the capital Prague) co-ordinate work at the local level. They are granted a certain independence in their decisions from the co-ordinator for the national level. In Estonia the AIDS Prevention Centre implements the policy at the regional level. Until recently Norway still had annual meetings of the medical officers of individual government districts with the Board of Health. Normalisation made these meetings obsolete. Meanwhile, the ministry of health plans to stage regular meetings of the representatives of involved institutions. In Poland regional co-ordinators are subordinated to the respective premier and report to the health minister. In Romania decentralised departments of public health represent public organisations at the local level.

The following barriers and problems have been described in the reports regarding the implementation of HIV prevention policies in northern, central and eastern Europe:

The Estonian ministry considers the supervision of funds its main responsibility and rarely deals with contents. And fear of contact still prevails between government institutions, in particular ministries, and NGOs. This is especially the case when they work in projects that seem innovative for Estonia. Lacking co-operation between individual programmes or projects also reduces the effectiveness of the overall programmes. The reasons for this are inadequate funding of social programmes in general and the fear, in this context, of further budget cuts.

In Bulgaria the integration of non-medical organisations is still very difficult.

In Norway there is a certain competition between beneficiaries of the public budget. For example, criticism has been voiced against preferential treatment of initiatives targeted at "men who have sex with men". The current stabilisation of the situation has diminished social and political commitment, which has led, among other things, to a reduction of human resources. Therefore, many projects were not continued after the funded term. Despite clearly defined responsibilities in the Norwegian plan of action, their distribution is still unclear. Unlike in the start-up years of AIDS prevention work, it has now become virtually impossible to test new initiatives without having to expect cut-backs elsewhere. In general, there are great uncertainties as to what changes will become effective after expiry of the current plan of action (2001).

The independence of Sweden's county councils means that the National Institute for Public Health does not have the legal authority to stop less effective prevention measures.

In general, in central and eastern Europe, and to a lesser extent in Scandinavia, the lack of available funds is seen as a great problem for the implementation of prevention policies.

3.4   Legal aspects

Since the early 1980s the consequences and effects of HIV infection and AIDS have faced the European states with new demands the full extent of which cannot yet be anticipated. After a certain time, this situation puts pressure on the state's political, administrative and legislative system to take action. In society we see the emergence of new assessments, a need for values and new values that are not yet mirrored in the judicial system. "The need arises to find regulations" (Prokop, 1990, p. 277). To solve the problem, one resorts to existing laws or tries to create new ones.

Dealing with HIV infection and AIDS calls for a social orientation and learning process, which must focus on the goal of optimising infection and disease-preventing behaviour. And so the problem arises what contribution, if at all, law plays in this process. As AIDS prevention mostly aims at behaviour modification, one must ask whether individual behaviour in potential risk situations can be influenced by laws. While, the compulsory wearing of seatbelts has established "safe" (driving) behaviour in most European countries for visible road traffic, the enforcement of "safer" sex by legal regulations is hardly imaginable for - mostly invisible - sexual intercourse.

In this chapter we shall discuss topics related to the positive or negative influence of legal framework conditions for HIV prevention. The considerable impact of legislation can be illustrated by simple examples: Repressive anti-drug laws reduce the possibilities of an addict to avoid risk-taking behaviour (NIH, 1997), and bans on distributing condoms in public have a very adverse impact on prevention. Likewise, claims that men do not have sex with other men and that drugs do not exist in prison, because both are prohibited, make it impossible to develop adequate prevention measures.

The legislative itself is dependent on the political system, be it democratic or socialist, and even similar social systems can show considerable differences, as some countries have a centralistic and others a decentralised, federal government. For example, Germany's federal government is essentially responsible for health insurance legislation and thus for securing funding and performance of the health system. In contrast, the federal states have major legislative powers regarding hospital planning and the public health service. In addition, local and city councils, as the providing bodies of local health authorities, have an influence on regional health care. In Switzerland, for example, the cantons are completely autonomous in the field of public health, and it is hardly surprising that there are great regional differences regarding drug-related prevention policies. They range from repressive policing measures through "harm reduction" approaches to the medically prescribed distribution of heroin to drug addicts (Kübler et al., 1995).

One specific feature of the social development of central and eastern European states is that, even though these countries now have democratically elected governments, laws from their socialist past may still continue to apply within existing legislation and may have an impact on HIV prevention polices, like compulsory testing of entire groups of the population, a common practice in the past, as an HIV prevention measure. Often such measures are only gradually rejected and laws modified due to WHO and UNAIDS intervention (in Ukraine, for example, only in 1996, Burban 1996), and sometimes, however, through close co-operation with western European states.

The experience of the European states shows that one cannot do without the supportive function of law for AIDS prevention. An exemplary legal system should clearly show, in view of prevention, what behaviour it condemns and what it demands of those affected and for those affected, if necessary. This includes eliminating discrimination against those involved, protecting their privacy, promoting tolerance and avoiding risk-taking behaviour (Gostin & Webber, 1998). The following country comparisons show to what extent these aspects are incorporated in the legislation of European states.

3.4.1 Western and Southern Europe

In general, in Western and Southern Europe, the laws, decrees, regulations and official guidelines in regard to HIV/AIDS do not represent particularly serious constraints on individuals.

Numerous laws, even though indirectly related to HIV/AIDS, are having a positive impact on some of the HIV/AIDS policies, for example to mention a few:

- In France, several steps, such as under the laws of 1987 the sale of syringes and condoms advertising are unrestricted; the "Civil Solidarity Pact", a contract legalising same sex or other non-married couples, has just been voted; in July 1990, PLWAs are given protection on the basis of their health or their handicap against discrimination, migrants who do not have regular status in France have access to medical treatments under the law regardless of their status, and the law favours granting resident status to patients who do not have it; the organisation of health care for prison inmates falling under the ministry of health since 1995, instead of previously under the ministry of justice, and a 1996 circular giving prison inmates unrestricted access to free screening, to condoms and to bleach for disinfection of injection materials.
- In Germany, the long overdue decriminalisation of homosexuality which was initiated in the mid-seventies and fully reached in 1994; in prisons, the distribution of condoms and lubricants, and the implementation of a needle exchange programme as pilot project in Lower Saxony; in working conditions, the HIV positives and PLWAs fall under the Severe Disability Law, with the right to take additional vacation time, and to be protected from unlawful dismissal, with further financial relief (special rates for public transportation, and low taxes for radio, TV, vehicle, and for telephone use).
- In Greece, adult homosexuality is accepted since 1950; people suffering from HIV/AIDS are provided by the state with a pension fund and treatment is free of charge for all Greek citizens.
- In Iceland, the recent 1997 legislation passed permitting the marriage between homosexuals, and the HIV antibody screening offered to prison inmates.
- In Ireland, the age of consent for homosexuals and heterosexuals fixed at 17 years of age under the Criminal Law Sexual Offences Act 1993; mandatory and available sex education throughout the school system; voluntary but not compulsory medical screening for HIV and Hepatitis offered to the growing number of refugees and asylum seekers.
- In Italy, a 1993 Law inserted in the Criminal Proceedings Code in which it was forbidden to keep PLWAs in precautionary custody in prison; people entering prison undergo a medical examination and an interview with a psychologist; the test for HIV cannot be carried out without the authorisation of the person concerned; IDUs can request to be entrusted to the health care service for drug addicts inside the prison; a law of June 1990 which states that confirmed HIV infection can in no way constitute a reason for discrimination.

- In Spain, the safeguarding of confidentiality is seen as the most important regulations part of the broad legal framework of the Constitution of 1978, and under that framework any health worker, prison inmate or migrant who might agree to screening and be detected as sero-positive is not subject to discrimination; HIV specific medicines are free of charge, and non-HIV specific medicine are charged 10% of the public sale price.
- In the Netherlands, a December 1998 bill approved by the Dutch Cabinet to allow partners of the same sex to marry; a bill introduced in 1997, still under discussion but should be passed in 1999 at higher level, on the control and regulation of commercial prostitution, the strengthening of the fight against involuntary prostitution, the protection of minors against sexual abuse, and the improvement of the prostitutes' position; foreigners entering the country are not subject to mandatory tests, following the unanimously accepted European decision; the early introduction in the early nineties of prevention and education programmes in the various types of penitentiary institutions (prisons, houses of detention and youth institutions); the protection of applicants' health in a newly revised law of 1997.
- In the UK, the asylum and immigration regulations requesting that the migrants' HIV status should be ignored as long as the person fulfils the normal requirements to enter or leave the country; the 1996 Education Act obliging secondary schools to provide sex education within the National Curriculum, including HIV/AIDS and STIs as a minimum.

Yet, some laws even though indirectly related to HIV/AIDS, and despite some positive development in relation to legal aspects, are having a negative impact on some of the HIV/AIDS policies, for example to mention a few:

- In France, an old law of 1970 still penalises the use of drugs without distinguishing between soft and hard drugs, and are classified as illegal, and penalises the possession of drugs for personal use; prosecution is dropped if a person accepts treatment; fines and prisons for sex workers for active soliciting in public places or from cars, despite the abolition of measures regulating prostitution and brothels.
- According to German law, prostitution is a social and immoral act, having as the consequence that prostitutes are not obligated, nor do they have the right to obtain a state or a private insurance, having therefore a negative effect on their social protection; for the migrants, Asylum Laws keep many questions open, especially for cases in which the illness is chronic or mental, or for more specific illness like AIDS.

- In Greece, users who possess a small amount of drugs are arrested; condoms and needles are not provided to prisoners.
- In Iceland, and in Ireland, no special access to condoms or clean needles and syringes in prisons. Although, in Ireland, a recent report commissioned by the department of justice, Equality and Law Reform recommended "a strictly controlled supply of clean needles and syringes", coupled with the provision for their disposal, and the provision of free condoms to all prisoners.
- In Italy, access to drugs or syringes are illegal in prisons but a recent Law on 12 July 1999 attempts to improve previous practices although the decree has not been issued.

In addition, certain practices are identified as ethically doubtful, or not facilitating positive policy developments, for example:

- In Austria, the lack of a satisfactory compliance, particularly in the hospital setting, with the AIDS Law specifying that the HIV testing is performed on a voluntary basis with the patients' consent; the lack of quality and effectiveness of condoms and lubricants distribution in prisons despite their availability in most prisons, and no needle exchange programmes.
- In Belgium, a screening test is done prior to hiring in the State police force, however, a positive result does not lead to rejection; some asylum-seekers are submitted to screening tests, although these are not compulsory; and tests are often carried out without patients' knowledge, in particular emergency services, during pre-operative preparations and in prisons; some fundamental rights are not applied to prison inmates: condoms, although authorised and supposed to be accessible, are very difficult to get in reality, as well as sterile injection materials and substitution therapy for hard drug users.
- In Greece, immigrants are not obliged to have a medical examination to enter the country whereas for those who apply for a green card, blood test for infectious diseases and a chest X-ray are mandatory.
- In Iceland, even if a law of sexual education in schools exists, it is known not to be universally done.
- In Italy, despite a low age of consent (14 years old) for heterosexuals or homosexuals, the Penal Code provides for public decency norms which have been used against homosexuals and date back to the Fascist period which have pushed the gay organisations to battle for the legal recognition of gay couples; prostitution is legal, but the Municipal Police has repressed it; an ambiguous law against discrimination for PLWAs which may become a mere statement of good intentions.

- In The Netherlands, despite the introduction of basic education in 1993-94 of sex education and information in the core goals of the curricula, those are vaguely formulated, and, finally, each school is free to use their own explanations and implement fully those or not.
- In the UK, despite the 1996 Education Act, many teachers feel that the older Section 28 of the Local Government Act, prohibits them from discussing lesbian and gay issues in the classroom.

The fact no laws exist in relation to some specific aspects can be detrimental too: for example, in Greece sexual health is not taught in schools, and in Italy, the ministry of education has never taken a stand on the compulsory schooling to educate young people before they become sexually active, letting the application to the discretion of each school and their directors or teachers. In Portugal, for drug addicts, no norms for AIDS/drug addiction were issued in the past few years despite the mounting problem among this vulnerable group, and the same among migrants.

Only two countries, among which the Netherlands, mention the EU treaties of Maastricht and Schengen containing regulations for a collective approach of cross-border drugs trade. In all EU states there is the possibility to replace or supplement punishment through therapeutic measures.

Despite the various legal aspects described here, what makes a difference, as reported in Ireland, is that underlying factors increasing the vulnerability to HIV/AIDS be identified and combated such as, poverty, discrimination, unemployment, abuse, educational opportunities, homelessness and other factors which result in marginalisation and disadvantage. For many people living with HIV, the virus is not their major or most immediate problem and working with PLWAs often requires a range of responses to an even broader range of problems. Community development approaches and outreach work may ultimately make the difference.

3.4.2 Northern, Central and Eastern Europe

Likewise, only few of the countries of northern, central and eastern Europe still have laws, decrees and regulations that restrict the freedom of individuals in the context of HIV/AIDS.

As in western Europe these countries have many official directives, laws, etc. that have a positive impact on the development of AIDS policies. In the following you will find a selection of such "laws" for each individual country:

Bulgaria:
- Nobody may be prosecuted for his/her homosexuality.
- Under the education plan health education is part of the national curriculum.
- Recognised asylum-seekers have equal rights in the health system.
- Since 1992 prison inmates have been offered voluntary tests.
- Regulations on the safety of medical staff are in force.

Czech Republic:
- Homosexuality is not a criminal offence.
- Procuring is penalised by law.
- Prostitutes are not obliged to undergo tests.
- A positive HIV test is expressly no reason to refuse an entry permit.

Estonia:
- Since 1998 IDUs are legally entitled to support.
- Since 1992 expressing one's homosexuality is not an offence.
- Sex education is part of the national curriculum.
- A positive AIDS test is no reason to refuse a residence permit.
- PLWAs receive a severe disablement allowance.
- Since 1997 regular tests have been legally prescribed for medical staff.

Finland:
- Homosexuality was decriminalised in 1971.
- The age of consent was lowered to 15.
- Discrimination against homosexuals became an offence in 1995.
- Prostitution is legal, but not for women from non-EU states.
- Voluntary HIV tests and access to condoms in prison
- Medical care is free for PLWAs.
- Laws against discrimination are in force.

Latvia:
- Homosexuality was legalised in 1992.
- Orders from the ministry of education to include health education in the curriculum.
- Each prison inmate must undergo an entry test.
- Persons who work in the field of medical care for AIDS patients receive an extra monthly bonus of 30 to 40% of their salary.

Lithuania:
- Since 1993 homosexuality is no longer an offence.
- HIV tests are permitted in prison.

	• Regulations to protect medical staff against infection are planned.
Norway:	• Prostitution is legal.
	• Homosexual partnerships can be officially registered.
	• Sex education is compulsory.
	• Examinations and tests are offered to immigrants but are not compulsory.
	• Prisons have needle exchange programmes.
Poland:	• Homosexuality is not a criminal offence.
	• Prostitution is legal, but procuring is not.
	• Condoms are available in some prisons.

Slovakia:	• Voluntary tests for prison inmates, accompanied by counselling and needle exchange programmes
Slovenia:	• Expressing one's homosexuality is a constitutional right.
	• Although there are no special regulations for immigrants, they are entitled to free treatment if they suffer from AIDS.
Sweden:	Gay couples in a registered partnership have nearly the same rights as straight couples.

Prostitution is legal within certain limits.

HIV tests are not compulsory for immigrants, but many of them take advantage of the offer.

If in need, PLWAs are entitled to a pension.

Medical staff are offered routine tests, but they are not compulsory.

Treatment, information and counselling are free.

The following laws have an adverse impact on risk groups:

• There are no laws that accord homosexual partnerships the same rights as heterosexual partnerships. This is neither anticipated nor planned (e.g. in Latvia, Bulgaria, Estonia, Slovakia, Slovenia, and Poland).
• No regulated check-up measures for prostitutes (e.g. in Norway, Slovenia, and Poland).
• No entry permit for HIV-positive persons (e.g. in Lithuania). Refugees seeking asylum are tested in Bulgaria. From 1986 to 1991 everyone who

went abroad for more than 30 days had to undergo compulsory AIDS tests. Immigrants must undergo an AIDS test (Slovakia).

- No specific laws to protect the rights of PLWAs (e.g. in Estonia and Norway).
- No needle exchange and/or methadone programmes in prison (e.g. in Latvia, Estonia, Romania, Sweden, the Czech Republic, and Poland).
- In densely populated or rural regions the right to anonymity is not ensured for AIDS treatment (e.g. in Finland and Bulgaria).
- Homosexuality is still a criminal offence (e.g. in Romania).
- Prostitution is a criminal offence along with procuring (e.g. in Romania and Slovenia).
- Prostitution is legal, but in Sweden soliciting prostitution has been an offence for punters since 1.1.1999, which has eliminated the positive aspect of legalised prostitution for HIV prevention.
- Since May 1999 prostitution has been illegal for women from non-EU countries in Finland and a reason for extradition.
- No screening offers for medical staff (e.g. in the Czech Republic and Poland)
- Sex education in school is still a controversial topic (e.g. in Poland).
- Those affected have the choice whether to inform their partners of a positive HIV test (Czech Republic) or not.

Some countries allege that it is illegal to expose other persons knowingly to the danger of HIV infection (e.g. in Poland) and this may be penalised by long prison sentences (Romania). From the preventive point of view such laws, which also exist in western European countries, are controversially discussed. Especially in the public opinion such laws are "only natural" and serve to prevent new infections, which makes them preventive. But from a sociological point of view these laws are counter-productive to prevention.

Apart from the negative examples, even in the countries of central and eastern Europe HIV/AIDS-related legislation is now more or less liberal - at least on paper - and hardly differs from that of western European countries, with a few exceptions (e.g. Romania). In the field of prostitution, some northern and western European countries have even more restrictive laws. But most states are more liberal in practice, as existing laws are simply not applied. Still, there are severe setbacks in the countries of central and eastern Europe: the factors of social deprivation mentioned in 3.4.1. such as poverty, unemployment, homelessness, etc., which may exacerbate the risks of HIV infection and should therefore be combated by corresponding laws, are much more pronounced in this part of Europe. Regardless of this legal regulation, which was not explicitly investigated in the reports, these factors may, sometimes to a considerable extent, impede the application of existing laws. For example, the right to optimum free medical care cannot be exercised, if the public coffers are empty. And if the police are poorly paid, for example, they are more prone to be corrupt, which may favour unconstrained human trafficking for prostitution and even child prostitution. Sex education in schools, which is prescribed by virtually all countries, frequently cannot be implemented because of lacking funds for corresponding training programmes for teachers or school workers.

Finally, one should point out that compulsory HIV testing of migrants - still practised by some countries - is definitely a feature of restrictive legislation and of very doubtful benefit for prevention. From the perspective of these countries, which still have a very low prevalence of HIV but are exposed to a huge influx of migrants from eastern neighbour countries with extremely high HIV infection rates, like Ukraine for example, such measures seem understandable.

3.5 Epidemiology

As of end 1998, Western Europe with an estimated 500,000 adults and children living with HIV/AIDS, and 270,000 in Eastern Europe and Central Asia, ranked together the second region of the world hardest hit by the epidemic, following closely North America, excluding developing countries (UNAIDS, Dec. 1998). As the trends go, the total number of cases in Eastern and Central Asia may in the next five to ten years surpass the one in Western Europe.

The present review, by the nature of the countries' selection, is limited to north and western Europe, to southern Europe, to a few countries of central and eastern Europe, and to the Baltic States. Nevertheless, epidemiological trends and pattern of other countries in eastern Europe (e.g. Ukraine and Russia) will be briefly mentioned because of their importance in the HIV/AIDS epidemic in the WHO European Region as a whole.

A recent publication from the European Centre for the Epidemiological Monitoring of AIDS (Hamers et al., 1998) documents the "Diversity of the HIV/AIDS epidemic in Europe," and with other recent publications constitute the basis of the present analysis (Dehne et al., 1999; Hamers & Brunet, 1998; European Commission, 1997; Cattacin et al., 1997; European Centre for the

Epidemiological Monitoring of AIDS First to Fourth Quarterly Reports; UNAIDS country fact sheets).

The standardised AIDS incidence data in Europe, including HIV seroprevalence studies among selected subgroups (IDUs, pregnant women, blood donations, prisoners) are processed through the European Centre for the Epidemiological Monitoring of AIDS (located in Saint-Maurice, France, and supported by the DGV of the Commission of the European Communities and by the French Direction Générale de la Santé). Those have been very useful for assessing the impact of HIV-related morbidity at the population level, characterising patterns of spread, monitoring long-term trends, and making international comparisons, as documented next. The complementary and added value of the European HIV reporting system being in the pilot phase in 1999 by the Centre is discussed elsewhere (ref. Para. 3.6).

a) Patterns of HIV spread

The early epidemic occurred in Europe predominantly among homo/bisexual men, and shifted subsequently to IDU cases due to the rapid and intensive spread of HIV through injecting drug use in countries of south-western Europe, particularly Spain (9.8 AIDS per 100,000 inhabitants), Italy, and more recently Portugal (8.2 AIDS per 100,000 inhabitants).

The distribution of cumulated AIDS Cases reported by the end of 1998 (CESES, Quarterly Report no. 60) according to the Modes of Transmission indicate the following patterns. The WHO European Region is presently characterised by AIDS cases with the largest proportion among IDU (40%), followed by homo/bisexual men (34%) and by heterosexually infected persons (16%).

Illustration 2: Distribution of cumulated AIDS cases declared up to 1998 in Europe by mode of transmission

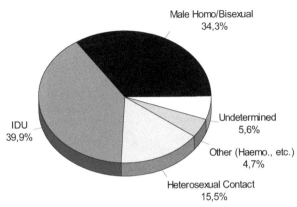

The modes of transmission are different between the three main sub-regions of Europe: in north and western Europe, male homo/bisexual transmission (54,5%) predominate, whereas in eastern Europe almost an equal mix of transmission is shared between male homo/bisexual (31,6%) and heterosexual contact (28,5%), and finally, in southern Europe the IDU transmission (61,6%) predominate. Different policies and strategies need to be tailored according to these different transmission patterns.

Illustration 3: *Distribution of cumulated AIDS cases declared up to 1998 in Eastern Europe by mode of transmission*

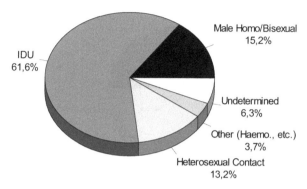

Source: Adapted from Euro. Ct. for Epidemiological Monitoring, Qtly. Rpt. 60

Illustration 4: *Distribution of cumulated AIDS cases declared up to 1998 in Southern Europe by mode of transmission*

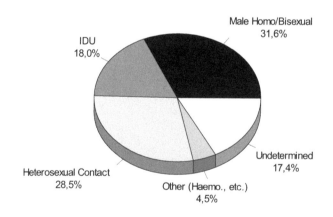

There is a sharp gradient of decreasing AIDS incidence from the south-west to the north-east of Europe. Geographical differences in AIDS cases are more markedly visible among IDUs than among homo/bisexuals, confirming the hypothesis that among the European countries, larger variations exist in the extent and practices of IDUs than in sexual behaviours, the latter found to be relatively homogeneous in a recent special study in western Europe. HIV prevalence vary considerably among IDUs not only by countries, but by regions within countries. The link with HIV infection between prostitution and toxicomania is high. In Europe, in contrast to Africa and South East Asia, the role of prostitution in the spreading of HIV seems limited due to marginal use of prostitutes, and the fact most prostitutes use condoms among their clients.

Comparing maps of AIDS incidence by transmission reveals that countries with a large epidemic in one sub-population generally have relatively large epidemics in the other sub-populations, illustrating the spread of HIV across different sub-populations (IDUs, homo/bisexual men, heterosexual vs. the "all cases" category). The diffusion of HIV in the population outside high-risk groups, although of major concern at the onset of the epidemic, appears to have remained somewhat limited. The low and stable or even declining prevalence (less than 5 per 100,000) in blood donations in western Europe, even though selected among individuals at low risk for HIV, indicates that HIV tends to have remained confined to high-risk population (UNAIDS June 26, 1998). While there are marked variations in the spread of HIV between countries, there are even greater variations within countries, with the highest prevalence generally found in large cities (e.g. England, Wales, Italy, Germany).

Illustration 5*: Distribution fo cumulated AIDS cases ut to 1998 in North and Western Europe by mode of transmission*

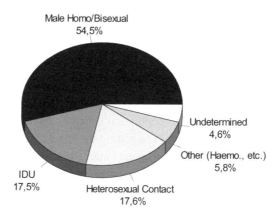

Male Homo/Bisexual
54,5%

Undetermined
4,6%

Other (Haemo., etc.)
5,8%

IDU
17,5%

Heterosexual Contact
17,6%

Source: Adapted from Euro. Ct. for Epidemiological Monitoring, Qtly. Rpt. 60

Illustration 6: 1998 AIDS incidence, per million population, WHO European Region

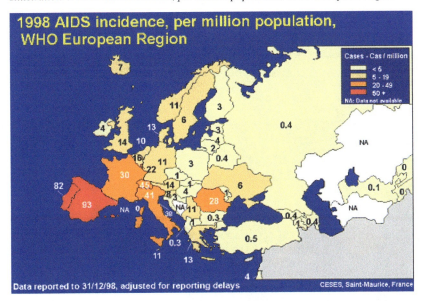

533

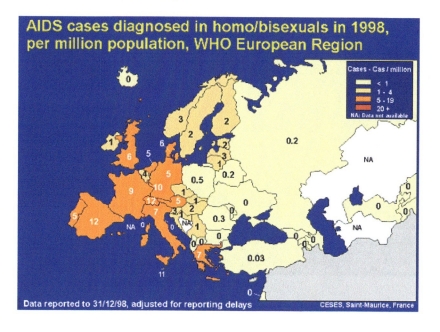

AIDS cases diagnosed in homo/bisexuals in 1998, per million population, WHO European Region

Illustration 8: *AIDS cases diagnosed in injecting drug users in 1998, per million population, WHO European Region*

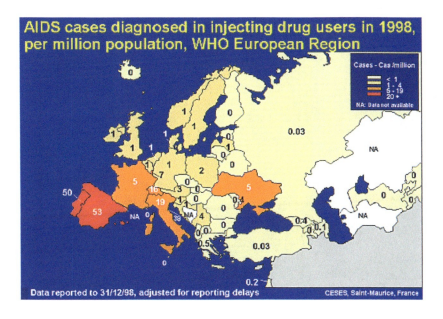

Illustration 9: *Heterosexually-infected AIDS cases diagnosed in 1998, per million population, WHO European Region*

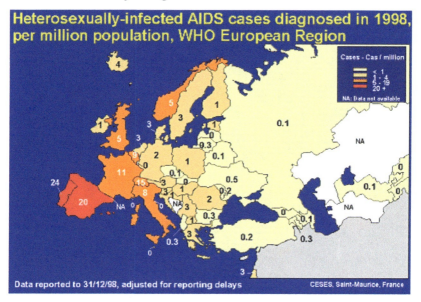

b) Recent trends

Recent trends in western and eastern Europe are discussed based on AIDS incidence data, whilst keeping in mind that those reflect patterns of infections which occurred on average ten years earlier and that HIV incidence peaked in the mid-eighties in western Europe.

For the first time since the start of the epidemic, the annual number of AIDS cases reported in the WHO European Region decreased (5% between 1995 and 1996), partly explained by the peak in HIV incidence in western Europe in the mid-1980s, and the recent rapidly increasing uptake of the new treatments (Hamers et al., 1996). As reported in the last Surveillance Bulletin (Europ. Ct. Qtrly. 60, 1998/4), the European Union accounted in 1998 for 92% (201 593) of all reported cases in the WHO European Region. AIDS incidence continued to decrease in the European Union, from 13, 986 cases in 1997 to 11, 071 cases in 1998 (-21%). The number of annual deaths declared among patients with AIDS has also decreased as well for the first time in 1996 (-10%), and in 1997 (-32%). The recent decline in AIDS incidence could thus be at least partly explained by the underlying HIV incidence curve (the recent and rapidly increasing uptake of new anti-retroviral therapies being one of the major reasons). AIDS incidences were highest in Spain (93.3 cases per million population) and Portugal (81.8) and lowest in Finland (3.2) and Ireland (3.6).

In Western Europe, the sharp decline in AIDS incidence which occurred in 1996 (-12%) was distributed among homo/bisexual men (-21%), followed by IDU (-10%), and heterosexually infected persons (-2%).

Table 2: Main epidemiological features in Eastern Europe

Sub-Region	Main epidemiological feature	Increases in reported syphilis rates*
Baltic States (Estonia, Latvia, Lithuania)	Few cases reported, mainly MSM, emerging epidemic among IDU	+++
Central Europe (Poland, Hungary, The Czech Rep., Slovakia, Slovenia, ...)	Low prevalence, mainly MSM, old IDU epidemic in Poland	(+)
Balkan countries (Romania, Bulgaria, ...)	Mainly heterosexual transmission reported, old IDU epidemic in Yugoslavia	+

Source: Dehne et. al., AIDS 1999, 13, p. 745

Eastern Europe benefited from a quasi absence of epidemic before 1995 with a few exceptions of different nature in Romania, south of Russia, Yugoslavia, and Poland. The epidemiological trends vary greatly between countries: increase in some such as the Baltic States, stable in others (e.g. Poland), and decrease in others (e.g. the Czech Republic). In the central and eastern part of the WHO European Region, AIDS incidence has increased by 14% overall (from 1,167 in 1997 to 1,236 cases in 1998). Romania has the highest AIDS incidence (2.8 per 100,000 inhabitants), followed by Ukraine (0.6). In 1998, the highest AIDS incidences were observed in Romania (27.6 cases per million), Slovenia (7.6). The large majority of AIDS cases in Romania occurred among children due mainly to 'nosocomial' infections (therapeutic micro-infusions and multiple injections with non-sterile equipment). The large increase in STDs cases reported in the region, especially syphilis with 100 per 100,000 population in the Baltic States (Dehne et al., 1999), is of concern for the direct impact on HIV transmission (UNAIDS Jun. 26, 1998). In contrast, a low number of syphilis cases is reported in central European countries varying between less than 1.8 per 100,000 in Slovenia, to 2.1 in Slovakia and 4.0 in Poland, and higher in the Balkan countries, with 27 per 100,000 in Bulgaria. It is anticipated that AIDS incidence will increase extensively in the future in several eastern countries, including Belarus, the Russian Federation and Ukraine where large outbreaks of HIV infection have occurred since 1996. In the Russian Federation, most infections were spread sexually until 1995, and infection in drug injectors was virtually unheard of, but in 1996 and 1997, drug users accounted for four out of every five newly-diagnosed HIV infections, and in Belarus 87% of HIV infection occur among drug injectors because many of them share injection equipment (UNAIDS June 1998). Several factors seem to have been fuelling the HIV epidemic among IDUs, including the demand, supply and consumption of drugs, migration, widespread local drug production, and shrinking resources.

The Balkan countries differ from the rest of eastern Europe in that heterosexual transmission is more frequently reported. Except for Yugoslavia (Serbia and Montenegro), IDU-associated HIV infection has remained the exception. Homosexuality is still severely stigmatised, probably much more than in central Europe, and is often legally restricted. Homosexuality transmission is therefore likely to be underreported. The Balkan countries with some of them among the least developed countries in Europe, and which are, in addition, becoming increasingly drug traffic routes between Asia and western Europe, may suffer similar developments than in the newly independent states in the near future, or than in Lithuania and Latvia in the Baltic States, where the pattern of infections is moving from homosexual men to IDU (Dehne et al., 1999).

Recent data on HIV prevalence suggest in 1998 that 80,000 new infections occurred in eastern Europe and central Asia, while 30,000 persons become infected each year in western Europe (CESES, "HIV Prevalence", 6.8.99). The number of HIV infections in Eastern Europe has increased nine-fold in just three years, from less than 30,000 HIV infections in 1995, to an estimated 270,000 infections by December 1998, with approximately 80% of infections in individuals who inject drugs. The most dramatically affected regions (falling outside the present study area) are Ukraine, Belarus, Moldova, Kazakhstan and the Russian Federation. The central European sub-region seems to be much less vulnerable to a large scale spread of HIV than the newly independent states. Economic performances are better and fewer young people are unemployed, with as a consequence less IDU or work in the sex industry. STD rates have remained at a low level.

c)   Vulnerable groups

In Western Europe, *homosexual and bisexual men* continue to be the most severely affected population group.

"HIV/ AIDS and the health of women" (European Commission 1997) illustrates how the European Commission can influence governmental policies with data-based evidence brought to the attention of the Governments and public through such an analysis: first, AIDS cases have increased steadily in the fifteen West European countries reported in this comparative analysis among *women* between 1986 to 1996; second, in 1996 women constituted 17% of the cumulated AIDS cases (and increasing yearly); third, the most frequent transmission routes among women in 1996 were IDU (51%), followed by heterosexual contact (37%), and others/unknown such as transsexuals (6%), and blood transfusion recipients (5%); fourth, the transmission routes vary between countries with Spain, Ireland, Italy, and Portugal which have the largest part of AIDS cases from the IDUs. The analysis concludes that despite the scientific evidence that women are at risk of getting infected, there has been up to 1996 few preventive measures for women, particularly young women in general. The HIV epidemic in Europe is considered a "concentrated epidemic" (UNAIDS terminology), justifying therefore measures towards specific vulnerable groups, but women are usually considered part of the general population. Campaigns have been more targeting the general population among whom women are considered to be encompassed, or the better defined specific vulnerable groups (e.g. homosexuals, IDUs, and prostitutes). As a consequence, women or young women are overlooked for messages tailored to their needs and interests. The lack of and need for tailored messages in general population campaigns adapted specifically to men or women, and in which the sexuality of men and women are taken into consideration, as well as power differences, were already pinpointed in a recent EU study on Sexual Behaviour and HIV/AIDS in Europe (Hubert et al., 1998).

An encouraging comparative reduction trend of the AIDS incidence in 1997 is visible in comparison to 1996 by countries by the three main transmission groups: among homo/bisexuals (1996, -22%; 1997, -37%), among the IDUs (1996, -10%; 1997, -33%), and among populations infected with an heterosexual contact (1996, -2%; 1997, -18%). This reduction is also mainly due to the opportunity of receiving Highly Active Anti-Retroviral Treatment (HAART). In addition, the incidence of AIDS among children infected by vertical transmission which had stabilised since 1990 has decreased significantly in 1996 (-37%), and 1997 (-24%).

A recent age-period-cohort analysis revealed large country differences in the dynamics of the HIV/AIDS epidemic among *intravenous drug users* (Houweling et al., 1999) as reported next. Estimates for hard drug use are difficult to obtain and specific estimates for injecting drug use are not available. Available estimates of hard-drug users produced by countries are based on very different methods and are subject to different types of biases, and range from (per 100, 000): 120-180 in Germany, 100-210 in Finland, 130-190 in Austria, 160-180 in the Netherlands, 160-230 in Sweden, 240 in Denmark, 280 in France, 330-550 in Italy, and 460-550 in Luxembourg.

Comparing incidence patterns in the 1965-1969 to 1960-1964 cohorts suggests the epidemic has reached a plateau at low to intermediate levels in Austria, Greece and the north-western European countries, and at high levels in France, Italy and Switzerland.

In Spain the epidemic was uncontrolled with a high incidence among recent birth cohorts. In Portugal the epidemic was still at an early and expanding phase.

Earlier introduction of the virus and higher prevalence of IDU may explain some of the generally higher incidence in Southern Europe countries, but the larger part of it is most likely explained by local characteristics of drug users, such as younger age and more frequent sharing of needles and syringes, and a less effective public health response.

In general, north-western European countries have more often endorsed needle exchange programmes, whereas France, Italy, Portugal and Spain, introduced them largely after 1993. The early adoption of needle exchange programmes in different parts of countries may explain how HIV prevalence has remained low in nearby towns surrounding some of the cities with major epidemic (Edinburgh, Amsterdam, Zurich).

In France, a study to evaluate the effects of liberalisation of syringe sales at pharmacies in 1987-1988 showed that the mere availability of needles and syringes, not embedded in a wider programme of HIV prevention, is insufficient to eliminate needle sharing: about half of the participants continued to share in a variety of ways (Ingold & Ingold, 1989).

d)   Potential factors accounting for the diversity of the epidemic

The diversity of the HIV/AIDS epidemic reflects complex interactions between several factors: the time of the introduction of HIV, sexual and drug-use behaviour (prevalence, types of practice, and social networks), and prevention interventions (mass media campaigns to raise awareness and interventions targeting at-risk populations). To determine the role of each of these factors, many of which are themselves hard to quantify and have changed over time, is difficult:

"...in particular, much as one would like to measure the specific impact of prevention interventions (which are a priority), *this is, in practice, very difficult."* (Hamers, Brunet, 1998, p. 68)

In western Europe, HIV was introduced in the early 1980s, resulting in rapidly rising incidence which peaked in the mid-1980s with many infections occurring before there was any public awareness of the threat of HIV. Declines in HIV incidence following the peak are probably due to both behavioural changes, under the influence of country policies, and to cohort effects with relative saturation of the population at risk not being replaced by a similar number of new susceptible individuals.

The major differences existing until recently between the epidemics in western and eastern Europe are probably due to the later introduction and to the lesser potential (until recently) for subsequent spread of HIV in eastern Europe: high levels of social control, relatively low prevalence of injecting drug use (with new pockets developing in some Eastern Europe countries), strict norms regarding sexuality, and unlawfulness of homosexuality including little opportunity for expression of homosexuality and limited development of sexual and drug use networks. External major disturbing factors which have occurred in the former Soviet Union may contrast with other more open and stable factors of other central and eastern Europe countries, including economic ones. central and eastern Europe may have benefited from lessons learned from the west and implemented timely prevention interventions (including the development of organisational support structures), or is in the process of implementing innovative preventive programmes, for example among drug users based on recent Guidelines (WHO Europe, 1998).

e)   Issues for prevention and control

Experience in Europe and elsewhere has shown the extent to which epidemics, once triggered, can develop extremely rapidly. The trend of HIV incidence in recent years (in contrast to AIDS incidence) is not really known, and (projections) in the future even less so, explaining the importance of maintaining the prevention and control efforts.

In the Eastern Europe and the Commonwealth of Independent States (CIS), economic migration, wars and the opening of internal and external borders have led to increased population mobility both within and between countries. It is still unknown how much these factors contribute to the spread of HIV (UNAIDS, Jun. 26, 1998).

Based on the above data, the European Centre for the Epidemiological Monitoring of AIDS concludes with a pledge to pursue further primary prevention efforts in western Europe by all means, despite the decline in AIDS incidence, as well as meeting the challenge of providing effective therapies to a maximum number of HIV-infected persons. In eastern Europe, preventing further spread of HIV through behavioural interventions and control of bacterial STD, and care of the many already HIV-infected persons are the major challenges in the context of political instability and economic hardship. The original wasteful and ineffective control policy of the former communist countries of Eastern Europe centred around mass HIV testing, mostly without counselling, with little attention to primary prevention, must be overcome.

The recent epidemiological analysis of the HIV/AIDS epidemic in eastern Europe includes purposefully the following implications for policy-making (Dehne et al., 1999):

- The Baltic States of eastern Europe: move away from the policy of drug supply and/or drug demand reduction to promote a harm reduction approach to HIV prevention among IDUs in order to balance the existing policy and programme mix, along the recommendations of the UNAIDS Task Force (UNAIDS, 1997). Create an enabling environment not only with HIV prevention among the most vulnerable segments of the population (e.g. IDUs, men who have sex with men, sex workers), but also programmes to sensitise the population at large and decision-makers.
- Central Europe: pursue the already started outreach and peer prevention programmes to prevent HIV among vulnerable populations, such as the example of the Czech Republic, Hungary and Poland.

- The Balkan countries which need further assessment to the vulnerability of HIV: priorities among IDUs, and among programmes and projects aiming to prevent infection among migrant population who have lived in higher prevalence areas and men who have sex with men.

f)   *Lessons learnt for HIV/AIDS prevention policies in Europe*

Epidemiological data have influenced national and international policies in Europe in some cases, or in other cases have been overlooked or abused (Cattacin, 1997). Policy analysts often conclude that HIV prevention activities are based on other factors and influences than epidemiological data.

The present overall review of HIV/AIDS documents, and our interaction with policy-makers, give evidence that the use of epidemiological findings in order to prompt or guide new policies in each country should not be underestimated:

- Epidemiological studies and analysis conclude and point to areas which need more attention and action as documented locally, or at national or international levels,
- Epidemiological findings presented at conferences, workshops, meetings, and newspapers influence in turn and are used by policy-makers in their countries,
- policy documents from international organisations for specific programmes (e.g. preventing HIV infection among drug users, or targeting young women) are justified and often based on epidemiological evidence,
- there is evidence that new orientations and emphasis in programmes (e.g. AIDS public education, targeting of more vulnerable groups etc.) follow, within a brief lapse of time, the epidemiological trends documented in publications, hence supporting the use of epidemiological data for decision-making.

More research is needed to understand exactly if, and how much, the epidemiological surveillance of HIV/AIDS is contributing to the national policy in each country.

Finally, the present review of various epidemiological Reports point to the following recommendations in order for the epidemiology of HIV/AIDS to even play a more useful and influential role than presently towards the development of HIV/AIDS policy in the European Region:

- to encompass more detailed analysis of the changes in trends among vulnerable groups,
- to address gender issues, particularly pointing to specific issues related to women,
- to distinguish the youth in a separate analysis.

We note that the present European Centre for the Epidemiological Monitoring of AIDS (CESES) is playing fully and with high standards its original role of "collection, analysis and dissemination of epidemiological data with the objectives of describing and better understanding the HIV epidemic and improving prevention and control" in Europe. In addition, the CESES is contributing directly to stimulate the improvement of the surveillance of HIV/AIDS in each country as well. In order for the CESES to contribute more to its second objective of improving prevention and control by recommending policies to the individual countries and the EU, we recommend that the data analysis be taken one step further to encompass the policy dimension which would in turn facilitate the policy-makers' present interpretation of epidemiological data. In order to accomplish this aim, the present small and efficient team composed of epidemiologists and a bio-mathematician could use the additional expertise of a policy analyst and/or social scientist.

3.5.1 Western and Southern Europe

The recent development of new therapies and the early diagnostic and prophylaxis policies have provoked a radical change in the epidemiological situation and policies development. For example, as reported in France, the enlargement of the "viral reservoir" due to the fact more people are living with AIDS than before, and the increase in the total number of PLWAs, combined with the steep decrease in the number of AIDS-related deaths. In addition, the numbers of socially disadvantaged individuals have expanded significantly, while screening and treatments have become increasingly complex and restrictive, particularly with their effects on vulnerable population groups. Finally, the decrease in the number of voluntary HIV screening tests leads to the situation of a significant number of HIV infected individuals are unaware of their infection until full blown AIDS is diagnosed, as is often the case for patients contaminated through heterosexual contacts and for foreigners, particularly from sub-Saharan Africa.

Control measures can be effective, but need to be interpreted cautiously, as large pockets of new infections may still exist in some part of cities:

- in Belgium, the successful control of IDUs transmission with a low proportion of transmission,
- the same in Ireland as well, with a drop from 45 to 22% between 1993 and 1998 of the new HIV transmissions, and services provision to gay men provided on epidemiological evidence
- in Italy, a net decline in the number of paediatric cases since 1997 due to the combination of an effective information campaign inviting pregnant women to undergo the HIV test, and the correct application of the guidelines on the anti-retroviral treatment of pregnant women with HIV.

Epidemiological data confirm new emerging vulnerable groups, such as:

- in Belgium, the largest group of non-Belgium women affected among the heterosexual transmission group; high percentage (55%) of new contamination cases among non-Belgian individuals,
- in Germany, from Patterns II countries an increase from 3 to 11% between 1995 and 1998
- in Italy, a more in-depth analysis, documents an increase among female adult AIDS cases from 16 to 23% between 1985 and 1997,
- in Portugal, the IDUs constituting the main forms of transmission,
- the UK which will place "greater emphasis in the future on developing national and local health promotion directed at vulnerable groups while continuing to maintain awareness of HIV in the general population" thanks to the "epidemiological connectiveness" and local health authorities to spend 50% of their prevention budget on work with the recognised target groups (An Evolving Strategy, UK Department of Health, 1995).

In the case of a nascent epidemic, e.g. Greece with more homosexuals and heterosexuals infected than IDUs, the lack of epidemiological evidence does not always facilitate the decisions for the prevention of the disease. But in the case of Iceland, in a similar epidemic pattern, epidemiological data and evidence are allowing to shift the original preventive work from the public in general and homosexuals in particular, to messages for the youth and heterosexuals. In the case of the Netherlands, low and stable figures do not give rise to much professional or political attention to the AIDS epidemic.

The data confirm an increase among heterosexual transmission:

- in Belgium, a 10% increase in approximately ten years among heterosexual transmission, or 47% of total transmission in 1997,
- in Germany, from 3 to 11% between 1995 and 1998,
- in Ireland, from 13 to 21% between 1993 and 1998,
- in Italy, as well, and Spain, principally among women.

Contrasting the various trends in the different transmission groups, there is evidence that it may be easier to change drug use behaviour, if clean needles are available, than sexual behaviours, for which the accessibility to condoms does not automatically result in their use. Hence, the increasing trends among the heterosexual population. In addition, women are affected more by the negative changes in trends than men. Besides biological and cultural factors, other contributing factors have been recently brought forward, such as sex tourism in Austria for men.

Austria reports a large group of AIDS patients who are categorised in the "unknown risk of transmission" and creates uncertainty for the interpretation of the statistics.

Due to the limited efficacy of the drugs available at the moment, the possibility that the number of AIDS cases start to increase again in the future cannot be ruled out.

Nevertheless, and despite some positive developments, we need to keep in mind that the epidemic situation of HIV new infections, with no drop in the number of new infections, may not have changed overall in different countries yet, taking the example of Germany.

The shift from epidemiological data focusing on AIDS to data on HIV, particularly the incidence of new HIV infections, is much needed, as well as data analysis focusing more on the emerging vulnerable groups, including youth. It may be more useful to move to the analysis of risk behaviours rather than limit the present main epidemiological analysis to the description of transmission categories (homosexual, heterosexual, IDU). The Netherlands documents the artefacts of reporting due changes in definitions, for example the definition of AIDS cases has increased the number of persons diagnosed with AIDS among IDUs.

In conclusion, there is strong evidence that decision-making on HIV prevention policies are influenced by epidemiological data available, but have not been determined by those. All countries report the wide diffusion of data or feedback in the country, including through scientific publications. Several countries report use at the local, i.e. regional, levels. Reporting delays, lack of data, incomplete coverage are all factors limiting the usefulness of some of the existing reporting systems.

Some evidence of control among some of the original vulnerable groups, e.g. homosexuals and IDUs, contrasts with the increase of transmission among the heterosexual population. This indicates a need to pursue continuing strategies aimed at the general population which in turn are challenged by the normalisation and medicalisation of AIDS, and resources constraints.

3.5.2 Northern, Central and Eastern Europe

In the states of northern, central and eastern Europe epidemiological data are made available to the corresponding political bodies and the public at large and generally (apart from Estonia) have a major impact on prevention policies, although HIV incidence in these countries is still mostly rather low, compared with western Europe. Only Denmark and Romania are in the European middle range. The low incidence rate of other Scandinavian states (Finland, Norway and Sweden) is comparable to that of central and eastern Europe.

In virtually all countries participating in the study, an institute that is mostly subordinated to the respective prevention centre collects HIV/AIDS-related data, evaluates them and makes them available in various forms both to those working in the field of prevention and to the public at large, as the following examples go to show:

The Finnish National Public Health Institute regularly sends info sheets to health institutions, ministries, regional administrations, NGOs and scientists.

In Norway the Surveillance System for Communicable Diseases provides weekly updates on the HIV/AIDS situation to health institutions, central and local administrations, and all others involved in the HIV prevention process, as well as to the mass media and to the public at large via its website. At least twice a year the data undergo in-depth processing, analysis and annotation. The Norwegian strategy plan for HIV/AIDS prevention is adapted to the current epidemiological situation every year.

Every quarter the Swedish Institute for Disease Control publishes its HIV/AIDS-related data, and once a year an in-depth analysis. Similar analyses are also performed at a local level. All of them are available to the public and serve as a basis for discussions on prevention policy measures.

In Denmark the Department for Epidemiology brings out a weekly Epidemiological Bulletin.

As part of the Latvian AIDS Prevention Centre, the Epidemiological Surveillance Unit is responsible for collecting, analysing, processing and publishing relevant epidemiological data. The public is informed, for example by the publication of a bulletin (ever year on World AIDS Day). The mass media are regularly kept up to date on the existing epidemiological situation. On the research institute's website visitors can retrieve information at any time. The results of study analyses that refer to specific risk groups are passed on to other organisations involved in prevention. The formulation of a basic national strategy for HIV prevention work in Latvia was based on the analysis of relevant epidemiological data.

In Poland the State Department of Hygiene is obliged to collect and analyse epidemiological data. They are passed on both to the National Office for AIDS Prevention and to other institutions at the regional and local levels.

In the Czech Republic institutions that conduct such tests, pass on their data to the National Reference Laboratory on AIDS. Once a month the data are statistically processed and fed back to the labs and all other organisations integrated in the process. Simultaneously, the data are published in print and on the website of the National Institute of Public Health.

The data provided by the Romanian ministry of health are considered highly unreliable, as hundreds of cases from some government districts are not reported.

Like the northern European countries the states of central and eastern Europe are now members of the European Centre for the Epidemiological Monitoring of AIDS in Paris. Information on the epidemiological situation is regularly sent there. In the same way they receive news of the situation in other European countries.

As the number of AIDS cases is very low in Estonia, corresponding statistics had no major impact on HIV/AIDS prevention policies there, except for the discussion on introducing combination therapy. In this context, the very short average survival time of AIDS patients in Estonia, compared with the two other Baltic states Latvia and Lithuania, was the decisive argument for making the corresponding medicines available.

Especially the emergence of new risk groups and changes to their priority status regarding HIV/AIDS frequency are unanimously rated as decisive epidemiological influences on prevention policies:

Since 1990 the infection rate for women has been rising in Finland. The same goes for the share of infections by heterosexual contact, while the number of infections by homosexual contact is falling. 20% of all cases are only diagnosed on developing full-blown AIDS.

In Sweden the target groups of HIV/AIDS prevention have hardly changed in the course of time. Recently the topic of sex tourism was given more prominence for the selection of prevention measures, as there have been relevant (minor) epidemiological indications. The development in Denmark is similar.

Although IDUs are already the most strongly affected group in Estonia, a further increase of their share among HIV-infected persons is anticipated. Moreover, the number of women among this group will also rise. The increase of female IDUs will also probably raise the incidence of perinatal HIV infections.

In Lithuania "men who have sex with men" were the main risk group at the beginning of the epidemic. They are now outnumbered by IDUs.

83% of those affected in Bulgaria became infected by sexual contact. 70% of them by heterosexual contact. Measures have been adapted accordingly.

As HIV/AIDS prevalence in Slovakia is rather low on the whole, measures focus on primary prevention and legal aspects. The rising number of IDUs and prostitutes makes these the main target groups of intervention programmes.

In Slovenia HIV prevalence is low at present and HIV/AIDS-related themes failed to draw public attention in the recent past. Still, it has a sound plan of action for HIV prevention.

Forecasts that the number of HIV-infected persons would rise dramatically after the collapse of communism in the Czech Republic (due to the breaking down of borders, increase of prostitution and migration, and easier access to drugs), has not held true so far in the epidemiological data. Still, these target groups are a focus of HIV/AIDS prevention.

The development of epidemiological trends differs greatly in the states of northern and eastern Europe: In the decade from 1987 to 1997 HIV prevalence and incidence were comparatively low in central and eastern Europe and the HIV virus spread mostly by sexual transmission. The situation drastically changed in the Baltic states (especially in Latvia and Lithuania) in 1998, which saw the first diagnoses of IDUs with HIV-infection. In Poland epidemiological trends show a rise in the number of new infections among heterosexuals aged 19 to 25, while the number of infected IDUs and men who have sex with men is falling. Correspondingly, prevention measures for young people now take top priority. In Romania the prevalence of HIV/AIDS is very high by European standards. This is mostly due to the very large number of infected children. Epidemiological trends suggest that in two to three years' time this rate will adapt to the European average. After the introduction of voluntary testing in Bulgaria, it has become more difficult to allocate the tested persons to specific risk groups, so that epidemiological data are no sound basis for the development of target group-specific prevention measures.

The introduction of new therapies (dual and tri-therapy) and the resulting epidemiological changes have had no adverse impact on prevention measures (e.g. Bulgaria, Poland) so far. In the Czech Republic one goes as far as to admit that the assumed existence of effective therapies could have an adverse impact on risk behaviour. In Denmark, the public at large now see HIV/AIDS not so much as a fatal, incurable but rather as a chronic disease. But we cannot derive corresponding indications from the epidemiological data yet. However, the number of people with AIDS has fallen in Scandinavia over the past few years, due to anti-retroviral therapies. Correspondingly, the statistical share of HIV-infected persons is rising. This means, among other things, that Sweden, for one, now focuses more on secondary prevention.

In summary, the impact of epidemiological data on prevention policies reported from central and eastern Europe is comparable to that reported from northern, southern and western Europe, although the observed epidemiological number of AIDS and HIV cases in these countries are much lower than in the rest of Europe.

3.6 Surveillance of HIV/AIDS being instrumental in guiding policies

A recent comprehensive study on "HIV Testing in Europe" (London School of Tropical Medicine and Hygiene, 1999) mandated by the European Union reviews in details the "HIV/AIDS Surveillance Strategies" (Chap. 3, pp. 50-58) in Europe. We summarise some of the main findings next, based on this study.

Different tools have been used to monitor the HIV/AIDS epidemic in Europe with a trend towards standardisation and co-ordination of surveillance systems between European countries, supported by recent changes in HIV screening policies:

- AIDS case reporting, with the European AIDS case reporting system in western Europe (European Centre for the Epidemiological Monitoring of AIDS) and the countries of eastern Europe (ref. section 3.5),
- HIV case reporting, with a European HIV case reporting system being currently set up (at the European Centre too) and existing already in the countries of eastern Europe,
- HIV prevalence surveys, particularly in western Europe.

The early 1990s policies in Europe, at least mainly in the west, north, and south, tended to arise out of growing opposition to compulsory HIV testing and mass screening. The introduction of the Highly Active Anti-retroviral Therapies (HAART) in 1996 has led to a new debate around surveillance strategies and HIV case reporting procedures, and a reconsideration of HIV testing in both primary and secondary prevention.

A recent comprehensive study (European Centre for the Epidemiological Monitoring of AIDS, 1998) revealed that out of 48 European countries, 36 already have nation-wide HIV case reporting systems (roughly half of which are countries of central and eastern Europe).

Four countries (France, Italy, Spain, and the Netherlands) have not yet set up a national reporting system for HIV, and are now planning to expand their HIV reporting programme. A few countries (Ireland, Poland, Latvia, Lithuania) have a small number of laboratories which perform serological tests, or a de facto centralisation of data. A few other countries (Austria, Belgium, Sweden) have a reporting system organised on a decentralised basis.

In the majority of countries, HIV cases reporting is mandatory with a few exceptions (in Germany, reporting of HIV positive confirmation tests is carried out by physicians on a voluntary basis; in France, the UK, and Portugal, reporting is voluntary). The choice of a voluntary or a mandatory HIV reporting often depends on the reporting of other infectious diseases in the country, and must therefore be considered in the context of the national health system of each country. The "HIV Testing in Europe" study found no relation between the nature of the report (voluntary/mandatory) and the quality of reported data.

In a few countries, HIV reporting is anonymous. In France, HIV case reporting is anonymous (no name, no code), therefore, the detection of duplicate reports can only be estimated.

In most countries the link between HIV and AIDS cases is possible, but it is not the case in several countries (France, Denmark, Germany, Hungary, Ireland, Italy and Romania) and, among those, some (Germany, Hungary, Ireland) are planning already improved linkages.

In conclusion, the surveillance systems are changing rapidly, with a recent emphasis on HIV reporting systems to adapt to the recent introduction of multi-drug therapies. These developments allow to strengthen both the primary and secondary prevention strategies and policies involved with an improved and early HIV case detection and reporting system, and to provide a more up-to-date picture of the distribution of HIV infection by population groups. Yet, the interpretation of data from HIV cases, and comparisons between countries, necessitate to take into consideration the various policies of HIV testing practices (overall rate of testing, choice of population group targeted, access to free anonymous testing, type of counselling, partner notification). Therefore in order to overcome these limitations, the "HIV Testing in Europe" study still recommends to pursue the anonymous sero-prevalence surveys in random samples of the population, independent of testing practices.

3.6.1 Western and Southern Europe

The surveillance systems set up in the second half of the eighties are largely centralised, and based on regional laboratories to carry out confirmation tests. Screening for HIV and AIDS is taking place on a voluntary and anonymous basis, with a few rare exceptions, e.g. sex workers in Greece, and in Bavaria in Germany. Data are usually aggregated by the main vulnerable groups and/or probable route of infection. Information on ethnicity is often lacking, although the various systems are starting to introduce this information as well. Different types of data and indicators are used, generally grouped into: the surveillance of AIDS cases (the oldest system), the monitoring of HIV/AIDS mortality rates, the surveillance of HIV infection either through routine reporting or sero-prevalence surveys conducted in different settings (e.g. sentinel groups), and additionally, in some countries, through behavioural surveillance data (KABP).

Original serological investigation, involving non-correlated, anonymous testing aiming to estimate the prevalence of HIV/AIDS infections in Belgium for researchers was abandoned for ethical reasons (sero-positive detected but inability to notify the person tested). A few countries, e.g. the Netherlands, have used seroprevalence studies conducted on a local scale to gain insights into the seroprevalence and behaviours among specific groups, e.g. IDUs. The nature of the studies based on convenience sampling precludes those from being called a surveillance or monitoring system.

The tendency is towards the integration or grouping of data collection, for example in Germany, the RKI encompasses the epidemiological surveillance of HIV and AIDS with other significant infectious diseases, such as Hepatitis, Tuberculosis, and vaccine preventable diseases. The data available cover not only patients ill with AIDS since the early eighties, but also HIV infected persons since the mid-eighties. Consequently, the establishment and improvement of the surveillance of HIV/AIDS is benefiting indirectly other diseases reporting as well.

With the introduction of anti-viral treatments, countries are reporting a national consensus to move from AIDS towards HIV surveillance, because the original AIDS system does no longer provide adequate information to determine the need for prevention and care services. Countries are introducing such systems slowly, careful that there is an absolute respect of privacy of people with HIV/AIDS, for example in Spain, through the sentinel groups surveillance strategies and a national System of Information of New Infections.

Compulsory and anonymous reporting of AIDS cases, or of HIV-positive status, varies by countries, and is being introduced gradually through different methods. For example, one of the first country to adapt the reporting was Germany, whereas France has just introduced this in 1999. In parallel, the collection and analysis of information by regions is also being more and more emphasised.

Systems have set up sophisticated reporting, for example to avoid double entries with the person's initials and date of birth, and to overcome the limitations inherent to anonymous basis of reporting. In parallel, the national agencies in charge of surveillance have set up mechanisms to avoid the duplication either of data or of sources of data.

Anonymous HIV test is most often offered free of charge in public health offices accompanied by counselling which can vary greatly in quality (ref. para. 3.12).

Iceland keeps a complete list of all HIV infection persons (around one hundred people since the beginning of the epidemic) in the hands of the State epidemiologist. The advantage of the system is to be able monitor the impact of treatment and make contact tracing easier, although the risk that the database becomes available is recognised.

Surveillance information are usually widely circulated and available through Epidemiological Bulletins to national and local health authorities, as well as to health care professionals, organisations and the media.

Some countries have also organised, in addition to the mere monitoring of numbers, some specific monitoring of needs and quality, with direct positive applications, for example:

- in Belgium, the sentinel practitioners ("médecins-vigies"), who form a national network overseeing the demand for screening, detection tendencies and demand, reasons and circumstances for testing; in the same country, an HIV prevalence surveillance network focuses on the more vulnerable groups of patients suffering from STDs,
- in France, KABP surveys were conducted at regular intervals both among the general population, and some vulnerable groups (i.e. homosexuals, drug users, migrant groups from Africa and French overseas territories, and prison inmates),
- in Spain, back calculations allow to estimate more precisely the number of HIV positive cases,
- in the Netherlands, the continuous monitoring of public sex campaign and behavioural cohort studies of HIV infection and AIDS among drug users (1985-1992), and among bi- and homosexual men (1984-1998) have had useful implications for prevention and education,
- in England, notifications of the recent rise in homosexually acquired gonorrhoea among men of all ages attending the GUM clinics, and the substantial numbers of HIV positive men who are aware of their infection but still acquire new acute STDs.; among IDUs, prevalence of HIV infection

falling amongst those participating in the monitoring programme but other sources indicating persistent risk taking through sharing of needles; among heterosexuals, the prevalence among pregnant women has risen, gonorrhoea diagnoses have risen substantially recently among men and women, and the prevalence of HIV among men and women born in Africa and attending GUM clinics is at present high.

The true situation is under-estimated (with the exception of blood donors now in all countries) because not all numbers of HIV positive individuals are registered. Reporting is incomplete or not fully valid or specific for different reasons, for example:

- in Belgium, one third of the declaration forms are incomplete in particular with regard to the assumed transmission channel,
- in Germany, among the migrant population, there are lower rates of testing among the migrants due to the lack of access, or fear of lack of anonymity, or other cultural or educational causes,
- in Ireland, the category "prisoners" refers to the number of HIV positive tests in prisoners rather than a specific risk category such as IDU or sexual behaviour; the data are collated on the basis of the year they are reported, instead of the current European CESES system of the year of diagnosis having the advantage of allowing retrospective analysis and overcoming the reporting delays; babies appearing in HIV statistics born positive, but not removed from the totals once losing the HIV status,
- in Italy, only 10 out of 20 regions actively follow-up mortality and routinely send the data to the central office, and an under-reporting of 10%,
- in Portugal, some sources of information, namely clinical laboratories, are still not part of the epidemiological surveillance system,
- in Spain, a sub-notification of AIDS cases estimated at 15% (1996 CESES study estimates), and the lack of useful data from behavioural monitoring,
- in The Netherlands, no continuous and systematic overview of the evolution of the HIV/AIDS epidemic -no general surveillance- in the country with a "vision of the epidemic getting more and more blurred" because there is no mandatory registration of HIV infection, and due to the impact of the new anti-viral therapies,
- in Austria, estimates between 12 and 15,000 of unreported HIV positive persons, in addition to the 6,903 reported HIV positive confirmed tests.

The epidemiological data provide enlightening and useful data for HIV prevention policies on some of the positive results and bottlenecks: "*the epidemiological data are the cornerstones of the practical focus of prevention work...(to) target the individual key groups or affected persons*" (Austria). Falling numbers of positive examinations for the past twelve years in Belgium give evidence of a lower transmission rates among the samples gathered for two specific STDs (N. gonorrhoea, C. trachomatis) in the network of laboratories thus an increased protection for the population. In Germany, the number of homo/bisexuals infections since 1993 have increased up to 1997 lightly, but the infections among migrants have clearly doubled over that period of time. In Ireland, the good medical management combined with the routine linked antenatal HIV testing in maternity hospitals introduced recently have reduced perinatal transmission based on no new HIV infections of babies born to know HIV positive women in the recent years.

3.6.2   Northern, Central and Eastern Europe

Generally, the HIV/AIDS surveillance systems in the countries of northern, central and eastern Europe are centrally organised and work according to the same methods as in western Europe. Some countries emphasise that their system is based on already proven surveillance methods for STDs (e.g. Estonia, Finland, Lithuania). Test practices meet western European Standards with Elisa and confirmation tests.

In Estonia all positive HIV tests are verified by the AIDS Reference Laboratory and, where appropriate, confirmed and reported to the National Health Inspection. Every reported AIDS patient is referred to Merimetsa Hospital in Tallinn, which is the only clinic in Estonia to offer the necessary treatment, medical surveillance and additional counselling. This is due to the fact that most affected patients live in the Estonian capital anyway and that their necessary anonymity can be protected in this way. We cannot assume that behaviour modification regarding risk behaviour is being monitored. Risk groups are only sporadically examined in Estonia. There are no long-term or repeat studies. So far, the target groups of surveys were school children, conscripts and sex workers. We cannot yet speak of an effective implementation of study-based conclusions at present.

Bulgaria likewise has only one authorised institute to ascertain "HIV-positive" status. Copies of the relevant records are sent to the ministry of health and relevant health authorities in compliance with safety regulations. The data are recorded and registered numbers allocated to the test subjects. Every year the ministry of health issues a corresponding report. There is a well-functioning voluntary test system. Anonymity and confidentiality are ensured by the personnel code. However, members of the affected groups suspect that in prison anonymity cannot be guaranteed and that people therefore fail to take part in voluntary tests. Currently, there are considerations whether to propagate the use of home tests. All patients undergoing antiretroviral treatment, are subject to regular medical surveillance. Bulgaria has only one (regrettably unsystematic) study on behaviour modification regarding the attitude to and use of condoms. Even here we cannot assume that risk behaviour is systematically monitored.

In Latvia the reference lab in Riga gives a final confirmation of positive HIV test results. The doctor in charge of treatment informs the affected tested person. All the essential particulars such as age, sex and mode of transmission are given a security code and sent to the AIDS Prevention Centre, which maintains the HIV register. Tests are voluntary except for blood, tissue and organ donors.

In Latvia the selection of prevention measures is based mainly on the assessment of epidemiological data. There are hardly any empirical studies on behaviour modification, hence prevention policies are not influenced by corresponding theoretical assumptions on behaviour.

Lithuania's surveillance system is more or less similar to that of Latvia. The first comprehensive Lithuanian KABP study, which examines the sexual behaviour of adolescents, is available now.

In Poland doctors report diagnosed cases to the Epidemiological Institute of the State Department of Hygiene in Warsaw. Until 1995 data in the AIDS register were not anonymous. Since their elimination (only the total figure is still known) all incoming data have been coded. A range of KABP studies have also been conducted in Poland. The target groups were first the general population (1993), then medical staff and social workers (1997 – 1999) and finally adolescents (1997 – 1999). The results of these studies are considered in the development of prevention measures. However, even these approaches constitute no systematic monitoring of behaviour modification.

In the Czech Republic all positive test results are reported to the National Reference Laboratory on AIDS at the National Institute of Public Health. Every month the data are sent both to involved institutions and to the European Monitoring Centre. And there are also anonymous studies within HIV risk groups. In a large-scale survey financed by the national Anti AIDS Fight

Programme, Prague University is examining the sexual risk behaviour of the general population. Also the individual HIV prevention target groups are observed in smaller studies on this topic. The studies do not overlap, as only one institute is authorised to monitor HIV/AIDS. The results of these long-term studies influence prevention policy developments.

Slovenia reports that, at least from 1995 to 1998, surveillance information did not lead to any changes in national AIDS policies. One of the reasons given for this is that HIV/AIDS rates are relatively low. At least at the local level there are reactions to corresponding data analyses.

Slovakia also has a central HIV/AIDS surveillance system. Test results are submitted on a voluntary basis with the exception of blood, tissue or organ donors. A few years ago compulsory tests for pregnant women were introduced, which are now voluntary again.

In Romania a reliable monitoring system was installed with the help of the WHO and CDC Atlanta in 1990. However, reporting of HIV/AIDS cases is not considered reliable in all regions of the country. Only a few KAPB studies have been conducted, and they constitute no adequate basis for prevention policy decisions, as they are not representative enough.

In Finland and Norway both the treating doctor and the corresponding test laboratory are obliged to report HIV-positive cases to the respective Register of Communicable Diseases, which is subordinated to the National Public Health Institute. This system is considered to be highly effective, as lacking reports of one institution can be identified with the support of the other the other and we can thus assume a 100% report rate. These data are collected and processed by the NPHI. AIDS cases are reported separately in Norway, quoting the name of the patient.

Sweden works with a similar system and was one of the first countries to install both AIDS and HIV registers in 1985. Together with the report to the Communicable Diseases Control Institute another report is submitted to the relevant federal state agency. When full-blown AIDS develops, another report is made, so that the course of HIV spread can be examined separately.

In the northern European countries of Denmark, Finland, Norway and Sweden KABP studies are regularly conducted both on the general population, particularly young people, and special target groups such as gay men or IDUs, and their results influence further strategy planning for HIV/AIDS policies.

The individual countries quote the following strong points of the respective surveillance systems:

- On a voluntary basis, the average number of tested persons has risen (Bulgaria).
- The strengths of the system lie in its effectiveness and immediate access to data (Estonia).
- As doctors and labs submit independent reports, coverage is assumed to be rather large (Finland and Norway).
- Norway justifies its submission of uncoded data on AIDS patients to the National Surveillance System for Communicable Diseases by the possibility of linking the AIDS register with other relevant registers for comparative surveys.

And the following weak points were mentioned:

- In some areas anonymity and confidentiality cannot be guaranteed (Bulgaria).
- Data that are crucial for prevention, such as particulars on the mode of transmission or sexual orientation are not included in the anonymous reports. The annual report lacks an analysis of the reported figures (Estonia).
- As the data of AIDS patients in Norway are not anonymous, no reports are sent to local health authorities in order to ensure confidentiality. This partly means that staff at this level are not involved in HIV/AIDS prevention work in the desired measure.
- Due to the anonymous data it is not possible in Sweden to compare the cases in the HIV register with those in the AIDS register.
- The number of target group-specific studies in Slovakia is too low.

The country reports all (with the exception of Slovenia) ascribe a major impact on the development of national prevention strategies to their respective surveillance system. In one aspect, the states of northern Europe differ clearly from central and eastern Europe: Alongside the purely medical HIV/AIDS surveillance system we find that in Scandinavia systematic surveys of sexual behaviour, for example, have a corresponding influence. Only few, if any, relevant KABP surveys have been conducted in central and eastern Europe, with the exception of Poland and the Czech Republic, where the results of such studies contribute to the development of prevention policies. In the reports the absence of such surveys is definitely seen as a lack and efforts to remedy this are called for. For example, the Estonian report sees an urgent need for in-depth studies on sexual behaviour. Anonymous surveillance systems have become largely established in the states of central and eastern Europe. In northern Europe, in contrast, Norway fails to record surveillance data of AIDS patients anonymously.

3.7 System of primary prevention

The primary prevention of HIV infection is probably one of the most successful case of public-related behaviour modification ("safer sex", "safe use"...) in the history of public health. The authors identifies the primary prevention of HIV infection with the new public health concept. It can be contrasted with the "old public health" less successful interventions in STD, or smoking, or nutrition (Rosenbrock et al., 1999).

Primary prevention of HIV infection is based today on a broad foundation of knowledge of different fields (sexual science, behavioural science, sociology, evaluation research etc.) which are often taking place with creative forms of co-operation between the communities concerned, public health professionals, social scientists, and state agencies. Numerous models of prevention in behavioural changes were developed with more refined concepts: original focus from risk groups (to vulnerable groups) to risk situations.

A review of ten years of lessons learnt in AIDS prevention in Europe point to the following findings and challenges based on the experience gained in Switzerland (Dubois-Arber, 1998). The four major lessons learnt are:

- the benefits and limits of prevention campaigns are known,
- it is possible to set up an efficacious targeted prevention,
- but the adaptation of individuals to risk varies, sometimes problematic and often remote from the principles of prevention,
- finally, preventive activities which are more "in-depth" or "non-specific" based on personal or lay interaction are developing, but at a slower pace, and are less known.

The author underlines that the transfer of experiences cannot be mechanistic but needs to be adapted to the different particular environments, particularly in light of the emerging problems in the East.

The future successful developments of prevention policies, taking into account the emerging budgetary constraints, will be dependent upon tackling the following issues:

1) The anchoring of routine prevention into normal activities to sustain the effort over time (among professionals, the youth etc.),
2) The integration of the contents, e.g. in reproductive health integrating HIV, prevention of other STD and contraception, or toxicomania, the stronger association of prevention of transmission by blood and by sexual transmission,
3) The challenge and largely unknown correct mix of the correct combination and dose of different types of prevention (general, targeted, individual prevention and counselling) in relation to their sustainability, efficacy, and costs,
4) The actors (institutional or individuals) mix to prevention and daily roles,
5) The policies of prevention addressing new emerging problems (inequality, lack of motivation of associations, mere medical or technical response to the epidemic, return to the old sexual education paradigm).

More research is needed on factors of risk to be used for prevention programmes (ref. for more details to section 3.11). Luger (1998) points to the fact prevention programmes seem not to have been as successful as intended, because they focused on risk behaviour and behaviour change rather than considering factors which may encourage risk behaviour, make individuals vulnerable to infection with HIV. This could be 'class' and socio-economic factors such as poor education, poor living and working conditions and poverty. Prevention programmes may not have taken into account possible class- and socio-economic differences and their implications on HIV/AIDS. "Little is known about socio-economic differences in industrialised countries (more in less developing countries), and their relation to HIV/AIDS. Most epidemiological information is on demographic factors, such as geographic distribution, gender, and risk exposure" (p. 13). As an example, the comprehensive comparative study on sexual behaviour and HIV risk reduction strategies among gay and bisexual men in eight European countries (Bochow et al., 1994), which gained important insight in risk behaviour and response strategies to HIV/AIDS, did not consider class-related or socio-economic inequalities within the study population.

More research is also needed to compare the effect of drug policies on the epidemiology of HIV and AIDS in different countries.

Furthermore, the accessibility and problems of adherence to therapy on the part of IV drug users, just like homeless or sex workers, are real barriers which new outreach strategies integrating medical and social care need to address, and present experiences remain to be evaluated.

3.7.1 Western and Southern Europe

The information to the population is the cornerstone of the primary HIV prevention system through efforts related to the continuous and adequate information of the disease, to minimising the risk of infection, and to action against social discrimination. Education, counselling, the use of HIV antibody test are all prevention strategies, but those encompass as well the provision of products and hygiene measures. Some countries include the offering of optimal counselling and care to persons living with HIV and AIDS as one of their goals in HIV prevention along a more global understanding of the prevention-care continuum. In Spain, there is a shift of HIV/AIDS prevention activities to be integrated into the national primary health care network. In January 2000, the former Health Education Authority (HEA) responsible among others for the direct public education will become the Health Development Agency (HDA) focusing more on the broader determinants of health.

The public health services were traditionally attached to fight communicable diseases, but were ill-prepared to include new important dimensions related to psycho-social, cultural, and environmental problems.

The countries have emphasised in the early years of the epidemic, information related to the disease, screening, transmission modes, non-discrimination messages, and protection measures. The varieties of messages accompanied or not by interventions to the public at large and/ or vulnerable groups make the measurement of impact almost impossible. In general, countries appear to have mastered the first four categories of information, but the last one on the protection measures becomes now the main focus. Evidence of success is not uniform for all populations, for example studies show that young people still lack knowledge of the disease and display behaviour deficits in prevention. The large proportions of AIDS patients in the 20 to 30 age group, particularly among females, give evidence of deficits in prevention messages in the teen ages when the infection most probably occurred. To address this deficit, countries such as

Austria recently who have taken special measures in and out of schools, by breaking down the triad of lacking knowledge, awareness of one's own risk, and skills, are rare.

The concept of risk situations or minimal risk is at the chore of the activities with a shift from moralism to persuasion.

The strategies chosen by countries are two-prone: information to the general population through media (radio, TV, cinemas, feature films and videos, posters, brochures, target group specific advertisements) and encouraging personal responsibility accompanied by supportive measures (i.e. prevention tools such as condoms, gels, syringes, and proximity activities to the vulnerable groups, counselling services). The former has been largely spearheaded by the public sector, while the second by the voluntary sector. The increase proportions of infections via heterosexual transmission show the need to reinforce prevention for the general population. In parallel, even if some countries document evidence of positive changes of behaviour among homosexuals and IDUs, there is evidence through new risk indicators that prevention efforts need to be maintained among those, particularly among homosexuals, as supported by data from France, and Germany.

Campaigns for the general public in France, integrating messages addressed to young people, to homosexuals and to drug users have been successful, whereas a similar recent experience in Spain was not well received. As a side effect to these campaigns, they have allowed the ordinary citizens to get a positive impression of the public authorities' commitment to tackle difficult issues. Countries have adapted general population campaigns to the seasons in order to break the danger of routine and audience fatigue. For example, in Belgium, in Summer, emphasis is put on prevention among the youth, and in Winter, on solidarity with sero-positive persons, or in Germany, the coloured condoms placards also changing with the seasons.

The availability of multi-drug treatments have become an additional important argument in favour of testing to start early treatment and prevent opportunistic infections. Some groups, such as migrants, do not have sufficient access either to testing or counselling, as signalled for Germany, most often because of cultural barriers. The HIV-Home tests are not promoted in Germany because of the lack of the necessary and important individual counselling linked to a test.

Prevention programmes are totally dependent of government subsidies which can create difficulties in time of budget constraints, priorities setting, and of additional subsidies for NGOs originating from the Government health insurance system as well. Often the programmes are designed and implemented by NGOs. In France, which also applies to a few other countries, the relationship between NGOs and state-run institutions is one of ambivalence, ranging between partnership and political antagonism. Until 1995, NGOs have plaid an important role in defining HIV/AIDS prevention policies. They have lost since power, however, vis-à-vis the State for reasons due to the decentralisation of prevention measures which favour local prevention policies, to the advances in the development of therapies which have redefined the stakes involved, and finally, to the radicalisation of certain organisations vis-à-vis governmental bodies and disagreements between them. We see the decrease in the NGOs' power and dynamism as one of the biggest threat to stimulate the nurturing of continuous and original HIV prevention policies. In Ireland, information campaigns on a national level have the advantage of keeping the public eye, but their high costs have decreased their numbers to particular times (e.g. World AIDS Day); their absence have resulted in the general public perception that HIV is no longer a problem. In the UK the funding available for general population work has reduced considerably since the beginning of the epidemic, reflecting a shift to a more targeted approach.

Some examples of campaigns and activities are listed below:

- the distribution of condoms through the first sales company in a large diffusion weekly periodical (Belgium),
- insertion of information pages on HIV prevention among the most vulnerable groups through large diffusion publications (Belgium),
- participation of the pharmacies in the low cost injection materials, particularly in the hot spot of the capital (Belgium),
- free and anonymous testing, accompanied by counselling, in the capital and a large town (Belgium),
- the Prevention, Action, Health and Work for Transgenders (PASST group) for transvestites and transsexuals and their involvement in the campaigns to overcome demarginalisation and integrate them as full partners in the response to AIDS (France),
- for the already infected persons, an understanding and informed environment, the creation of equal conditions for all chronically ill people, anti-discrimination measures and recognition of privacy (Austria),

- the Vienna's AIDS Hilfe 1998 safer sex campaign combining both meanings of a normal and safekeeping behaviour in the use of condoms, with motives on the posters adapted for the hetero-, bi.- and homosexual populations (Austria),
- carefully specific messages in Germany aiming to motivate young people to talk about sex with humorous tones, normalising condom use and removing barriers of use, or to address irrational fears and avoid stigmatisation of AIDS (Germany),
- the development of a set of new "early" indicators to allow to focus on the intention for or against safer sex, and willingness to accept protective measures, as assessment of one's own or a partner's behaviour (Germany),
- the focus on groups of mobile populations, such as asylum seekers, refugees, gypsies, sex workers, mobile injecting drug users, etc., to include activities in the national strategic plan and define the co-operation between national organisations responsible for mobile populations, and the information of high school students in a participatory manner (Greece),
- a large media campaign organised in 1998-1999 stressing the preventive value of using condoms to prevent STDs has been successful in increasing awareness (Iceland),
- the shift from an educational orientation form HIV disease prevention to sexual health promotion in schools through the Alliance Centre for Sexual Health, and a community approach to the drug related problems among youth through the Ballymun Youth Action Project (Ireland),
- a travelling exhibition to inform the youth in playful, pedagogical and interactive manner to erase taboos and convey correct concepts on AIDS, while approaching sexuality, reproduction and the use of condoms in a broad-minded way (Portugal),
- the close monitoring of performance of the local public health authorities through the minimum of 50% allocation they should spend on the recognised target groups in their areas(UK),
- the national safe campaigns have integrated the objective of HIV prevention with a safer sex approach with regard to all STDs since 1994 (the Netherlands).

Activities working with vulnerable groups are essentially supported through NGOs, for example:

- an NGO in charge of prevention among IDUs recruits ex-IDUs to carry out small field surveys and tailor and promote as a consequence minimal risk strategies (Belgium),
- condom distribution to the youth in large mass youth assemblies (Belgium),
- anonymous telephone counselling (Belgium, Germany),
- working with specially trained women to become prevention agents for women (France),
- programmes for migrants and for the socially disadvantaged groups who are often not reached by other prevention messages and who have no access to care (France),
- giving the means to drug users to get involved in prevention activities and consequently demystifying that the drug sub-culture and behaviours among IDUs cannot change and facilitating the development of their own group identity (France),
- the long experience of applying a combination of measures to prevent HIV infections among IDUs, e.g. harm reduction work through low-threshold institutions, with needle exchange programmes, distribution of free condoms, substitution programmes, and AIDS education and optional HIV tests (Germany),
- in complement to AIDS-Hilfe encompassing a large spectrum of activities, numerous self-help organisations (*PositiHIVCafe, Positiv Leben, Positiver Dialog, Menschen und AIDS-Club plus*, women's initiative *H.I.V.*, the *Buddy* Association, AIDS service of the Maltese organisation and pastoral work of the Catholic church) contribute to improve the quality of life of people living with HIV (Germany),
- following a research study on prostitution, a multi-agency approach and a safe environment for drop-in services with a comprehensive women's clinic and outreach work have succeeded through active local Health Boards in building trust and on-going relationships with female prostitutes in Dublin (Ireland),
- the gay men are far from being an homogeneous group, and the primary group of gay men to be targeted for HIV health promotion, recognise the need to reach young gay men, and those outside the major urban areas, the bisexual men as a hard to reach group, and those who do not identify themselves as bisexual or gay (UK),

Post-Exposure Prophylaxis following exposure to HIV (HIV PEP) is not widely publicised because of the fear to be detrimental to prevention activities.

On the continuum between prevention and care, sound alternatives to hospitalisation have developed, for example in France home hospital care, home nursing care, household help services, housing assistance. Despite this, HIV prevention in France, acknowledges that the country does not have a culture which encourages patients to take their day-to-day care into their own hands, and that counselling is underdeveloped with a number of clients who lack access to this service.

There is evidence throughout the countries that care and psycho-social support are unequally accessible, with a clear advantage for the HIV positive homosexual groups with a history of well-organised and strong lobby organisation.

Countries with a long and strong tradition of public health have fared better than others in enforcing early prevention policies not directly linked to Information Education and Communication (IEC), for example, in Belgium, safe blood collection and transfusion, or the policies facilitating the sales of condoms at low prices through tax measures, or early prevention measures among the homosexuals and IDUs with a close collaboration between the public sector and the NGOs. In Belgium, the national Flemish co-ordination agency (IPAC) stimulates the exchange of information and experiences related to primary HIV prevention between associations through organised meetings; whereas, the French speaking community suffers from the lack of means to work, with objectives not translated into operational objectives and lack of tasks definition.

Gradually, other Ministries than the Health Sector have been involved with various degrees of involvement, e.g. ministry of education, justice, women's affairs, labour and social solidarity, science and transport, defence. The non-governmental sector often pushes for more commitment for this intersectoral support. In the background of effective HIV prevention policies, in addition, a complex organisation of the health system, and the lack of integration of programmes (e.g. STD programme not connected to HIV/AIDS prevention) for example in France, may render the co-ordination of various medical specialisation areas and of activities difficult. In Austria, medical counselling for HIV tests in hospitals is subject to much criticism bringing uncertainties on an effective prevention of HIV/AIDS among people with STDs.

Some groups are not optimally addressed. For example, sex workers in Austria do not yet have any specific information material developed for them, or often mentioned by almost all countries, the migrants and disadvantaged populations, who in contrast to original vulnerable groups, such as the homosexuals or IDUs, do not have any history of social movements which could in turn facilitate the adaptation of prevention measures to the specific conditions of each group. Sex tourism is known to be a problem, for example in Germany or United Kingdom, but seldom addressed on a permanent and sustaining manner with the difficulty of overcoming cross-border issues. It is too often a subject which is largely ignored or not addressed adequately, often to avoid any negative impact on the tourism industry. Iceland mentions that no specific education is organised by the authorities for immigrants, sex workers or prisoners. In Ireland, despite the NASC report recommendation that the departments of health and education should be responsible for developing materials for young people in school, each school is left to devise its own policy on implementing the programme resulting in the more conservative schools providing quite a narrowly-based programme, and particular attention has been highlighted for early school leavers. Although the National AIDS Committee has emphasised the importance of informing the youth through the school system, the ministry of education has not yet taken up the challenge, and the same applies to young people who do not attend school and/or come from poor or marginalised social backgrounds.

Despite, positive outcomes in a prevention project among IDUs in the Province of Milan, Italy, the experience has not yet been scaled up in other urban areas of the country by lack of the local administrations' support. In Spain, despite 23% of prison inmates having HIV/AIDS, and despite the efforts of NGOs, professional health workers, lawyers, and pharmacists to implement prevention measures in prisons, the prison administrations have not been supportive with the exception of two prisons; for the lack of sexual education in schools due to full curricula, fragmented teaching of subjects, incomplete training of teachers, with lack of information sources for out-of-school youth at sixteen and beyond; for MSMs and WSWs a recognised feeling that a certain nonchalance has emerged about taking precautionary measures during sex, and an emerging problem of the lack of access to HIV/AIDS information and care for migrants. For people living with HIV and AIDS, prevention work in the UK is not well developed up to now, despite the fact it is a recognised target group. In the Netherlands, extra attention needs to be paid to migrants, ethnic minorities, asylum seekers, fugitives and illegal persons, with emphasis on behavioural change,

and people with HIV. For the latter, no structural attention is given to prevention of HIV transmission among HIV infected persons (re-infection).

Germany is signalling less access to information due to strong reduction of resources for campaigns between 1992 and 1997. As a consequence, indicators are alarming: the proportions of singles under 45 who had no contact at all with any different media campaign almost tripled to 18%; the extent of interpersonal communication declined from over 50% in 1991 to less than 24% over six years, and regular condom use of persons with several sex partners has declined by 3% between 1996 and 1997, in comparison to positive trends from 1988 to 1995. Such early signs and consequences of less attention to prevention campaigns may be an early warning signal for other European. The reduction in funding may also affect in turn research activities related to HIV and AIDS which are still much needed for some of the new difficult issues related to reaching better emerging vulnerable groups, as signalled in The Netherlands. Action research for activities related to work with vulnerable groups has been found quite useful in Belgium.

Countries are commonly acknowledging, and tackling with different degree of commitments, the new emerging vulnerable group of migrants, particularly originating from sub-Sahara Africa, and of the increasingly larger group of socially disadvantaged populations (ref. para. 3.12). The fear of stigmatising migrants by targeted campaigns is big, as well as the lack of know-how on how to reach them effectively (e.g. cultural, language, economic barriers). Prison inmates represent a high priority group, but despite good political will at the national level, the accessibility to prevention programmes are still highly dependent upon each prison policy and wardens' good will.

Countries are moving HIV prevention messages will be more acceptable and sustainable in the long run when integrated in global health and sex education concepts.

In conclusion, sustainable minimal behavioural risk-taking is the challenge of any kind of public health programmes, particularly for HIV/AIDS in relation to sexual behaviours, be it among the general population or among vulnerable groups. Countries have recognised in common the priorities needs related to emerging vulnerable groups, such as women or migrants or disadvantaged populations, yet, surprisingly, large scale commitments (vs. small programmes or interventions) are still lagging behind.

3.7.2 Northern, Central and Eastern Europe

Virtually all reports from these regions agreed that the following three fundamental primary prevention goals take priority:

a) Prevention of sexual transmission of HIV,
b) Prevention of HIV transmission by blood and blood products,
c) Prevention of pre- and perinatal HIV transmission.

For the individual countries the following additional aims, resulting from their respective national situation, are also essential:

Increase of condom use, application of safer sex practices and hence limitation of HIV spread (Bulgaria), provision of information on the virus itself, its transmission and protection against infection (Estonia), as well as information on test methods and institutions that offer tests (Czech Republic) are explicitly quoted as chief prevention goals.

In Estonia IDUs have become the most severely affected group and thus the main target group of intervention programmes within a very brief space of time. Moreover, work with specific ethnic groups takes centre stage. In Estonia young Russians face much greater social problems than Estonians. Their share of drug addicts is 95%, and they account for 85% of sex workers. However, politicians and other decision-makers often neglect or ignore this situation.

In Romania medical staff are one of the main target groups of prevention measures. Many of them still work without any safety measures. Hence, corresponding regulations are urgently required.

In the Czech Republic prostitution in the borderlands is a major problem for prevention work.

Finland emphasises that the key principle of HIV/AIDS prevention lies in informing the public as effectively as possible. All groups must have the same possibilities to access information.

The focus on different risk groups shifts along with epidemiological developments. But, due to the essentially informative nature of primary prevention work, all countries invariably concentrate on adolescents and young adults as their main target group for intervention.

The different risk groups are listed in the following, along with the respective key goals of measures tailored to them. This applies largely to all countries of northern, central and eastern Europe. Measures that are only performed or quoted by some states, are attributed accordingly:

General population

- Voluntary and anonymous tests
- Provision of information, especially in co-operation with the mass media

Adolescents
- Education and information measures, peer education
- Teacher training
- Popular events
- Access via mass media

Sex workers
- Find right approach, decriminalisation
- Counselling, test offers, training offers, peer education
- Prevention or treatment of STDs

IDUs
- Low-threshold programmes, streetwork offerings
- Needle exchange programmes
- Methadone programmes
- Counselling
- Rehabilitation

PLWAs
- Provide access to combination therapy (Estonia)
- Guarantee psycho-social support system (Estonia; Latvia)
- Free treatment
- Provide sufficient quantity of antiretroviral drugs (Slovakia)
- Active integration in prevention measures

Men who have sex with men
- Find right approach (Bulgaria)
- Promotion of co-operation between local and international gay organisations (Estonia)

- Distribution of info material in relevant clubs
- Test offers
- Monthly publication of magazines
- Streetwork offerings

Ethnic Minorities and mobile populations
- Use of communication forms tailored to target group (Bulgaria)
- Entitlement to health services (Finland)
- Information in the relevant national language

Prison inmates
- Debates on legalisation of sexual contacts between prison inmates (Bulgaria)
- Personnel training
- HIV/AIDS and hepatitis test offers
- Access to clean needles and condoms

Medical staff
- Additional training
- Corresponding safety and hygiene regulations

Pregnant women
- Voluntary tests and information offerings

Street children
- Projects in co-operation with UNICEF

Factors with a negative or obstructive impact on prevention differ between the countries:

The lack of uniform methods and sporadic selection within target groups are quoted as obstacles for providers and recipients of primary prevention in Estonia. Lacking funds also impede work considerably. For example, it is often difficult to persuade musicians to give free performances at charity events. Co-operation with other programmes of the same calibre (e.g. alcoholism and drug addiction) is inadequate. Antiretroviral combination therapy is not available yet.

In Romania there is a lack of co-operation between individual institutions and organisations. Moreover, frank discussions on sexuality between adolescents and their parents or teachers are rather unusual. Some teachers even disapprove of such projects.

In the Czech Republic immigrants with a certain status are not integrated in the health insurance system. An alternative financing model has to be found here.

In small towns and rural areas of Finland it is difficult to meet the demand for anonymity. There are not enough health counselling centres and the training and expertise of medical staff vary considerably from region to region.

The following campaigns are quoted as examples of HIV/AIDS prevention work from 1995 to 1999:
- Annual campaigns for World AIDS Day (Bulgaria, Finland, Latvia, Poland, Slovakia, Slovenia)
- Information stands at erotica fairs and exhibitions (Estonia)
- "Summer rubber" – an annual campaign propagating the use of condoms (Finland)
- Publication of Sixteen magazine with a condom inserted in each issue (Finland)
- Valentine's Day campaigns, with info materials and condoms distributed at discos and clubs or at concerts (Bulgaria) and "I wish you safe" campaigns for Valentine's Day, propagating the use of condoms (Slovenia)
- Broadcasting of video and audio clips (Bulgaria, Latvia)
- Safe sex campaign with disco, bar and night-club visitors as a target group (Latvia)
- "Say NO to Drugs" and "Living for Tomorrow" (Latvia)
- Concert campaign under the motto "No Drugs, No AIDS" (Bulgaria)
- Annual rock summer, rave events (Estonia)
- Football tournaments in schools "Soccer against AIDS"
- Information campaign "What you should know about AIDS" with school children as a target group, conducted by teachers and doctors (Poland)
- "Safe Vacation" – information material to make school children and students aware of the topic; lots of copies were issued in tie-in lessons and during the holidays on the most heavily frequented train and bus routes (Poland)
- "Coming out of Hiding" is directed at MSM: With the co-operation of NGOs the project is not just rated as an information measure but also helped improve integration of the target group noticeably (Poland)

- "Women in the age of AIDS": a project conducted in close co-operation with public broadcasting stations. The topic of HIV/AIDS was increasingly integrated in programmes specially targeted at women (Poland)
- A nationwide 24-hour phone hotline, where doctors and psychologists offer advice (Poland).

And one ought to mention the following, particularly beneficial examples of completed or ongoing prevention projects in individual countries:

- Bulgaria: The work of the "Health in Schools" network, which organises both teacher training and peer educator instruction. An analysis of needs and available funds was made in advance. However, no scientific assessment of the project is available yet. One result of the measure is a text-book on methods, which is now used nationwide. In Bulgaria new intervention methods such as peer or self-education were used for the first time. This was a good indication of their effectiveness.
- Estonia: The "Stop AIDS Marathon" project, which aims to provide information and concentrates above all on individual government districts and not, like its predecessors, on the capital of Tallinn. Specialists work locally with target groups and are financed by the APC. No evaluation is available yet.
- Latvia: The "STOP AIDS" campaign, which familiarised the general population with safer sex methods and was initiated by AIDS Prevention Centres with the support of UNAIDS.
- Norway: The "Bussen" project in Oslo. A bus calls at IDU hang-outs, distributes clean needles and condoms free of charge and offers counselling. The measure was evaluated in 1998 and rated as beneficial and cost-effective.
- Sweden. Annual "Summer Campaigns" conducted by the National Institute of Public Health and NGOs and targeted at adolescents. Measures include poster campaigns, distribution of info material and condoms, music festivals, etc.
- Slovenia. The "Gaflon" project - anonymous telephone counselling for homosexuals. The publicly financed hotline is open for calls every night and has good publicity. There has been no formal evaluation so far.

Only few country reports characterised the currently prevailing prevention approach: In Estonia prevention work has shifted from pure information to an approach based on the conviction that changing behaviour is essential. The methods used by Norway to approach risk groups are marked by dialogue, discussion and co-operation. In general, the Norwegians are very open to the HIV/AIDS problem. In the Romanian report the current prevention approach was characterised as pragmatic and moralistic. In the Czech Republic all interviewed experts described the prevailing prevention concept as pragmatic.

Probably because of the rather low number of infected gays in central and eastern Europe and the complete lack or gradual emergence of NGOs with a homosexual identity (except in Slovenia), there are hardly any prevention measures for this group, unlike in western Europe. Owing to the rising number of infected IDUs more offerings in this field are being created and expanded. There is an encouragingly large number of prevention campaigns in northern, central and eastern Europe that target adolescents and young adults. This is accompanied by the trend to expand or introduce sex education in schools. In some countries this still meets with the disapproval of some parts of the population and of the involved teachers (see Romania), still it has come off to a promising start. However, many planned and practised prevention measures are threatened by a lack of funds and need the support of international and European institutions.

3.8   Social and economic support measures for HIV positive persons

World-wide, AIDS has led to interesting major innovations in the field of health services. Efforts were stepped up to implement a system of integrated and continuous care in the service structure. "The spread of AIDS put the political machine into a state of intense fear of a possibly uncontrollable disaster. This made politicians very willing to take action and offer funds" (Schaeffer et al., 1992, p. 11). This willingness to offer funds, which was true at least in wealthy western European countries, changed the health services landscape for good in many states, with an impact not just on hitherto medically focused services but also on social and economic support measures for those affected. From the point of view of UNAIDS (UNAIDS Report 1999), such measures should include both emotional support for HIV-infected persons and their families/partners and social measures to cushion economic and other hardships caused by AIDS.

Psychological support is a key factor of care and support for persons living with HIV and AIDS. It can help those affected to come to terms with HIV, develop a positive outlook on life and learn how to cope with anticipated or currently occurring consequences when others learn of their HIV infection. Alongside economic measures that may include free public transport, rent allowances, free medication, pension, etc. as part of social assistance, others are needed to combat discrimination. Combined with medical services, these measures generate major financial expenses. Even in countries with a low prevalence of HIV we can observe a definite increase in health service costs. So, in view of scarce funds in individual countries, priorities must be established in prevention policies. Alongside decreasing budgets, the normalisation of AIDS, observed in many countries and caused by new forms of therapy, has again led to a stronger "medicalisation" of HIV treatment and a decline of specialised treatment and care services that emerged in the phase of 'exceptionalism' (Rosenbrock, 1999). The time gained by new therapies often calls for psycho-social support for the problems of living with HIV/AIDS: "Many have problems making it through therapy and cannot cope with the essentially contradictory challenges of medicalisation and normalisation of their lives." (Rosenbrock, 1999, p. 30)

The following chapter reports on the available support offerings of secondary prevention under these conditions in the surveyed European countries. It runs the whole gamut of offerings from financial support through psycho-social counselling and home care to residential shelter units. Moreover, it looks into what areas were given priority in the individual countries, depending on available funds and the epidemiological situation. And another important issue where the countries in Europe may differ - be they wealthy or not - is to what extent these measures are supported by public institutions or NGOs and whether they are financed mainly by the state or also by donations, foundations, etc.

3.8.1 Western and Southern Europ

In general, AIDS is considered a disease like any other, and as such it is covered by the federal social security system. Optimal counselling and care of persons with HIV and AIDS, and the promotion of an accepting and supportive treatment have become the two political priorities of governments.

The financing is carried to the greatest extent by the state, the insurance companies, and to a lesser extent by churches and foundations financed through donations. NGOs have been largely supported by state funds, but also have raised funds for their own service provision.

The NGOs are often the first source of information and offer direct assistance quickly and without any red tape. They emphasise the individuals' central involvement in their own health care as a policy priority. NGOs have sometimes been centrally involved in compensation cases against the Government on behalf of its members (e.g. the Irish Haemophilia Society). In Portugal, both through ministry support, and their own financial resources, the Private Social Solidarity Institutions (PSSIs) carry out psycho-social care and follow-up centres, home care services, and residential shelter units. Systems to support psycho-social services in Belgium have provided an annual lump sum allocated per patient to each of the seven AIDS Reference Centres to finance a multi-disciplinary team, including a social worker and a psychologist to counsel patients in psychological, social, legal and other matters. In addition, volunteers have been trained to provide support services, through, for example in Flanders the "buddies". Those have dropped unfortunately due to the loss of interest in AIDS and because of the sensational nature of information on new treatment methods.

Care in sanitary institutions differ:

- In Belgium, care in sanitary institutions cannot be refused to persons not covered by health insurance. Social and economic assistance can be problematic though for the destitute patients or illegal migrants. A recent development is an increase of affected persons originating from underprivileged environments and who display depressive tendencies. The psychiatric structures are not eager to accept patients with a combination of social and psychological problems, in addition to the medical ones.
- In Germany, the state-run organisations like the Social Welfare Offices as well as Social Centres offer not only social, but also financial support; social support, besides medical care, is financed by the health insurance for those not in need of a hospital stay.
- In Iceland, the ministry of health and social security, the Institute of Social Services, and the outpatient clinics cater for services and social support.
- In Portugal, the ministry of health covers all costs of hospital admittance and pays all anti-retroviral therapy expenses.
- In Greece, a hostel combines psycho-social and care of HIV positive people: residential care and nutrition free of charge, home care, psycho-social support, financial and social rehabilitation.
- In Italy, the council administrations tailor the cost of assistance and care to give the necessary economic support.

Social work related activities, often handled by NGOs, address in addition to financial security, the reintegration into the job market and/or preserving jobs. For example, in Austria, due to the often precarious situation of the clients who are often on social welfare, debts settlement, housing assistance, sick pay, early retirement, social benefits, fee exemptions for medicine are also a compounded problem which need to be dealt with. Beyond the traditional sense, social work supports genuine talk and support of the clients without having to think about possible consequences or prejudices. In France, through the home assistance programme, the accommodation programme including therapeutic co-ordination, and a programme to ensure access to the handicapped adult allowance scheme, the day-to-day needs of HIV positive persons in their environment are fulfilled. In Greece, a new home care programme has just started, covering the broad Athens metropolis. In Portugal, through the ministry of labour and solidarity, a specific social protection programme entitles patients to a disability allowance, and a minimum national income general programme allows a non-taxable allowance to fight destitution on one hand, and specific allowances programme allow to re-establish a functional balance for families facing very serious economic hardship. In Spain, the Local Councils can either manage the social services structure themselves, or establish working agreements with NGOs and religious organisations; the development of a basic social service infrastructure is attempting to work more in conjunction with primary health care services, and there is an increase in demand for services, principally for day-care centres, shelters and centres for professional reintegration.

Other new patient education programmes have been set up in France by NGOs financed by the State and by the Government health insurance system to facilitate compliance with treatments via the support of psychologists, health professionals, social workers, representatives from organisations and from the patients' own environment members.

Positive initiatives have developed, e.g. funds raised for holidays for some of the clients of AIDS-Hilfe in Austria; the participation in sport programmes for people living with HIV and AIDS are paid by some insurance companies (e.g. AOK Hamburg) in Germany; drop-in services and housing projects and help with holidays are all accessible services provided in Ireland which people with other diseases do not benefit from; among others (state disability pension or accompaniment allowance) free of charge use of the urban transport network in

Italy as civil invalids; a 0.52% of the State's income tax revenues to programmes of social interest in Spain; the uninsured or illegal persons who fell through the safety network in The Netherlands are now offered solutions through a recent legislation.

In conclusion, countries are still struggling to provide comprehensive attention and care to the people living with HIV or AIDS, particularly for those who live in precarious conditions. The absence of a global vision of the social problems, and of grasping the HIV/AIDS infections problematic beyond the new therapies, combined with shrinking budgets for AIDS activities, have often resulted in poor co-ordination and the lack of comprehensive and effective services.

3.8.2   *Northern, Central and Eastern Europe*

In their prevention policies for PLWAs all states have given priority to enabling free access to all necessary treatment and therapy measures. Reducing the economic, social and emotional effects of HIV/AIDS on the individual and on certain population groups or society as a whole also takes centre stage. As another further-reaching priority, only Bulgaria mentions the attempt to centralise existing offers and Estonia quotes encouraging self-help and the active integration of PLWAs in HIV/AIDS prevention work as further essential goals.

In all countries of northern, eastern and central Europe basic needs such as free treatment and therapy are borne by the national social insurance systems. Poland and the Czech Republic expressly mention that almost 100% of the total costs incurred are met by the state.

In addition to covering the cost of medical treatment, the state provides funds for financial support, accommodation and transport of PLWAs in Bulgaria. The national AIDS programme (Estonia, Lithuania), the national pension fund (Estonia) and the district governments (Finland) also dispose over the corresponding funds. The Polish National Office for AIDS Prevention provides NGOs with funds that are to benefit HIV-infected persons suffering the worst social and economic hardship.

Some help offerings are also supported or entirely financed by decentralised sources: For example, in Estonia donations, foundations, and contributions of international organisations and box office proceeds from charity concerts are used for self-help promotion. In Finland the National Slot Machine Association (which has a monopoly for slot machines) finances most NGO activities. In Bulgaria NGOs have been offering both financial assistance and psychological and social counselling for the last 3 to 4 years.

The executive organs of the corresponding support measures in all countries of northern, central and eastern Europe are generally the social, health, labour and legal authorities, along with public AIDS information centres and NGOs.

PLWAs and their relatives, the Central Clinic for Infectious Diseases (Estonia), local social and health authorities, the Red Cross (Finland), the State Infection Centre (Latvia), church-run hospices (Poland), the county councils and welfare organisations (Sweden) are also mentioned in the individual reports as providers of support measures

Here is a list of typical PLWA support measures reported from the individual countries:

Bulgaria:

- Financial support is offered to registered haemophiliacs with HIV or AIDS.
- Antiretroviral therapy and transport to the only clinic that offers it are free of charge.
- Free accommodation is offered under certain circumstances.
- Help with the creation of more suitable working conditions.

Estonia:

- Payment of pensions and severe disablement allowances.
- Medical and psycho-social counselling in clinics.
- NGOs provide immediate help to PLWAs in particular crisis situations.
- NGOs offer support in kind (clothing, food).

Poland:

- Accommodation and care of AIDS patients in hospices.

Romania:

- Projects, mostly in university towns, that offer support to families with HIV-positive children.

- Antiretroviral therapy and transport to the only clinic that offers it are free of charge.
- An NGO-operated and financed day care centre for PLWAs in Bucharest.
- Free use of telephone services.

Slovenia:

- Registered haemophiliacs with HIV and AIDS and their infected partners and possibly orphaned children are granted financial support.
- Legal assistance, arranged by NGOs and financed by private donations.

Czech Republic:

- "Lighthouse" project: accommodation for patients with day care and rehabilitation offerings.

The Scandinavian countries mention no specific measures for PLWAs, and Norway explicitly claims that such special measures do not exist, as they are integrated in the general health service available to everyone.

In Slovenia no PLWA self-help group has been founded yet. The reasons quoted are the comparatively low number of infected persons and fear of stigmatisation.

The range of economic and social support measures for people with HIV and AIDS in central and eastern Europe does not differ from that of western Europe. But there are major differences in their implementation. Due to the comparatively low incidence and therefore even lower number of affected persons the specified measures are demanded to a much smaller extent and can therefore be provided by the states, although many of them are already pushed to their financial limits. Poland, for example, with its rather high HIV incidence can still provide the promised care and support for PLWAs, but partly only because many publicly financed NGOs continue to work even if they haven't received their money for months and face an uncertain future. In other countries, like Romania, the support work of NGOs is only possible because they receive funds from foreign foundations and international organisations. On the whole, one must highly appreciate the commitment of NGOs, which developed rapidly in some countries after the collapse of communism and now work in all states of central and eastern Europe, although they have no comparable tradition to look back on like their role models in the west.

In the northern European countries the "normalisation" of HIV/AIDS is obvious in the field of social and economic support, as it has been fully integrated in general health services.

3.9   HIV/AIDS treatment and care

World-wide, medical treatment and care are attributed a decisive function in secondary and tertiary HIV/AIDS prevention. "People with HIV or AIDS have significant health care needs. HIV infection slowly progresses to ever-more serious complications and most often to an untimely death, even for the minority of HIV-infected people with access to the latest antiretroviral drugs" (UNAIDS-Report, 1999, p 44). Over the last few years interest has focused mainly on the availability of new therapies. Since the mid-1990s there has been considerable progress in the treatment of people living with HIV and AIDS. HAART, highly active antiretroviral therapy, uses drugs that inhibit virus reproduction on their own, but even better when combined in tri-therapy. Meanwhile there is evidence that HAART can long postpone the occurrence of serious fatal infections. However, the newly available and highly effective drugs are patented and very expensive, which makes them unaffordable for parts of the Third World and even for some countries of central and eastern Europe.

UNAIDS and WHO were able to convince some of the most well-known pharmaceuticals firms to facilitate access to adequate treatment in the context of research programmes in some developing countries, but only to some extent and not universally. Of course, these programmes are not aimed at Europe and not even at the countries of central and eastern Europe, which partly have great problems financing adequate treatment of AIDS patients. However, UNAIDS supports these countries in the development of adequate national strategies: "At country level, as part of national strategic planning on HIV/AIDS, Theme Groups encourage communities to set their own locally-relevant standards of care with the involvement of people living with HIV. While taking resource constraints into account, community standards of care should be technically sound and satisfactory to those served. The standards should cover palliative care (the alleviation of pain and distressing symptoms), access to drugs for HIV-related opportunistic infections, such as tuberculosis and fungal infections, and, where resources permit, more sophisticated treatment such as antiretroviral therapy" (UNAIDS-Report, 1999, p 45).

However, access to new treatment methods may have an adverse impact on care. While medicine started to focus on the patient in the early days of HIV/AIDS treatment, it has now often shifted back to treatment needs again. Priority has moved from 'care' to 'cure' (Schaeffer 1998). "The disease and its curability again take centre stage, more or less shifting the focus of attention away from the patient" (Rosenbrock, 1999, p. 27).

On the whole, the spread of HIV/AIDS has led to a modernisation and liberalisation of health services in many countries and great efforts were undertaken to develop systems of integrated and continuous care in the entire service network, with different countries applying different solutions. According to Kirp & Bayer (1992) the strategies of patient treatment in the industrialised countries differ much more than the methods of primary prevention. This is due to the different systems of general medical care and social security for illness. The countries also differ in their respective medical cultures. However, in their goals, most countries commonly accept the WHO's "Health for All" strategy, which means that patient treatment is composed of co-ordinated medical, financial, social, psycho-social and care measures, so that each patient receives adequate treatment for his particular disease (WHO, 1981).

In most countries in-patient and ambulatory treatment for people living with AIDS is provided mainly by hospitals and university clinics, and in some countries GPs play a decisive role in outpatient care. In addition, there is a variety of psycho-social and care offerings, which are financed partly by the state or NGOs. The following chapter describes the differences and common features of patient care in the surveyed European countries.

3.9.1 Western and Southern Europe

The spectrum of HIV/AIDS treatment and care is vast, and comprises counselling and partner notification, advice services, out-patient monitoring (compliance) and medical treatment, treatment information, in-patient medical treatment, and palliative care.

Care is provided through first level services represented by a variety of outlets: General Practitioners and non-hospital-based specialists, and through hospitals or specialised clinics, or special units such as the ones found in clinical psychiatry of University hospitals as part of the treatment for drug addicts (e.g. Vienna), or infectious disease outpatient clinic in the University Hospital (e.g. Reykjavik), or the HIV priority private practices or the Co-operation of Ambulatory Care (AGAV) of the Deutsche AIDS-Hilfe in Germany among others, or diagnostic clinical centres and psycho-socio-sanitary centres among others in Italy, or support centres for drug addicted persons and social solidarity institutions and NGOs and State anti-Tuberculosis ambulatory services among others in Portugal, or ambulatory clinics in Spain carrying out intensive care of diagnosis, treatment, prophylaxis, screening and health education, or AIDS treatment centres which are hospital-based, nursing homes called "AIDS beds" and buddy projects in the Netherlands, the GUM clinics (over 200) in the UK quite popular in comparison the General Practitioners which have not been the main access point because of different concerns (confidentiality within small communities, concerns over competence and attitudes of some GPs and fear of forced disclosure of HIV status due to insurance applications).

The teams are composed of a mix of different professionals (doctors, nurses, pharmacists, biologists, dieticians, etc.) based on the level of care and the different countries.

Protease inhibitors have been used widely since the mid-nineties in the region. The sources of provision of the anti-retroviral agents are changing, for example in France, they were originally dispensed only in hospital pharmacies from hospital budgets, and since October 1997, they are now distributed through normal pharmacies and covered by health insurance. In Italy, drugs are now accessible through pharmacies. In contrast, in Portugal for example, those are still exclusively provided through the hospital system.

To safeguard compliance to treatment, different schemes have been set up, e.g. in Spain therapeutic commitment units, the national Plan on AIDS campaigns, and various NGO projects, with the example of the monitoring of patients' hospital visits to collect medicines for HIV treatment, usually every three months.

An obstacle to high quality of care by first level physicians reported in Belgium, and which can be transposed to other countries as well, is that the relatively low number of HIV/AIDS patients, combined with the high density of physicians, make the ratio patients per doctor very low, consequently, leaving few opportunities for the physicians either to apply or to improve their expertise.

In Spain, despite the material designed for health care workers, and accessibility to in-service training in HIV/AIDS care, services are still inadequate at the primary level, because health professionals are generally reluctant to do this kind of work, and because of the poor co-ordination between specific and primary care programmes.

Some countries or regions have designed their own Guidelines for General Practitioners (e.g. French-speaking part of Belgium, the Netherlands). In the Netherlands, the guidelines are part of a new programme (Sept. 1998) on "HIV test and HIV treatment", encompassed in the comprehensive AIDS control programme 1999-2002. The care and support needs and demands of the people with HIV themselves allow to shift current policies and care towards a more need-oriented care. In addition, the needs of vulnerable and socially weaker groups are also taken into consideration with prevention and education. For other countries, there are no guidelines, on the basis that scientific knowledge is evolving so quickly that any recommendation would rapidly be obsolete (e.g. Flanders in Belgium, Iceland), and that the delivery of HIV treatments services has "evolved with increased knowledge of the disease" (UK). This does not preclude on-going up-dated guidance through regular organised meetings and discussions with colleagues for updates, as organised in Flanders.

In Austria, a self-help manual has been developed on topics related to medicine, self-help resources, legal aspects, and nursing primarily for the use of medical and psycho-social professions. It has been provided free of charge through AIDS-Hilfe organisations.

In Germany, the findings of a model project on "Medical Ambulatory Care" have been instrumental to develop specific training courses for Medical Doctors working in private practices.

The costs of care are covered usually by the countries own well developed social security system. In some countries, the destitute patients have access to public centres (e.g. the Social Welfare Centres in Belgium). A movement in Greece favours the restriction of the provision of drugs free of charge to HIV positive patients who are Greek citizens only in order to avoid draining the country health care resources. For opportunistic infections, patients may have to contribute to a share of the amount (e.g. in Portugal).

In general, we can state that the access to care for HIV positive or AIDS patients is adequate in Western and Southern European countries. .

In France, the medical system is based on a town and hospital network system to facilitate the continuity between the hospital and non-hospital care, for HIV care (100 networks), and also adopted for the care of drug users (200).

Ireland reports on the difficulty for the hospitals to liaise with the General Practitioners for the co-ordination of patient care.

In the UK a recent survey of over 2,000 HIV positive patients showed that overall, satisfaction with clinic services was very high. The median travelling time was 30 minutes only, but a significant minority (14%) needed more than an hour to access their clinic, and a small proportion (3%) more than two hours, or three hours (1%). Only 6% of the sample who reported having difficulties in getting treatments in the past half a year due to interruptions in the drug supply or lack of complementary therapies, professional insensitivity to individual needs, and trouble in getting appointments, and 0.5% only who reported having been refused treatments or told that treatments were unavailable.

Despite existing services, some vulnerable groups fall through the systems though, as reported next. The political and socio-economic conditions in south-eastern Europe have recently aggravated the situation of illegal migrants which in turn has a direct impact on the HIV/AIDS treatment and care for that population group in particular.

For example, in Belgium, the illegal migrants are afraid that using either public or private organisations, their status will be disclosed to the Federal Bureau of Foreigners; the same in Austria. In France and Germany, social vulnerability remains the main cause of lack of access to care for HIV patients, as well as for any other diseases. In addition, despite the existing free, anonymous tests, anonymous treatments is limited and only exists in some counselling and information centres for Venereal Diseases which are offered by individual health centres. Illegal immigrants also find themselves in a more difficult situation in Greece; the social allowance received at the local welfare department does not protect the anonymity of the patients in rural areas. Foreigners who have not been granted a permit to stay in Iceland cannot receive the treatment without getting a special permit from the Institute of Social Services. In Ireland, the issues of stigma and fears of lack of confidentiality often mitigate against people with HIV to access the full range of community services available from NGOs, such as home support, counselling, help with retraining and social supports, resulting in some people feeling very isolated. In Portugal, the absence of an articulated and effective network of support services, with no legal counselling support to facilitate the immigrants' legalisation, compound the immigrants' barriers of the access to treatment. In Spain, two groups are at disadvantage: the migrants living outside the national legal framework are only attended to in case of emergency; and the present or former IDUs are not prescribed medicine because their levels of adhesion to basic health necessities are considered to be low. In the UK, people from African communities access services late, regulations set out in the new Asylum and Immigration Act exacerbate the issue further, and illegal residents have open access to testing, but treatments are not available for them.

A recent law (1998) in Italy makes explicit reference to take into care illegal immigrants affected by infectious diseases.

The trend of the HIV/AIDS affected persons is to be taken care of in their homes, instead of in the hospitals, hence the rise of ambulatory care.

As part of a supportive environment to care and treatment, NGOs (e.g. AIDS-Hilfe Austria and Germany) have pioneered efforts in social communication through their centres. Support encompasses a variety of activities: e.g. in Austria, day and evening meals, massage and exercises; activities related to the (re)integration into gainful employment; self-help centres with basic infrastructure and services (office, telephone, photocopies, secretarial support).

A number of "best practices" are reported in the different countries, as documented next. In Belgium, experts have arrived to good practice consensus: systematic prophylaxis after a recent sexual risk, or a recent intravenous injection, is rejected to avoid negative repercussions on primary prevention; in contrast, it is practised in cases of potential contamination in connection to occupational conditions; the seven AIDS Reference Centres provide answers to technical inquiries from physicians or organisations.

In Austria, the Red Cross has performed comprehensive in-house training courses and information events to meet the organisations capacities to be able to match the growing needs of home assistance and care, and nursing services.

In France, efforts are being made to improve the application of the law on the legalisation of resident status for all HIV patients for them to benefit from full access to social security services. Migrant associations are struggling to make the law better known and applied, with no restrictions, in all towns of the country, with the full support of the local administrative authorities.

In Germany, the "AIDS and children" model programme based on interdisciplinary workgroups tailored optimally different components (clinical research, in-patient treatment and ambulatory medical, psycho-social care) to respond to individual needs. Most of the forty jobs supported have now been taken over by the States. The financing of the successful model programme "Expansion of ambulant help for AIDS infected persons in the scope of social stations" with 3,000 HIV and AIDS patients taken care of through the provision of an additional two hundred jobs in the old Federal States, is being pursued further through an agreement between the States and the Communes.

In Ireland, counselling initiatives have been pioneered at the St James' Hospital Social Work Services for pre-test counselling to promote primary and secondary HIV prevention for clients who are vulnerable or at risk of future infection. Participants have found it useful, supportive, accessible and non-judgemental. The Open Heart House provides day care services for people with HIV in Dublin, and provides support to people in taking control of their lives while challenging the isolation in which many people feel.

In Italy, the Villa Glori managed by the Caritas Diocesana in Rome has now for ten years welcomed men and women with HIV/AIDS who live under difficult economic and family conditions and are unable to deal with their situation adequately.

In Spain, the number of initiatives led by hospital outpatient units, or primary care programmes, or NGOs (ex. of the Catalan NGO Actua with the SIDA programme) to cater for home care is growing.

In the Netherlands, a project on standardised training and school materials on HIV/AIDS which started in 1993 has allowed to develop a training manual for home care workers, social workers, and drug abuse counsellors, and is useful for other institutional care workers and the staff of penitentiary institutions. The initiative followed the model of a successful "trainerspack" from Scotland.

3.9.2 Northern, Central and Eastern Europe

In most of the reporting countries the national strategy for handling HIV/AIDS comprises medical treatment for those affected and psychological, social and economic support. This policy is generally based on the National AIDS Prevention Programme, which specifies all legal and financial aspects. In practice, everyone is entitled to medical care, even those who are not insured. Illegal immigrants are an exception (e.g. in Poland, Sweden, and Norway). However, in acute, life-threatening cases these patients are also granted assistance (e.g. in Sweden).

Treatment itself is generally not prescribed by the state. In Sweden, for example, there are no national recommendations or guidelines that regulate certain procedures. Instead the county councils, clinics and treating doctors take responsibility for the treatment of HIV-positive patients, based on their long experience and scientific findings. However, Slovakia is an exception here, as its report says that it has guidelines for HIV/AIDS treatment developed by experts from relevant scientific fields of medicine.

Treatment offered in all states of northern, central and eastern Europe includes ambulatory and inpatient clinic treatment, psychological and social counselling and out-patient treatment. In the following we have listed national characteristics regarding existing and lacking offerings and problems with their implementation:

In Bulgaria necessary treatment and therapies are currently provided only by the Clinic for Infectious Diseases of Sofia. Discussions are ongoing on whether to extend treatment facilities to further institutions, at least in conurbations, but there are no concrete plans yet. Only since purchasing the corresponding drugs in 1999 can the clinic offer suitable conditions for tri-therapy. In compliance with existing regulations, HIV-positive persons in Bulgaria are automatically referred to the Clinic for Infectious Diseases for further treatment. For various reasons this offer is rejected by some of those affected. For one part, they fear losing their anonymity and, for the other, medical treatment is only considered necessary when the patient develops full-blown AIDS.

Medical treatment of HIV infections in Denmark is generally covered by the social insurance system, so that no costs incur to those affected. All citizens and people with a residence permit are granted free therapy. Combination therapy generally starts before the immune system is severely damaged or before opportunistic infections occur.

Until 1997 AZT was the only therapy offered in Estonia, after the introduction of alternative drugs, combination therapy has been offered since 1998. Basically, in Estonia both patients covered by the social insurance system and those without insurance are entitled to the necessary therapies. Obstructions to optimum treatment are generally caused by the patients themselves due to lacking compliance.

Although all Finnish health institutions are involved in the early detection of HIV/AIDS, treatment and therapies are generally performed in the departments for infectious diseases of the university clinics. Psycho-social counselling is offered by the local health centres, the AIDS council and the Red Cross. There are no national guidelines and participation in the measures is voluntary.

In Latvia all relevant costs are borne by the national budget. For the prescription of combination therapy a corresponding indication is necessary. Necessary treatment and counselling is only provided by the National Centre for Infections in Riga.

In Poland there are no special AIDS wards. The patients are treated in wards for communicable diseases. As the medical staff already has to meet special safety regulations for handling patients, HIV-positive persons are not forced to reveal their illness to them or other patients. In Poland it is very difficult in general to be granted a place in a hospice. PLWAs are not accepted everywhere. Neither do any home care or out-patient programmes exist.

In Lithuania home care and other alternative care practices are organised mainly by NGOs.

The report for the Czech Republic points out that problematic compliance (and hence diminished efficacy of treatment) has been observed mostly in IDUs.
In Romania some hospitals still refuse to accept HIV-positive patients, claiming that they cannot observe the necessary safety regulations for lack of protective gloves or disposable syringes.

On the whole, the countries of northern Europe offer comprehensive in-patient and ambulatory treatment facilities and support care for people living with HIV and AIDS. The offerings are decentralised, easy to reach in general and freely accessible to everyone, with the exception of illegal immigrants. But even they receive help in life-threatening situations, for example in Sweden. They have unlimited access to anonymous test and counselling offers. These are no HIV/AIDS-specific rulings but apply to the entire health service. The applied therapy methods meet modern standards.

Likewise, the surveyed countries of central and eastern Europe largely offer adequate treatment facilities, especially in in-patient care, while ambulatory treatment and care lags way behind western standards in most states. In-patient care is only provided centrally in big cities, in some countries it is limited to a single clinic in the capital. This has advantages and disadvantages for PLWAs. The disadvantages are obvious: people living far away from these centres have considerably restricted access to treatment facilities, they may have to pay high travel costs or move near the centre, which is virtually unaffordable for many. One advantage of the centres in big cities is their anonymity. HIV-positive persons from remote, sparsely populated areas often fear that they will be unable to maintain their anonymity there and try to move to big cities for fear of discrimination, which simultaneously puts them closer to better treatment facilities. However, if, like in Bulgaria, treatment is only offered by a single institution in the country, those affected also fear losing their anonymity in big cities, as they already expect stigmatisation on entering the clinic. Modern antiretroviral therapy is now available in all states and free for the patients. However, the costs incurred are a huge burden for most countries and can partly be cushioned only by the corresponding support of international organisations and the pharmaceuticals industry.

Below you will find examples of treatment quoted in the country reports and of support and care facilities:

- On the introduction of tri-therapy in Bulgaria the ministry of health initiated a broad-based, popular information campaign, which was able to reach hitherto uncooperative patients.
- The Stop AIDS Campaign in Denmark features a buddy service, with voluntary helpers visiting AIDS patients and lending them a helping hand.
- In Denmark patient groups meet every month in larger hospitals nationwide and discuss the situation in the respective ward with medical staff and social workers.
- "Positive Outlook" in Estonia is a self-help project organised by and for PLWAs and their relatives.
- The Finnish Slot Machine Association finances a project that offers home care as an alternative to in-patient hospital care in Finland.
- Latvia's State Infection Centre successfully offers so-called post-test counselling. In the case of a positive test result, it provides counselling and support, where needed, during a one-week stay.
- The Phare LIEN Programme at Bucharest's Victor Babes Hospital in Romania is a training programme for employees, voluntary NGO staff and affected parents that is to give infected children a better quality of life and longer life expectancy.
- In Sweden some clinics for infectious diseases have specially trained nurses, who can manage the organisation of home care offerings, where necessary. They liaise with local nursing staff, prepare them, where needed, for special requirements, and can be contacted at any time, thus creating a direct link with the clinic.
- Slovenia likewise has a network of around 700 district nurses who offer home care.
- The "Lighthouse" project – a self-help programme organised by the Czech AIDS support organisation

- 1999 the Contact Centre for People with HIV in Norway added a hospice to its day-care centre, supported by funds of the city mission and the city of Oslo.

3.10   Overall expenditures

"HIV/STD prevention spending is among the best investments countries can make, returning billions of dollars in health care savings, production   and   income."
(Principle formulated in a WHO meeting on Prevention, Geneva, 5-7 October, 1999)

"General access to high-quality health services is one of the basic principles. The state should take a leading strategic role – by establishing priorities – and recognise that there are limits to what the state can spend on health care – limits that every country must define for itself." (Dr. Gro Harlem Brundtland talking to the WHO-Regional Committee for Europe, 17.9.1998). These basic principles are recognised by the members states of the WHO region Europe. And we must keep this in mind when reading the statements in the country reports on the assessment of overall expenditures caused by HIV/AIDS. The figures tell us something about the countries' willingness to provide funds for combating HIV/AIDS both by care and prevention, but also about the financial limits of each country. Hence, if a country's overall economic situation deteriorates, this generally leads to immediate cuts in the health system. Moreover, a change of attitude to the disease may also generate cuts in prevention measures and research.

If, like in many western European countries, the spread of HIV lags far behind the rapid development of the epidemic predicted in the 1980s, this may also reduce the willingness to provide resources for corresponding prevention measures and research projects, as do new therapy methods that allow us to hope that AIDS will become a treatable disease. On the other hand, a sudden increase or first emergence of HIV infections within certain groups or countries may reinforce the willingness to make more funds available.

Alongside the increase and reduction of available funds, the experts of the country reports were asked to assess the total cost of the HIV/AIDS epidemic, which should comprise both public and, where available, non-public expenditures. In particular, they were asked to quote the costs of prevention and information/education measures. In practice, it was rather difficult to answer these questions for many countries, as central public expenditures for prevention, screenings and research were easy to assess, but often only incomplete estimates could be given for decentralised expenditures down to the local level under this survey. It was virtually impossible to gain a complete overview of all non-public expenditures. In many countries it was difficult to access information on total actual treatment costs that are borne by health insurance, social insurance, and pension providing bodies, but account for a large share of costs caused by HIV/AIDS. For example, for Germany we only have an estimate of total costs incurred by prevention, treatment, rehabilitation, care, administration, training and research of the Federal Statistics Office for the year 1994. According to this information the costs incurred by HIV/AIDS in 1994 amounted to DM165bn (ca. 83 billion euros).

3.10.1 Western and Southern Europe

In general, even in a period of national budget constraints, the overall global costs of the endemic in each country are not known, either at the national or federal level with a few exceptions. The reasons can be one or several, among which: the lack of definition of terms, difficulties to calculate direct costs (prevention, diagnosis, treatment) and indirect costs and aggregate costs despite various types of costing studies, different budget headings and different Government departments (e.g. Ireland), national taboo on analysing expenditures in the field of medicine and public health (e.g. Austria), backlog in expenditures data (e.g. Germany reports comprehensive resources allocation up to 1995), unknown voluntary sector financial resources.

The bulk of the resources for HIV/AIDS activities are provided by ministerial budgets (national, regional and local authorities, national health and pension insurance fund), and the smaller part by private donations. Large contributions through fund raising for the past few years have been earmarked more for direct assistance to the people affected by HIV and AIDS, than for prevention activities (e.g. Austria).

In France, the global costs of the AIDS epidemic are estimated at more than 5 billion French francs per year. Public funds are earmarked for anonymous free screening, epidemiological studies, prevention, training, non-hospital treatment, hospital care and research, with the largest share going to non-hospital activities and prevention measures. France documents less funds for studies and training, while more was spent on anonymous and free screening centres.

In Italy, since the beginning of the epidemic, emphasis has been put on allocating funds to hospitals to the detriment of prevention activities as documented by the National AIDS Plan budget (80% to infectious disease clinics, 15% to first, second level care structures and research centres, and 5% to primary prevention of infection with information campaigns and training and to the voluntary associations).

In The Netherlands, the total expenditures for HIV/AIDS education and prevention amount to 6.5 million NLG per year with the bulk (5.0) for national prevention and education tasks, and the rest for public safe sex campaigns (1.5).

In Portugal, in spite of the increase in the number of anti-retroviral treatments, the global costs per patient have stabilised, explained possibly due to the positive impact of HAART. At least half of the budgets from the National Committee for AIDS (45%), and from the ministry of health (50%) are earmarked to health promotion and AIDS prevention.

In Spain, one third of the funds budgeted in the national plan are earmarked since 1998 for HIV/AIDS prevention programmes of the regional health authorities of the Autonomous Communities, in addition to their own budgets. 1997 data on the cost of HIV/AIDS prevention in the country came up to a total of 700 million pesetas (including human resources costs). Each region receives a minimum sum (10 million pesetas) and the remaining funds are allocated according to the population size and the HIV infection incidence. In addition, NGOs working in prevention and psychological care receive 7.5% of the Secretariat's budget.

Despite the funds allocated in each country for HIV prevention activities, the trend and concern reported in general is that spending has decreased significantly in the global area of HIV prevention, and in communications in particular. In Iceland, the budget had been reduced by half for the past two years with a reduction for prevention programmes. The reasons invoked by the countries are the gradual slowing of the epidemic, combined with the introduction and impact of the new combination therapies.

A few exceptions exist to these negative trends. In Greece, the funds allocated to prevention, including information and other activities, have increased five fold in the last years. In Spain, a three fold increase in the overall budget for AIDS, and consequently in prevention activities, occurred between 1997 and 1999. In England the budget allocation for prevention activities was 53 million Pounds in 1998/1999, with the same amount allocated in 1999/2000. An "allocation formula" allows an equal share to the one hundred English health authorities.

The budget allocation for treatment and care was more than four times more, or 228 million Pounds in 1998/1999, with an additional 7 million in 1999/2000.

The support for services of the large NGOs (e.g. AIDS-Hilfe in Germany and Austria) are known.

But the majority of countries do not have available costs of communication or of social support (e.g. Belgium). In Italy, the allocation of funds for campaigns has decreased by two third between 1992 and 1998. In Spain, the HIV/AIDS prevention campaign was supported by 22% of the Secretariat's total budget, and the campaigning costs doubled in 1999 in comparison to 1998. In The Netherlands, between 1987 and 1998 13 million NLG were spent, or less than one Guilder per Dutch for the campaigns.

The cost of tri-therapy treatments are in general better known, in Belgium, for example, it amounts to approximately EUR 1,000 per person per month. The total cost of tests in Belgium amounts to approximately EUR 3 million.

Original positive initiatives have developed which in turn can have an impact on HIV prevention policies funding. In communication in the Netherlands, since 1994 a prevention fund has taken over from the ministry of public health the financing of the public safe sex campaigns. In Spain, funding through the Foundation for the Advance of Spanish Research into AIDS has been initiated by the ministry of health with the private sector pharmaceutical companies for interdisciplinary HIV/AIDS studies in basic, clinical, epidemiological, economic and social, including preventive matters.

The introduction of tri-therapy methods in the mid-nineties have significantly reduced the duration of hospital days. Consequently, the costs to the social security systems have decreased. The financial advantages of lower hospitalisation costs appear to be significant, even when compared to the additional costs of introducing costly new therapies. Greece, points to the urgent need for developing alternate models of care, for example "managed care programmes" aiming both at the control of cost, and the quality improvement of the services provided. Although anti-retroviral treatment and prevention should not compete for scarce funds, the gap may increase in the allocation of funds for these two components, as brought up with the example of Spain. Of the total ministry budget for HIV/AIDS, the annual prevention expenditures represented a small amount (8%) of the total amount spent on anti-retroviral treatment.

In conclusion, HIV prevention policies reflected particularly through communication activities are in danger if budgets and expenses are not more transparent, for whatever reasons (e.g. integration of activities into the ministry of health, or other factors mentioned above).

3.10.2 Northern, Central and Eastern Europe

The quoted figures for costs incurred by AIDS generally refer to expenses for preventive measures, tests, research and treatment. In virtually all cases these are funds provided by the respective government. Information on NGO expenditures is only rarely available. No further distinctions were made between expenditures on a local or regional level. Actual financial expenditure is very hard to identify, if at all, as there is no access to relevant data and a monetary calculation of certain parameters is extremely difficult. Moreover, most of the expenses incurred are covered by health insurance, social insurance and pension providers, and specific information on them is hardly accessible.

According to the available country reports the following picture emerges for the origin and composition of annual budgets available in the respective countries:

In Estonia the government provided funds of EEK1,710,000 (around 109,600 euros) each year in 1996, 1997 and 1998 for the national AIDS programme. However, the assumed inflation rate is 8-10% a year, so that there is a downward trend in financing. Of the EEK1,500,000 (around 96,000 euros) earmarked for prevention, around EEK600,000 (38,500 euros) were spent on information and education measures.

Lithuania's national AIDS prevention programme had a budget of 120,000 litas (around 30,000 euros) in 1996, of 204,000 litas (around 51,000 euros) in 1997 and 180,000 litas (around 45,000 euros) in 1998. Expenditure for information measures amounted to 51,100 litas (around 12,500 euros) in 1998. Data on NGO expenditure is not available.

In Romania estimated annual costs amount to 300 billion lei, with the ministry of health contributing fifty per cent. However, over the last two years only 10% of the earmarked sum has actually been paid. No financing of prevention measures is intended. They are funded by the NGOs alone, which receive financial support from other countries and international organisations.

In Slovakia costs are covered mainly by public institutions. UNAIDS and the Czech-Slovak-Swiss Health Society are also mentioned as major financial backers. Of the total budget of SK52m (approx. 1.2 million euros) actual therapy costs account for SK12m (approx. 276,000 euros). The remaining SK40m (approx. 920,000 euros) are spent on tests and screenings. The Institute for Health Education also organises and implements AIDS information campaigns as part of its activities.

As Slovenia has no national AIDS council, there are no corresponding funds. Relevant measures are integrated in the national health service. No estimates of the total costs are available, just figures for individual examples.

In 1999 the amount provided by the government of the Czech Republic was CZK41.3m (approx. 1.16 million euros). No exact statements could be made on regional distribution patterns. Around half of the sum was earmarked for treatment costs and medication. Preventive measures account for approx. one-third of expenses.

The Polish national budget earmarked spending of almost €10m for HIV/AIDS in 1999. Two-thirds were used for antiretroviral treatment and one-third for HIV/AIDS prevention. Another €5m were made available for drug prevention.

Latvia can only provide concrete data on the costs of preventive measures, which amounted to LS167,349 (approx. 280,000 euros) in 1999 and have remained almost unchanged for three years. Additionally, NGO-financed prevention projects were supported by UNAIDS with a total of $100,000 in 1996/97.

In contrast, HIV/AIDS spending in the Scandinavian countries is much higher:

In Denmark most of HIV/AIDS prevention is publicly financed. In 1999 total expenditures amounted to approx. DKr31.3m (approx. 4.2 million euros). DKr13.3m (approx. 1.8 million euros) of this sum went to the National Board of Health and activities of public institutions on a regional level. The remaining 18 million (approx. 2.4 million euros) went to NGOs such as the AIDS hotline, the Association of Haemophiliacs and self-help groups of PLWAs. In addition to the national budget, the individual government districts have separate financial resources. The costs of tests and therapy amount to an estimated DKr65,000 (approx. 8,700 euros) per year and patient, with an alleged patient figure of approx. 1,250. Moreover, there is an AIDS fund fed by donations, foundations, membership fees and charity proceeds.

Finland had a total budget of FmK28,100,000 (approx. 4.8 million euros) in 1998. More than one-third of this sum was spent on treatment costs, a similarly large portion on preventive measures. The remainder was shared between expenses for tests, counselling and research, among other things.

The budget provided by the Norwegian ministries of health and social affairs in 1999 amounted to NKr16.6m (approx. 2 million euros). The National Institute for Public Health had NKr.2.5m (approx. 308,000 euros) at its disposal for information and education campaigns.

Sweden's government made an amount of more than SKr160m (approx. 18.8 million euros) available in 1999. Of this sum, information and education accounted for SKr3.5m (approx. 411,000 euros). Estimates showed that treatment costs of SKr100,000 (approx. 12,000 euros) per HIV patient incur every year. For AIDS patients the costs amount to approx. SKr130,000 (approx. 15,300 euros) due to tri-therapy.

Unlike in many western European countries, there are no reports of a reduction of funds spent on HIV/AIDS prevention in northern, central and eastern Europe yet. Among the Scandinavian countries, only Sweden reports a slight reduction in provided funds, which are on a high level. The amount of reported HIV/AIDS-related expenditures ranges from €18.8m in Sweden to around €50,000 in Lithuania, and these sums are solely public expenditures. Of these amounts an average share of one-third is earmarked for prevention measures. The annual amount of approx. €4m quoted by Denmark seems rather low at first, but must be put into perspective in view of the fact that the country only has a population of 5.3 million. Among the central and eastern European countries, Poland has both the highest incidence and the highest public spending on HIV/AIDS by far, amounting to approx. €10m. On the whole, the public funds provided for HIV/AIDS in central and eastern Europe are hardly adequate and prevention measures can often be realised only thanks to financial assistance from the EU or UNAIDS (e.g. in Romania and Latvia). However, this is not an HIV/AIDS-specific phenomenon in these countries but a reflection of the general economic situation.

3.11 Research on risk behaviour and behavioural changes

Right from the start the HIV/AIDS epidemic has posed a major challenge to society and an extraordinary task to research, which faced completely new questions with this first retrovirus epidemic. As a priority, biomedical research was stepped up to find promising cures and an effective vaccine. As those involved soon realised that such solutions could not be found in the foreseeable future, the modification of risk behaviour became one of the top-priority tasks of prevention policies. Responsible behaviour of the individual has lost none of its importance for individual protection against infection and is still the most effective means against a further spread of AIDS. "This goal can be reached by two, on the face of it, stunningly banal behaviour modifications: the use of condoms for penetrative intercourse outside monogamy and of sterile needles for intravenous drug consumption" (Rosenbrock & Salmen, 1990, p. 13).

As these modifications affect the individual sexual behaviour and techniques of drug use of IDUs, and thus intimate, taboo and emotionally controlled behaviour, this field is much more complex and more resistant to changes than, for example, risk behaviour on the road, where the "safe" practice of wearing seatbelts has become established in virtually all industrialised countries. Hence, the social sciences were and are required to analyse this field in depth. This includes the identification of relevant sexual behaviour in the general population and in particularly vulnerable risk groups as a basis for targeted prevention measures and the evaluation of corresponding measures in relation to actual behaviour modification.

"In Europe, the lack of basic data on sexual behaviour in most countries means that behaviour change, condom availability and use are all difficult to monitor" UNAIDS claimed in Geneva back in 1996, although detailed surveys on sexual behaviour were available at the time for some countries of western Europe, and the EU-funded broad-based study on "Sexual behaviour and HIV/AIDS risk in Europe" had already been conducted from 1991 to 1995. The following chapter will show to what extent studies on sexual behaviour of the general population and key risk groups have been performed in the European countries under review.

The effects of prevention measures on changes of risk behaviour in intercourse and drug use are the subject of another group of sociological studies that are of major importance for the further development of prevention strategies. These are the so-called KABP studies (Knowledge, Attitudes, Behaviour, Practice), which examine to what extent prevention messages improve people's knowledge and actually change attitudes and behaviour in reality. The study focus is on whether the individual takes in the necessary information on health risks through HIV/AIDS, whether the respective person changes his attitude, by realising the degree of his own vulnerability and accepts the necessity of a behaviour modification. Only this process will lead to an individual attempt to change his behaviour. For prevention it is then decisive for what term the modified "safe"

599

behaviour in sex or drug use is consistently maintained. Such KABP studies are highly complex and particularly the survey of sustained behaviour modification entails numerous methodological problems, as this field is generally not one of observable behaviour but has to be determined by elaborate interview methods. However, well-structured KABP studies are an excellent tool for the evaluation of prevention strategies.

3.11.1 Western and Southern Europe

Countries have combined surveys to examine levels of knowledge, attitudes and perceptions, and practices in relation to behaviour patterns (KAPB) with regard to HIV infection. Those have been more frequent in the general population, but also carried out among some vulnerable groups (e.g. male homosexuals, IDUs, prison inmates). Some countries have yearly surveys, others, once every four to ten years. Only Iceland reports a national survey conducted more than five years back (in 1992), while Ireland and Spain do not report any country wide study at all. However, Ireland reports some ad-hoc studies on risk and behavioural changes among the youth in urban environments, and Spain has carried out local research.

A recent study carried out in Austria among the youth showed that they still lack knowledge of the disease and display behaviour deficits in prevention. The country lacks a recent gay sexual behavioural study as well.

In Belgium, a large national sample among a population aged fifteen years and more in 1997 documented that a large proportion of the population had partially inadequate knowledge, with severe information gaps, and a number of false believes. False believes were more widely spread among lower income groups, and among older people. Discriminatory opinions towards HIV positive people were often expressed, particularly among less educated or older people, and among non Belgians. There were marked differences by Provinces. The survey will be repeated in 2001 to monitor these knowledge and attitudinal indicators. Specific studies were carried out among high risk population groups, and have shown a decrease in risk taking among homo- and bisexuals, and IDUs. However, the highest priority group, i.e. sub-Saharan Africans based on epidemiological data, is the less known of all.

In France, in 1998, despite the fact that most of the population (98%) is familiar with the main HIV modes of transmission, in comparison to 1994, there was an increase in false information on HIV (26% believed AIDS can be transmitted in public toilets, 23% by insect bites, and 22% in the same hospital ward as an HIV positive person). This is explained by previous communications that were prevention oriented within the scope of sexual and blood transmission, instead of naming actions and situations where there is no risk of transmission. Experts fear presently that the improved knowledge of therapeutic progress since 1997 gives rise to fears that HIV prevention could be relaxed. The survey also showed that sexual activity and the use of condoms have remained stable, but major changes occurred in the peoples' perception of AIDS:

- a decrease in demand for medical control and a more medicalised perception of AIDS,
- confidence in physicians remains high, but there is a decline in the confidence to anti-AIDS organisations, research personnel and to teachers,
- greater indifference, less compassion to HIV positive people,
- a lower level of personal interest in AIDS information campaigns,
- diminished fear of AIDS (from 32% in 1994 to 21% in 1998).

On the positive side, in France, surveys among young people (15-18) show that this age group seems better informed and more tolerant towards HIV-positive persons than adults. Condom use has increased substantially in this group since 1990. The age of first sexual experience (17 years old among males and females) has remained stable, declining only slightly over several decades. Among homo- and bisexuals safer sex practices appeared to be holding, although some sub-groups evidence more risk-taking than others. Drug users overall did not share syringes any longer, but, however, no change was observed in the practice of drug users reusing their own syringes, and sharing injection materials other than syringes; in addition, condom use remains low among this group. Prison inmates were less informed and tolerant of HIV infection than the general population with medical and social care remaining difficult among that group. Furthermore, in France, in 1998 there was a decline in screening tests, particularly among young people, singles, and people with multiple partners. In parallel, there was a declining number of calls made to the free AIDS Info Service Hotline since 1995, which is partly explained by the decline in AIDS concern in the population as a whole. The improved knowledge may be another reason too.

In Germany, like in France, recent studies show that the majority of the population (98%) know the main transmission routes, as well as the means of protection. The acceptance of condoms has increased both among males and females, and all studies prove that changes in attitudes and behaviours have taken place in this intimate area of life. There has been no increase in anonymous AIDS testing.

In Ireland, a recent study has provided information on HIV prevalence and on the inmates' sexual and drug using behaviours.

In Italy, a large study carried out in 1997 show that one fifth of the population (11 to 30 years) did not know precisely the transmission routes of the virus, and where to go for an HIV test. Almost two thirds (60%) aged between 11 and 16 years did not know that they could not have the HIV test free of charge and anonymously. One third of the population sampled felt uncomfortable about using condoms, although the vast majority (91%) agreed on the mutual respect it entails. In another study among a sample of 324 homosexual men 15 to 55 years, 39% mentioned the theme of AIDS with a new partner before sex, and only one fourth (27%) claimed always using a condom; 13% claimed not using one because they did not have access to it at the time of need, and 6% were convinced that having sex once without protection cannot result in an HIV infection.

In Portugal, there were several nation-wide KAPB studies since 1987. The latest findings document that even though there were positive changes of public awareness of the AIDS problem, and knowledge on how to prevent HIV transmission, condom use is still at a relatively low rate, and the level of risk of the sexual behaviours is still high, based on the significant number of extra-marital relationships and of unprotected occasional intercourse.

In Spain, condom use among Men who have Sex with Men (MSM) increased from 63 to 81% between 1993 and 1995. Among IDUs with occasional partners, condom use increased from 36 to 63% between 1993 and 1996.

In the United Kingdom, a National Survey of Sexually Attitudes and Lifestyles took place in 1991 and a new one is taking place presently with results expected in 2001. A National Gay Men's Health Survey carried out in 1998 found out that 50% homosexuals had taken the HIV test among whom 6% were tested positive, and 43% had never taken it. A WHO cross-national survey has also been carried out among the children 11-15 years old. Some one-off surveys have taken place which allow to measure perception and attitudes among adults aged 15 and older in England. For example, in the most recent one (March 1999), the majority of respondents (85%) agreed that there is still a great deal of stigma around HIV/AIDS, almost one fourth (23%) didn't know enough about the risk of HIV/AIDS to people like themselves. Only one fourth (24%) agreed that HIV/AIDS had made them change their lifestyles in some way, and encouragingly, among the 15-24 years, they were more likely to have changed their lifestyles (43%). In addition, many in-depth research on behaviours associated to HIV transmission are being carried out among prisoners and other groups. Through an unlinked anonymous survey of HIV prevalence among genitourinary clinic attendees, between 1990 and 1993 of the 1,752 homosexual or bisexual men with an HIV diagnoses, almost one third (30%) had an STD which indicates recent unprotected sex, and among those more than half (53%) were unaware of their HIV infection.

Condoms sales as an indicator of behavioural change show the following:

- In Austria, the Durex condoms sales have increased more than three fold in less than ten years, to 22 million in 1998.
- In Belgium, condoms sales increased by 5% a year until 1996. They have stagnated in 1997-1999 though, explained by the public relaxed prevention behaviours due to the misunderstanding that the endemic has been successfully controlled thanks to the success of the tri-therapies.
- In France, a 4.4% drop in condom sales in pharmacies between 1997 and 1998, with stable sales in supermarkets, and no data on sales from other sources.
- Germany reports a growing sales of condoms.
- In Greece, preliminary findings of a recent study (Summer 1999) placing emphasis on sexual behaviour in a new relationship showed overall an increase in condom use, with three fourth of respondent using condoms in their new relationship started in the past 12 months, and among the condom users, the vast majority (99%) having used during the last sexual intercourse.
- In Iceland, condom sales have been stable.
- In Italy, approximately seven condoms per year per sexually active male with 100 to 150 million sales per year, with 80% being users for contraceptive reasons, and not to prevent HIV or other STDs infection.
- In Portugal, the figures are available from market surveys of specialised companies, but the National Commission is designing two new studies on the risk and prevalence of HIV and condom accessibility.
- In the Netherlands, sales rates of condoms have increased yearly at around 155% since 1995.

- In Spain, in 1995-6, the average number of condoms used by each sexually active (15-49 years) member of the population was 8.5.

The sales of syringes can also be used as indicator of behavioural change among IDUs:

- In France, there has been a rise since 1996, with 13.8 million sales reported for pharmacies in 1997, and an estimated 200,000 Stéribox kits (low-priced kit sold in pharmacies and containing injection material, sterilisation and condoms) are sold monthly in pharmacies.
- In Iceland, syringes sales and needles have been stable.
- In Portugal, the syringes collected country-wide increased by 33% between 1994 to 1997, to 3,250,185, but decreased by 6% in 1998 in comparison to 1997.
- In Spain, needles share dropped from 57 to 30% between 1993 and 1996.

The relative success of the response to HIV/AIDS among IDUs in Belgium is due to a number of factors: from the start of the endemic an easy access to injection material and to substitution treatments, a rather low level of needle sharing, easy access to social protection, and low contacts with high prevalence areas.

Figures on HIV testing and analysis are not so well documented and leave room for various interpretations as it stands.

In conclusion, many countries are carrying out a number of sound research allowing to document risk behaviours and behavioural changes. Several of those have documented positive changes over time. In a few countries, research has shown positive and encouraging changes in condom use among the youth in particular, but this vulnerable and essential group is not sufficiently known. The countries who have been carrying out national research, or research among vulnerable groups, show areas of weaknesses which need to be urgently addressed, for example, to mention a few only: the important stigma still surrounding HIV/AIDS and a greater indifference or less compassion to PLWAs, lower level of interest or a general fatigue in AIDS information campaigns, still insufficient or low condom use among some of the vulnerable groups (i.e. homosexuals, prison inmates, IDUs, STD patients) and similar evidence in a few countries among the youth, syringes still shared among IDUs.

3.11.2 Northern, Central and Eastern Europe

Representative studies on HIV/AIDS-related knowledge, attitudes to risk behaviour and behaviour modification have been conducted in virtually all northern, eastern and central European countries. Studies in northern Europe already started in the mid-1980s, and in central and eastern Europe some five to ten years later in general. The target groups of these studies were invariably the general population and chief risk groups such as MSM (men who have sex with men), mostly in Scandinavia, or adolescents (especially in central and eastern Europe). Research findings are generally used for the planning and implementation of prevention measures.

In Bulgaria a UNDP-financed KABP study from 1995 was being evaluated at the time of writing the country report. According to this and other studies, condom sales increased tenfold from 1991 to 1999. The number of voluntary HIV tests is rising. Among CSW (commercial sex workers) the number of those who claim that they always or nearly always use condoms increased from 63.9% (1987) to 92.1% (1999). Expert analyses on adolescent sexual behaviour showed that in Bulgaria the average age for first-time pregnancies is well below the European average, that condom use is very low in this age group, that alcohol and drug abuse is very often combined with sexual contacts, and that adolescents frequently change partners. Information is available on the use of safer sex practices in the MSM group. Using condoms has already become standard practice for anal but not for oral sex. Drug users are very poorly informed of infection risks and protection measures. Around a third employ used injection materials.

From 1993 to 1995 Estonia conducted a study on sexual behaviour and corresponding knowledge of pupils aged 12 to 15. The results were rated as alarming. Evaluations showed that 20% of informants could not remember ever having been informed of HIV/AIDS in school. Around fifty per cent of adolescents quoted television as their main source of relevant information. In the context of another recent study, 336 teachers for health education claimed that the lack of uniform methods was a decisive obstacle to an effective transfer of knowledge at school.

In the context of the "Reproductive Health and Behaviour" study conducted jointly by the UNPD and the Latvian ministry of social affairs in 1997, 4,586 people aged 15 to 45 were interviewed on HIV/AIDS-related aspects. One of the striking findings of this study was that first sexual relations were comparatively late. For example, 70% of women claimed that their first sexual experience had been after their 18th birthday. In contrast, half of the men were younger than 18 when making their first sexual contacts. There is a great lack of knowledge on the modes of transmission of STDs. Around a third of informants claimed that insect stings or using public swimming pools were possible modes of transmission. One-fifth thought that shaking hands was a source of infection. 93% of condom users gave contraception as their reason. The rate of condom sales is not documented. In the "Public Survey of AIDS Issues", a UNAIDS-financed study, a selection of the general population were asked about their behaviour and attitudes. Although, according to the findings of this survey, 98% of the population know that HIV/AIDS is transmitted by sexual contacts, only 63% see condoms as an effective protection measure. The attitude towards HIV-positive persons must be rated as rather discriminatory. 75% of informants believe that infected persons should not work in medical institutions. 7% would like to bar patients completely from public institutions and places.

So far, KABP studies in Lithuania have mainly focused on adolescents as a main target group but also on health care staff. Studies on further risk groups are still ongoing or are being evaluated. Interviews of adolescents clearly showed that knowledge of the modes of transmission and protective measures is rather good but has hardly been put into practice yet. It is rated as alarming that in a survey of medical staff, 52% of interviewed doctors showed a lack of knowledge of HIV/AIDS aspects.

Since 1993 there have been several KABP studies in Poland. And there have been interviews with doctors (1997), nursing staff (1998) and social workers (1999) on their knowledge and attitudes regarding ethical and legal aspects of HIV/AIDS. Since 1996 affected persons have been interviewed at annual meetings on the emotional, social and economic effects of the disease and asked to evaluate the existing care system.

Studies performed in Romania on HIV/AIDS include the "Romanian Reproductive Health Survey" (1993), "Young Adult Reproductive Health Survey" (1996), "Survey in Bucharest on HIV/AIDS Knowledge" (1995), and qualitative "Research on Behavioural Determinants among Vulnerable Groups" (1999). A study that accompanied the "HIV/AIDS & Sex Information for Young People, Parents and Teachers" project in 1997 showed that teenagers are well informed of the modes of transmission. However, they are not so well informed of safer sex practices.

In Slovakia there have been regular surveys on sexual health and sexual risk behaviour since 1993. They showed a significant increase both of the condom use rate, the number of exchanged injection materials and the use of offered tests.

Although recognised as an essential basis for prevention work, Slovenia has conducted no comprehensive studies so far. However, questionnaire campaigns have been performed, although their results are not necessarily representative. In a study conducted in 1996 students were asked about their sexual experience, habits and knowledge of HIV/AIDS. Data on condom sales, issuance of injection materials to drug users or the use of offered tests are not systematically collected. Still, according to importers' claims, we can assume an increase of condom sales of approx. 850,000 a year before 1994 to 1,300,000 in 1998. In 1998 the NGO STIGMA, reported a 200% increase in the number of exchanged injection materials compared with 1997.

In the Czech Republic 2,003 people aged over 15 were interviewed on their sexual behaviour in 1998. A similar study was already performed in 1993 and allows for corresponding comparisons. There were no major changes in the age of first contact and the number of sex partners. In contrast, condom use behaviour has changed significantly. In 1998 62% of men and 54% of women claimed that they used this form of protection, compared with only 41% of men and 35% of women in 1993. Only 9% of CSW, down from 41% in 1993, did not use condoms. No data were collected on condom sales. Data on needle exchange programmes were only available from the state-run public health institutions, while NGO data are lacking. The number of persons who took anonymous tests rose from 661 in 1990 to 13,836 in 1997.

Initiated by the National Board of Health, KABP studies in Denmark have been conducted both on the general population and on HIV/AIDS risk groups nationwide. Until 1997 they were performed regularly every two years. According to these studies, the population is rather well-informed on HIV/AIDS. A rising number of people claim that they have modified their sexual behaviour for fear of an infection. 90% of informants showed acceptance and tolerance for those affected. In 1998 the number of gonorrhoea patients rose among MSM. No other information was provided on indirect indicators.

Under a WHO project, Finland investigated the experience, knowledge, attitudes, and sources of information regarding the sexual behaviour of adolescents aged 13 to 15. The investigation identified a high level of knowledge on HIV/AIDS, with the mass media taking a backseat as a source of information to personal contacts (medical service at schools, teachers). Another study focused on changes in sexual behaviour among the general population. This can be compared with studies from 1971 and 1992. One question concerned the influence of HIV/AIDS risks on personal behaviour. 2.8 % of women and 1.8% of men claimed that they had changed to a celibate lifestyle for fear of AIDS. For the same reason 5.5% of women and 8% of men had changed their sex practices. Moreover, there were studies on MSM and young adults. In Finland condom sales fell drastically within a year (from 1998 to 1999). The same trend could be observed in other northern European states. This could be due to the lower number of women of childbearing age but also to the reduction of sex education in schools caused by budget cutbacks. The number of performed HIV tests has been rather stable since 1987.

In Norway KABP studies have been regularly performed since 1987. Evaluations showed that sex habits and practices have hardly changed and that there is no direct relationship between knowledge and attitudes and risky sexual behaviour, which is still widespread. There are no reliable data on condom sales. Only the import figures of wholesalers, which were rather stable from 1985 to 1990 at around 9 to 10 million condoms a year, provide information. In view of study results, we can assume that information campaigns in school have a positive effect on the condom use rate of adolescents. Extensive outbreaks of hepatitis A, B and C within the IDU group since 1995 show that needle-sharing is still widespread. The fact that the number of chlamydia infections since 1990 is stable at 12,000 diagnosed cases a year indicates an unchanged sexual behaviour of under-25s. No exact data on the acceptance of offered anonymous tests are available.

In Sweden the first KABP study was conducted in 1986. Annual surveys up to 1989 complete this survey. Initiated by the National Institute of Public Health, similar studies followed from 1994 to 1997, where 4,000 people aged 16 to 44 were interviewed on their knowledge, attitudes and sexual behaviour. Later studies also showed a rather high level of knowledge on HIV/AIDS. A constant decline in the number of HIV-infected IDUs is seen as an indicator of achieved behaviour modification and thus as a success of effective prevention measures. However, over the past few years STDs such as chlamydia, gonorrhoea and genital herpes have been on the rise, which indicates unprotected sex practices.

In summary, the country reports from northern, central and eastern Europe show that in all states large efforts are made to examine the sexual behaviour, knowledge of HIV/AIDS and relevant behaviour modification by sociological studies, in order to evaluate the effect of prevention measures and to gain a sound basis for further targeted prevention strategies. Findings from northern Europe show a high level of knowledge among the Scandinavian population and behaviour modification towards safer sex and safer use over a long term. The latest findings such as lower condom sales and an increase of STDs would suggest a decline in behaviour modification, which has not been mirrored by the number of new HIV infections yet. In these countries discrimination against people with HIV and AIDS seems to be very low.

In many central and eastern European countries, but not so much in the Baltic states and Bulgaria, prevention campaigns have quite successfully changed behaviour without any downward trend so far, unlike in northern and western Europe. These countries show a rise in condom acceptance and particularly safer use among IDUs - the main risk group in most of the states. This seems to be the successful result of prevention measures for specific target groups such as IDUs, CSWs and adolescents, as some countries that see corresponding behaviour modification in these groups, also report major information deficits on the modes of HIV transmission in the general population. And anti-discrimination messages issued in all countries have not reached the population everywhere yet (e.g. in Latvia and Romania).

3.12 Perception of the system, current debates and likely policy changes
The surveys (ref. Section 2 Materials and Methods) conducted by the country collaborators have brought new updated insights from some of the main public and voluntary sectors representatives for some of the key issues related to HIV prevention policies:

- in relation to the changes in the general perception of the disease and the current debates on HIV prevention strategy,
- presently, what are the gaps or obstacles regarding HIV prevention policy and support of PLWAs and regarding the quality of counselling and access to treatment,
- in relation to the future, the most important HIV/AIDS prevention policies and the main challenges for the future HIV prevention policies,
- and examples of outstanding HIV prevention measures.

3.12.1 Western and Southern Europe

a) Changes in general perception

Normalisation of the disease: The disease is better known and less feared for different reasons: the panic of the eighties is over, the public awareness of a stabilised epidemic, a disease which can be mastered and is not fatal anymore, a life prolonged and a chronic "treatable" disease, a false perception that treatment has become more effective because of the multi-drugs therapy, less fear of contagion because HIV is no longer a terminal illness, more remote in the people's preoccupations scale than before and a relatively normal problem, some changes in the organisational structures (i.e. closing of the public prevention agencies in some countries) have also influenced the public opinion that the threat is over.

The normalisation of the disease has nevertheless an unknown impact on changes in risk behaviours.

Medicalisation of the disease: The focus of HIV/AIDS work has changed over the past few years, since the mid-nineties, from prevention to cure, therefore medicalising the disease.

Less media coverage: Either the social or political coverage of HIV/AIDS have decreased with the consequence of having less public interest than before. Some countries feel there is more interest on cure than prevention, while others say that attention towards AIDS in general, and not only towards its prevention, are decreasing. In Belgium, there is even an impression that the media focus on Africa is leading to a general feeling that the problem is shifted elsewhere, and as a consequence affects negatively the attention to prevention. The introduction of the new treatments have led to an excessive optimism of the press with the negative consequences of a false sense of security among people who are lowering their guard. The media reflects a mounting concern on poverty questions.

Mix reviews on campaigns: Prevention campaigns have covered HIV, AIDS, sexuality, sexual behaviours and led to higher awareness of HIV/AIDS, to improved knowledge of HIV transmission, to less discrimination and more solidarity in general. The UK signals that stigma may have staid the same than ten years ago, with the exception of the gay community.

However, despite these successes, campaigns have difficulties to address and impact on behaviours. As expressed in Portugal: *"People are informed, but not educated..."* AIDS is still often perceived as a problem of others with the risk taking behaviours reported both among the heterosexual population (e.g. the youth), and among vulnerable groups (e.g. IDUs). Several countries are indicating that prevention messages need to be renewed because the public is getting tired of what they hear or see, that often messages are not adapted to the vulnerable groups (e.g. migrants), and that the absence of communication with vulnerable groups is leading to living the disease in a silent and a culprit fashion. The question remains whether large campaigns have as a side effect the increase of indifference with the consequence of people speaking less about AIDS, as noticed in France in relation to the relative quiet phase which followed the large "Sidaction 96" campaign.

More tolerance and openness: PLWAs are more accepted, less discriminated against, and less marginalised than before, e.g. the known cause of the disease has led to less fear, or no fear of getting closer to a sick person anymore, for example. Countries are nevertheless ambiguous in relation to full tolerance and openness, and they report pockets of resistance. France notes for example that one finds *"either solidarity or indifference"*, and Greece, despite positive developments, note that the fear is still present as illustrated by a hostel for HIV/AIDS patients which never opened because of the public negative reaction in the town where located.

b) Current debates

Lack or low debates: Countries in general note and regret the lack or low debates in relation to HIV prevention in comparison to before, because of the normalisation and less media coverage just discussed. They are presently addressing multiple issues concurrently, some country specific. The Netherlands point to the challenges which most country face, i.e. to keep the general public informed and committed, and at the same time avoiding the stigmatisation of the PLWAs.

Prevention vs. care: The duality of prevention vs. care has propped up recently, instead of normal continuum of services. Care is the new emphasis, with the consequence that either the public sector or the populations are overlooking prevention. This is reflected in the following different views:

"The leitmotiv addresses what is the impact of new treatments on preventive behaviours... prevention is too often narrowed down to condoms use and nothing else... prevention strategies have not taken enough into consideration the people living in a situation of excluded." (France)

"To pursue sustainable behavioural changes and prevent the fatigue of "Safer Sex" are more difficult in the rise of HIV infection which, in turn, is not taken so seriously anymore due to the availability of medical therapies." (Germany)

"Need to conduct prevention work with a stronger evidence base and by the groups most affected themselves, with funding earmarked for the process." (UK)

Integration is a common trend found in all countries which occur at different levels and involve different aspects, as a consequence of a combination of different factors (e.g. scarcer resources, a search for a sustainable response, the development of new therapies). As examples, if countries like Germany or the Netherlands have detached part of their responsibilities from the public sector and/or funds to agencies, other countries are tackling new issues. France is presently reflecting whether prevention should be kept in the present specific structure or be encompassed in the global policy at the Government level. Belgium is searching presently how to improve the integration of HIV prevention in STD Control and health promotion. UK feels a stronger co-ordination between HIV prevention and treatment and care is needed because *"...they are largely conducted in separate universes."*

Youth, women, migrants or other vulnerable groups (e.g. IDUs, prison inmates etc.) are at the centre attention in almost all countries. Each country has its own priority vulnerable group based on epidemiological facts, with the following examples. Increasingly, the youth and women are reported as vulnerable groups, although countries do not wish to alarm the general population with such an identification. France notes the lack of targeted communication for women, homosexuals, drug users, migrants with the impact of HIV/AIDS increasing on women and migrants. In Portugal, prevention needs to focus on the youths, women, drug addicts, and prison inmates. Belgium notes the present lack of priority actions for the populations originating from Africa, particularly requesting asylum.

Countries are commonly attempting to answer which preventive strategies to use for these populations because as it stands presently, they are not reached sufficiently, and the problem is further compounded with the fact they lack access to health care in general.

Communication: Showing the disease has helped making it more common and better known, and has contributed to have the PLWAs be more accepted. Yet communication needs to address still: the existing pockets of resistance on negative attitudes leading to discrimination, more emphasis on the fact the risk still exists, the promotion of healthy life-styles accompanied by no morality judgements. Some of these concerns are best reflected in Italy by the fact that despite positive increased knowledge, there are still some people with an image of AIDS linked to transgression, to a terrible disease and death, and some social categories are affected by cultural stigma, in turn leading to distancing, if not discrimination, of PLWAs.

The question remains, why people are still not protecting themselves in a context of information. Reaching consensus on prevention strategies is a difficult issue which each country needs to address. In light of the present development and limitations in the field of prevention, questions arise still in some countries on the role of the State vs. the voluntary sector in national campaigns, and whether the focus in communication should be at the national vs. local level?

Full-scale risk reduction strategies and sustainability: Countries are searching for ways to tackle the development of risk reduction group specific strategies and to sustain those. France reports on the *"failure of prevention among homosexuals presently."* On the other hand, Portugal reports too much emphasis on risk groups to the detriment of the general population approach, including the neglect of the older generations.

The search for best approaches in the context of budget constraints is best reflected with the question raised in Ireland: *"Where to adopt a disease prevention or a sexual health promotion approach?"* or in Germany: *"HIV prevention is moving into a long term perspective but scarcer resources have made the work challenging and more difficult... Need for long term strategies: integration of HIV prevention in the pedagogical teaching in schools about sexuality, embedding HIV prevention in health promotion in general, and pursuing education campaigns that are not moralising and adapted to the different age groups and social classes, and their languages (e.g. migrants)".*

Various country specific issues: Many country specific debates are arising, particularly in light of the testing, or new therapies, for example: to improve the specific definition of people eligible to HIV testing, to clarify the advantages and disadvantages of the "HIV home tests", to improve therapies for better compliance, to inform correctly (passing the message without impacting negatively on prevention efforts) about the "treatments of tomorrow" or of the early post-exposure prophylaxis. Some countries need to address in parallel the legal gaps, for example, in France, the law of 1970 on drugs need to be changed so that people can speak openly about drugs.

c) Gaps in HIV prevention and support for PLWAs

The perceptions differ between the public partners who appear to be more content or satisfied of HIV prevention and support, and the partners from the private sector who are dissatisfied and thriving for improvements and are playing the role of the movers.

Insufficient response to vulnerable groups: Countries commonly report the lack of addressing sufficiently and adequately these groups. The following remarks illustrate some of the points:

> *"Insufficient sensitisation of the general public, particularly the youth".* (Belgium)

> *"For the vulnerable populations, not enough consideration of their lives as a whole to avoid dichotomy between prevention speeches and personal life style".* (France)

> *"The cultural variety (language, religious, sexuality) of the vulnerable groups is not enough taken into consideration in the prevention measures... The same is true for the youth who are not a homogeneous group but composed of a variety of subcultures, and do not use the services for institutional or psychological barriers".* (Germany)

> *"Prostitutes' clients negotiate unprotected sexual intercourse by offering more money...Occasional interventions only among IDUs..."* (Italy)

> *"Lack of prevention campaigns directed specifically to youth and to IDUs".* (Spain)

" Lack of systemic and properly structured programme of sexual and affective education for youths... Lack of participation of target group representatives in the definition of preventive strategies... Lack of prison activities (app. 11% of inmates HIV positive) and Hep. C..." (Portugal)

"The sexual health needs of People Living With HIV have been ignored... and need to address the prevention needs of people living with HIV because secondary infections are demonstrably harmful in terms of drug regimes". (UK)

Quality and specificity of messages: Countries report an insufficient quality and specificity of messages for the various vulnerable groups. The difficulty in modifying the types of risk behaviours that facilitate HIV transmission (neglected use of condoms, shared use of needles) are well known.

In France, the public sector does not know how to address sero-positive people because they are afraid of stigmatising them. The communication on the living of sero-positive situation is insufficient.

Iceland notes the need for more peer education, including from HIV infected people.

Spain acknowledges the need for the raising awareness of the population at large.

Failures regarding campaigns and messages can be of a different nature, as reported by Portugal. There is a fear of shock inducing campaigns, abusively referring to youth sexuality and negative aspects of disease. Messages presently selected have a political slant instead of a technical one. There exists a lack of information on the early detection of HIV positive status. Some campaigns (either public or NGOs) are ineffective or even fail by missing their target groups. There are no campaigns for HIV positive persons. AIDS patients do not feel included in prevention campaigns.

Issues related to the lack of political commitment in prevention, prevention policy and supportive structures, and decreasing resources: Countries report a combination of factors which are detrimental to HIV prevention policies and their implementation.

Belgium reports on the insufficient political commitment in prevention, the absence of the decision-makers' public health perspectives, and of the co-ordination between those, and the insufficient decentralisation and close-by support.

In France, representatives from the Governments state that the present policy of prevention is very attentive to different targets, that there are no political obstacles to set up a prevention programme, as reflected with the fact that one can work with the most stigmatised group in full liberty. But those from the voluntary sector, on the other hand, finds that "*the obstacles to prevention is that prevention policy is complicated.*"

In Germany, the decrease in resources impact directly on the counselling, care and nursing services which in turn exacerbates the lack of solidarity.

In Ireland, safer environments, such as needles to be allowed in hostels, is needed.

In Italy, there is an increase in attention to HIV/AIDS, but a decrease in attention to STD.

Portugal notes the deficient articulation between private and public entities, and the need to restructure support policies for specific target groups (e.g. migrants) taking into account their socio-economic problems and difficulties in accessing information and health care. The country suffers from chronic backwardness in the health system with the lack of adequate articulation between primary and secondary care. This in turn impedes well-articulated multi-annual, periodically assessed programmes. The system needs decentralisation.

Social and informational support for PLWAs: Substantial efforts have been made in this area by the different countries, and yet some gaps persist.

In Belgium, one still finds an important continuous discrimination and social exclusion combined with the lack of solidarity to PLWAs. Budgets for home-care are insufficient.

France signals false believes still which must be combated, and an ill-adapted system today for PLWAs with a reinsertion problem for them at the work place. They need a policy which works for PLWAs and that is implemented through the associations with the support of the public sector.

Germany and Ireland signal the need to improve the social support because of the larger number of PLWAs due to the effectiveness of treatments. Ireland also underlines new needs of social support, and resolving issues of homelessness for positive children reaching adolescence and the age of sexual relationship. These children need to improve their skills to re-enter into the labour market.

Portugal reports on a number of gaps related to: home care networks providing medical and psychological support, human and technical resources in the district hospitals (central hospitals only for the PLWAs), institutions providing food, lodging, and follow-up, institutions for terminally-ill patients without family support, precise and adequate information to direct to those who can support them psychologically.

d) Gaps in counselling and access to treatment

Lack of qualified health care personnel in counselling, or bad attitudes, or lack of confidentiality: Countries report multiple, and sometimes serious deficiencies in this area. Even the countries which appeared to be better off in the past have a growing gap again due to the decrease of financial support (e.g. Germany). A frequent complaint is the lack of competence or of support found among the General Practitioners. In the UK the nature of the problem lies in *"largely structural"* obstacles and the way the *"services are configured"*. The various points brought up in France illustrate the vast array and depth of the difficulties:

> *"'Medical Doctors' resistance to speak about risks and sexuality with the people, except in the specialised centres... A real culture of counselling does not exist in France....Counselling does not have a global approach to people... does not exist for all, the most precarious people do not have access. Not enough trained people... Counselling pre- and post-test must be systematised... For the African community living in France, counselling needs to be adapted. Need to create in France a school for counselling."* (France)

Attitudinal problems are reported: *"Little emphatic attitude of some care-takers".* (Belgium)

Germany is suffering from a decrease of involvement of counselling offices. The consequence is that many experienced counsellors are leaving the field with the effect of a neglect of psycho-social care. General Practitioners are not at ease with the subject. Counsellors need more qualifications. Services need to be more anonymous, and the language barrier has to be overcome.

Greece has an inadequate counselling due to staff shortage, to doctors' incapacity to provide counselling, and only two hospitals which provide counselling with only one before the test as well.

An HIV positive woman reports in Ireland that the *"medical profession is dealing with bodies instead of people as a whole."* There is unequal access to counselling with the exception of an improved access for the two main cities. PLWAs express reservations using services in their locality because of the fear that confidentiality is breached.

Italy identifies the need for different kinds and levels of educators (General Practitioners, social workers, and employee representatives).

In Spain, the public sector notes an improvement of the public care workers in counselling, while the NGOs note in contrast the lack of qualified health care personnel to give counselling and the lack of time to dedicate to the care of PLWAs.

Heavy costs of treatments or of opportunistic infections are reported by all countries both for the public sector and the patients. Even though the anti-retroviral therapies are free of charge, the patients must also bear the cost for treating opportunistic infections and the secondary effects of the multi-drug therapies (Portugal).

Unequal accessibility to treatments for rural populations, or for specific target groups are reported by several countries.

In Belgium, there is poor knowledge of support and care references by some patients, particularly for the illegal residents.

In France, despite the accessibility for all to counselling and treatment, the social level determines access to care for all the diseases. Lodging for the most precarious is a problem, despite two months stay at the hospital because they do not have any other places than the street to live, whereas it would be cheaper on the long run to pay for lodging.

In Germany, the counselling services are identified as being too middle class or homosexuals oriented. Care-takers offices, in particular ambulatory nursing due to the lack of nursing insurance reimbursements, have closed. In-patients mental or psychiatric services are insufficient. Geographical access to special clinics is difficult because of long journeys. Too little institutions offer therapies for specific target groups.

Ircland suffers form unequal access to treatments beyond the good access for the two main cities. There is a need to tailor information for illiterates, to involve counsellors and disseminate information in a targeted fashion in prisons.

Italy needs to increase the accessibility to services for PLWAs in the rural provinces.

Portugal reports on the inadequacy of hospital care for the drug addiction problem.

e) Future prevention policies

Prevention policy and sustainability: The importance of having at least a policy of prevention and to sustain activities in prevention are some of the most common concerns of the countries for the future. Policies need to be better tailored for specific groups (e.g. IDUs on the streets, or in prisons). The public sector needs to be more involved hence to show more commitment in special sectors which need urgent attention (needle exchange programmes, rooms for safer injections, heroin maintenance programme, distribution of needles in prison). A few countries acknowledge the difficulty to sustain prevention on the long term, and emphasise therefore the need to speed up the vaccine development to the benefit not just of the developing world but of all countries.

Vulnerable groups and strategies: The recent newly developed strategies proven to be effective need to be strengthened. On one hand the growing number of People Living With HIV/AIDS calls for improved responses for this population, for example: the threshold of services for PLWAs needs to be lowered, accessibility of new diagnosed HIV infected to trained social workers, generalised and well-organised good treatments, improved AIDS reference centres to carry out counselling and support of PLWAs and meeting their new requirements. On the other hand, prevention strategies need to address the needs of the vulnerable groups better, for example, taking care of people in prisons, or improved accessibility to clean syringes for IDUs.

The following countries report distinct strengths and weaknesses, because of different factors, such as the programmes maturity, present perceptions and needs to mention a few.

France notes the importance of continuing the "safer sex" messages without moralising. Innovative and participatory methods using peer involvement and peer group education are proven to be effective, as well as the increased self-empowerment and assertiveness, and the involvement of each vulnerable group in the concept design and interventions.

Germany sees the legal measures as a major barrier for asylum seekers to access any services, in particular HIV/AIDS. Migrants lack access to health services.

Italy wishes to pursue massive, continuous campaigns directed to different target groups for the use of condoms linked not only to AIDS but to STDs in general.

Portugal will strengthen prevention activities and policies to match the target groups' needs (drugs addicts in social context, heterosexuals and diversity of behaviours, customs and habits, new-borns of infected mothers). The country wishes to shift the emphasis on policies erasing the notion of risk for particular groups to emphasise the risk in the whole community.

Structural matters such as integration, health care reforms, co-ordination, co-operation, task forces: HIV prevention policies and their successful implementation do not fall into a vacuum, but are linked to different matters related to structures and systems. Countries report the need to improve the integration of HIV/AIDS prevention into general prevention activities. HIV has to be more embedded in the "Sexual Health" concept. A shift from vertical to more horizontal and community approaches is commonly acknowledged. Care and support should be integrated with prevention. To avoid HIV prevention occurring in a parallel system, tying resources not integrated into the current health promotion measures. Various other supportive developments are proposed such as an improved co-ordination between different sectors (schools, prisons...) in prevention, the co-operation with new partners (e.g. migrants' representatives or associations), the establishment of a Task Force on Discrimination, National Committees with stronger roles in co-ordination and monitoring.

Scarce resources and competition: Countries are commonly grasping the challenge and question of how to tackle the issue of competing for scarce resources and prioritise interventions at the local level between current People Living With HIV/AIDS, and other emerging vulnerable groups.

f) Main challenges for future policies

To keep HIV/AIDS as a relevant and important theme among the general population, and the politicians, all confronted with the normalisation of the disease, is a main challenge for all countries, particularly with the new treatment options which have developed for the past four or five years.

These common issues to the countries can best be summarised with Ireland expressing the need *"to keep the issue alive... to avoid complacency"* , and Germany *"keeping the political support and interest, as well as the momentum..."*

Policy priorities and choices: Countries have gained knowledge of assessing their situations which helps them to predict changes and apply timely measures. The challenge lies in defined policies, centred around clear choices when countries are torn presently between multiple choices, and to make funds for prevention available.

France acknowledges the lack of experts in prevention. Spain supports an appeal to the public's sense of solidarity and justice to continue to support the free access to treatments and health care. Countries feel a common solidarity and need to tackle a global epidemic to co-operate with the societies in transition from central and Eastern European more deprived countries. The idea of setting up a special fund for those was even highlighted by Portugal.

Prevention integration and level of response: Countries feel commonly the need to integrate prevention in a more global context, and decentralise information to the regions and prefectures, and to redefine practice on a multidisciplinary level.

Yet as reported by France the challenge lies in *" how to overcome now the fall of the alliance between patients, professionals and social actors which had catalysed up to now the prevention activities, and will prevention survive through this?"*

Accessibility to prevention for vulnerable groups (youth, women and the marginalised): All countries are aware of new emerging and changing primary vulnerable groups who are difficult to reach. Those are far from being homogeneous, for example: women as a group; school students and pre-teenagers; young homosexuals, MSM who not identify themselves as gay, and lesbians; migrants, clandestine people, asylum seekers and prostitute migrants; couples with one of the partner from high prevalence HIV countries (Pattern II countries); young women, young teenage girls infected with HIV through drug use in the context of third generation of unemployment (specific to Ireland); poorer social classes, unemployed, and illiterates.

The diversity of these vulnerable groups calls for different prevention policies and approaches, adapting specific messages with campaigns or materials tailored to them, showing without dramatising or stigmatising, showing more respect of women's' rights and some of the marginalised groups.

Improved methods, and relevant and effective tools: As an already known cornerstone of successful prevention, there is a need for improved participatory interventions, and of official entities recognising the communities as partners. Tools need to be developed which enable people to find their own choices of prevention. The gap between the experts' risk assessment and the public to reach an agreement on priorities to reduce risk should be bridged.

The methods of communication need to be adapted to each community. Safer sex messages need to be updated and relevant to the present situation, and be specific to vulnerable groups. Wider access to condoms and more forceful information on the use of condoms are essential prevention methods which need to be widely promoted too.

Country specific needs and priorities are different. In France, among others, IDUs need to adapt messages to the French users and their particularities (e.g. injecting crack instead of smoking in England). Portugal focuses, among others, in the improvement of education measures to combat Tuberculosis.

The offering of special services (e.g. women with HIV who wish to have a child, sperm lavage, involvement of self-determination of PLWAs in order to increase their rights), and their accessibility to those in needs should be further strengthened.

A greater collaboration between organisations in and between sectors will facilitate this process further. Create multidisciplinary teams to improve the effectiveness of primary prevention information.

Portugal reflects much of the gap existing in the countries still to implement effective and adequate prevention measures. There is still a *"lack of valid indicators to measure prevention... and a need for improved knowledge of epidemiological and behavioural situation to tailor effective and adequate prevention measures..."*

3.12.2 Northern, Central and Eastern Europe

a) Changes in general perception

Like the western European states, the Scandinavian countries explain the changed perception of HIV/AIDS with the fact that certain procedures and organisational processes have become routine and that AIDS has become less "dramatic" since the introduction of HAART therapy.

A better understanding of the problem - due to the now adequate level of knowledge - has also led to this normalisation and demystification. The modes of transmission, corresponding protective measures, relevant terminology and, not least, knowledge of the difference between HIV infection and AIDS have made the disease seem much less alarming.

In the former socialist states this new attitude to HIV/AIDS is only a further indication of the revolutionary changes these countries have been undergoing for the last ten years. The reasons for a changed attitude to AIDS are definitely more objective media coverage and a more liberal view of the affected risk groups (e.g. MSM, CSW, IDUs),

Public appearances of people with HIV and AIDS have given the disease a "face" (Finland).

During or as a result of major campaigns there were more debates on AIDS-related moral, legal and lifestyle issues (Slovakia, Poland).

b) Current debates

The Scandinavian countries have reported a stagnation of debates on various levels due to normalisation.

"The most striking element (of the current debate) is the absence of debates regarding HIV prevention strategies." (Denmark)

"The debate has come to a halt. There is an absence of debate on which target groups it is most important to reach." (Sweden)

"Infection abroad, persons travelling abroad, immigrants from high endemic areas and continued new infection among homosexual men." (Sweden)

"It is still not clear whether a move should be made from major campaigns to information based more on the individual and attempts to influence habits based on studies of individuals' risk-taking and risk assessment." *(Sweden)*

Despite the implementation of numerous prevention measures and increase of knowledge on modes of transmission and protective measures, as demonstrated by KABP studies, expected changes in the sexual behaviour of certain target groups did not occur In central and eastern Europe. Therefore the question of the effectiveness and search for new forms of prevention is decisive for the debate of current strategies.

"The most prominent topic of current debates on AIDS prevention is the question of its efficiency, that is the possibility to change and influence risky sexual behaviour." *(Czech Republic)*

In eastern European countries, which witnessed a dramatic increase in the number of IDUs and CSWs, the resulting adjustment of prevention strategies is the main topic of current debates.

In Slovakia the legalisation of commercial sex work is being discussed, although, from Slovakia's point of view, this practice rather shows counterproductive effects on an international level.

c) Gaps in HIV/AIDS prevention and support for PLWAs

In many central and eastern European countries, prejudices and a lack of understanding for the worst affected risk groups such as IDUs and CSWs lead to their stigmatisation and isolation. The fact that prostitution and drug abuse are illegal in Lithuania, for example, makes it much harder to approach these risk groups.

"Prostitution and drug addiction in Lithuania are illegal and prevention towards this subgroups is very difficult and some preventive measures do not reach the target group and is therefore not effective." *(Lithuania)*

"Work with target groups is not very popular and is often not included in the HIV/AIDS prevention work. Some do not find any achievements in the work done during the past few years. Projects which address the population as a whole are accepted." (Estonia)

"The stigmatisation of these people by the general population can be considered as a potential problem. For example a Gypsy woman, addicted to drugs and earning an income by prostitution, is the subject of multiple discrimination from many members of the general population." (Czech Republic)

Discriminating attitudes, even on the part of responsible actors at the state level, are the reason for the partial lack of interest and financial aid for measures and projects dedicated to these target groups.

"One of the most important issues mentioned was activities with high risk groups, however officials stated that one of the biggest problems is not being able to reach these groups, NGOs stated the biggest problem being a lack of supporting attitudes among officials. Discriminating attitudes are mentioned as being the largest obstacles for the attraction of financial aid and implementing various projects within the country." (Latvia)

Generally, the main responsibility for work with and for the above-mentioned risk groups has been assigned to the NGOs, who constantly face the problem of inadequate or limited financing themselves.

The differing approaches of involved actors often make it difficult to find a common basis for the most comprehensive support. While doctors concentrate on the problem of finding the most effective therapy, NGOs focus on adequate methods of social and economic support (Bulgaria).

The normalisation of AIDS and reduction of public funding are obstacles to good and effective prevention work (Sweden).

The lack of funds is the reason why Slovakia cannot regularly monitor the effectiveness of HAART therapy.

The fact that PLWAs are only treated in clinics for communicable diseases, is rated as further proof of discrimination in the Slovakian report. Instead, the actual symptoms should be treated in the corresponding wards.

Of course, Finland's lack of an official HIV/AIDS strategy also generates poorly co-ordinated public prevention work, of which NGOs have to bear the brunt.

d) Gaps in counselling and access to treatment

While the northern European states do not see securing funds for therapy measures and counselling offers as a key problem, virtually all eastern European countries mention the constant battle for financial resources as a central task for ensuring these services.

Often the budget provided for AIDS therapy does not cover actual needs (Romania).

Uncertainties in financing terms are another frequent problem. In the Czech Republic costs caused by STDs are borne by the health insurance system. This also goes for uninsured persons. In the case of HIV/AIDS the national AIDS programme covers these expenses.

In view of the general economic crisis, the fact that treatment and medication are free is seen as an achievement, albeit with an uncertain future (Latvia).

In Slovakia guidelines for HAART therapy should be changed, so that it is also fully covered by health insurance for ambulatory patients.

Training measures are urgently needed for health service staff due to lacking experience and motivation (Latvia, Romania).

Slovakia does not have enough qualified teachers, sociologists, psychologists and doctors for prevention work with adolescents.

The range of counselling offers differs in quality terms in cities and rural areas. There is a strong urban/rural divide in counselling quality:

> *"It is said that there should be as good counselling and treatment opportunities in the countryside as there are in the big cities. One respondent says that a small number of those infected do not dare to seek medical care for fear of confidentiality." (Sweden)*

"Counselling is provided by few professionals in the central public health or research institutions and infectious clinics." (Slovakia)

Migrants who do not speak the language, often cannot benefit from counselling offers. (Sweden)

e) Future prevention policies

Many reports point out the necessity of a re-orientation of intervention measures, i.e. fewer measures for the public at large and more specific measures tailored to individual risk groups (Bulgaria, Romania, Slovakia, Slovenia).

"The most important lines for preventative policies in the next few years is the development of purposeful preventive educational measures for each risk group separately, planned and developed beforehand with co-ordinated work of various organisations." (Latvia)

Changing or adapting legal regulations (e.g. homosexual partnerships, access to injection materials) is a further goal of future prevention measures (Bulgaria).

Lithuania still has to create a legal framework for HIV/AIDS prevention policies.

The Czech Republic and Sweden point out the importance of pursuing empowerment strategies, i.e. enabling the individual to take personal responsibility for his or her own health.

"Empowerment and participation are prerequisites for being able to carry out preventive work successfully." (Sweden)

"Helping HIV positive persons in their very difficult life situation to become secure, strong and responsible people, who do not to be afraid of invention by authorities and compulsion." (Sweden)

While Slovenia does not expect to deviate from the prevention policies specified in its national programme in the near future, Slovakia sees securing financial resources for HAART therapy and establishing open sex education without ideological prejudices as new tasks for the next few years.

f) Main challenges for future prevention policies

Improving and intensifying co-operation between all involved experts, institutions and organisations is seen as a key aspect of future HIV/AIDS policy. In some countries, like Romania, there has to be a balancing of interests between public organisations and NGOs, in order to avoid further conflicts.

> *"The greatest policy challenge appears to be the cross-sector collaboration: the need to incorporate and bring closer to the HIV/AIDS problems experts and representatives from widest circles of institutions and organisations including Ministries, NGOs, businesses and the media."*
> *(Bulgaria)*

HIV/AIDS is often wrongly viewed as an illness that is "under control". Therefore the struggle to maintain promised public and financial assistance is another key factor of activities on a political level (Czech Republic, Romania).

According to the report, Slovakia lacks tolerance and understanding for the marginal population groups that are most vulnerable to HIV/AIDS. Greater efforts in this direction are to increase their acceptance.

More studies are essential to provide data confirming the necessary forecasts for the planning of measures (Slovakia)

In Slovenia strengthening NGOs and self-help groups takes even greater priority than efforts of state institutions.

Better management is to help avoid the misallocation of resources in future. (Sweden)

3.13 Examples of good practices in Europe

Following a critical review of the various dimensions of HIV prevention policies (3.1 to 3.12) in Europe, the countries have experienced many outstanding measures, or "good projects" or "great interventions", labelled in the present summary report "Best Practices", which were identified as a special question by the key informants of each country, in addition to the country collaborators' own sources.

Informants reported many best practices, on a small or large scale, in relation to HIV prevention and care or treatment. The limitations of the findings are that those, as specified in France, are biased towards reporting on his or her own organisations. This indicates also that best practices are not so well known, even among experts in the field, although many experiences would gain to be widely disseminated within a country, and the European community by and large.

The following best practices are not an exhaustive listing reported by all countries, but provide mere examples of the originality and wide spectrum of those. They merit further documentation and promotion in the future.

3.13.1 Western and Southern Europe

Information, education and communication

- Insertion of a condom in mass distribution weekly magazine, sponsored by the country's top condom manufacturer (Belgium)
- Distribution of various publications to the two main communities on each World AIDS Day, with one of them receiving 200,000 copies of a free newspaper with leaflets designed by organisations working with vulnerable groups (young people, Africans, homo and bi-sexuals, IDUs, etc.) (Belgium)
- National Summer mass campaign of 1995 by public authorities focusing on risk situations dealing with topics such as homo and bi-sexuality and drug use with an impact on the general population, including young people, 15 to 25 years old (France)
- Campaigns for the risks reduction among drug users getting involved and assuming responsibilities with a significant drop in HIV incidence (France)
- The Zone Afrique Centrale (ZAC) project by Afrique village NGO to develop and implement health education activities, and HIV/STD prevention campaigns among Central Africans living in France (France)
- The prevention campaigns on the community radio local stations for the Muslim community during Ramadan by Arcat-sida (France)
- The "3000 scenarios against the virus" short prevention films made by the CRIPS (France)
- The fast product control scheme for socially acceptable drug users at rave parties by ASUD (France)
- The posters and stickers national "*mach's mit*" campaigns to normalise the use of the condoms in the general and some vulnerable populations by the Federal Centre for Health Education, AIDS Programme, and recent large

- participation and enthusiastic response of a public contribution to design the campaign via the internet (Germany)
- The local initiative on prostitution and cross-border groups, youth and AIDS in Hamburg, and the German-Czech AIDS project "Jana" (Germany)
- All tourist and rural areas visited since 1995 by the KEEL information mobile unit for prevention, and information of high school students based on participatory techniques, students' mobilisation, peer education, trained school teachers, development of self-made audio-visual materials, and the support of psychologists mainly (Greece)
- Initiatives addressed to homosexuals with special information materials for men and women, and to sex workers, particularly foreigners, with information pamphlets distributed to their work places (Greece)
- The AIDS and Mobility project related to immigrants, e.g. trained teacher from Albania for the prevention aspects (Greece)
- The Winter 1998-1999 national campaign stressing the value of using condoms to prevent STDs targeting young people via newspapers, cinemas, bus stations, radio stations provoking a boost in visits to STD clinics, and considerable debate in the community (Iceland)
- The sexual health promotion approach in schools by the Alliance Centre for Sexual Health designed on responding to the participants' needs with an art based initiative and a peer education approach with the production of a sexual health promotion video and a peer led help-line (Ireland)
- The numerous initiatives (Sauna Project, Waterford area partnership project, Eastern Health Board involvement...) by the Gay HIV Strategies developing a partnership approach to target gay men for HIV prevention (Ireland)
- The development of a community response to drug use through the Ballymun Youth Action Project (YAP) through community action organisation and participation (Ireland)
- Changes in national information and education campaigns from technical/ guiding approach with hints of morality, to more persuasive campaigns, and more targeted to vulnerable groups, i.e. the mini television series for people to be self-conscious and assertive in the fall of HIV/AIDS interests, or for the youth the "AIDS – We intend to beat it" campaign, or for pregnant women to undergo the HIV test (Italy)
- The AIDS/Citizenship ("SIDANIA") Project: a travelling exhibition to schools and youth associations to inform the youth in a playful, pedagogical and interactive manner in order to erase taboos and convey correct concept on AIDS, while approaching sexuality, reproduction and the use of condoms in a broad-minded way (Portugal)

- Nation-wide programme of "AIDS Prevention in Schools" for 11-14 years old (Portugal)
- The "School for AIDS, Health and Coexistence" by the NGO FASE has been notable for its imagination and slant (Spain)
- The national 1998 safe sex campaign by the STD Foundation assisted by a creative team with a focus first on STDs, and second on improving the determinants of safe sex behaviour using a multimedia campaign (The Netherlands)
- The adaptation of the successful Scottish "trainerspack" for the "HIV/AIDS Standardised Training and School Materials" project which developed a standardised packed for HIV/AIDS training and schooling for health care and workers in home care, social work and drug abuse counselling (The Netherlands)
- The Philippine sailors project in Rotterdam where the prevention workers and the sex workers visited the ships... the holiday campaign for the youth who raised their consciousness about risks and condoms... education programmes in a multicultural environment... the "negotiated safety" campaign in which condom use was differentiated... the AFAPAC project for and by the African community living in the country (The Netherlands)

Access to services and counselling

- Establishment of anonymous and free screening centres also offering counselling services in Brussels and Liège since the late eighties (Belgium)
- Participation of the national pharmacists' participation, particularly in the "hottest" districts of the capital, to the programme providing low-cost injection materials, establishment of a few syringe exchange counters, sensitisation campaigns by former users, relaxation of rules for the sale of syringes (Belgium)
- The needle exchange pilot programme in prisons in Lower Saxony (Germany)
- The Province of Milan first prevention project among IDUs to encourage the use of syringe-exchange machines installed by the municipal administration, to facilitate the access to social services, and to provide a telephone counselling service on AIDS and related topic (Italy)
- The "Say no to a second-hand syringe" Programme which is a nation-wide project, supported by the National AIDS Control Programme (NACP) and mediates partnership between the ministry of health and the National Pharmacies Association to prevent HIV infection among IDUs in which 80%

of the national pharmacies participate, and the participation to the "Syringe Exchange Programmes in Southern European Countries" (Portugal)

- The opening of voluntary, confidential and anonymous HIV testing centres (Portugal)
- The pharmacist exchange needle programme (Spain)

On-going training and information of health professionals

- Monthly publication of information (2-4 pages) for General Practitioners in a bi-weekly newspaper, scientific information, updates on epidemiological data or on behaviour patterns, physicians' accounts (Belgium)

Treatment and care

- Concept of systematic prophylaxis after a recent sexual risk or a recent intravenous injection rejected by experts to avoid negative repercussions on primary prevention, and avoid the lack of compliance among low motivated patients. But for occupational conditions, including industrial medicine, systematic prophylaxis is applied (Belgium)
- Early prophylaxis in the case of accidental exposure, e.g. torn condom, contaminated syringe or accidental occupational exposure, as a true innovation (France)
- The Villa Glori home care project for men and women under difficult economic and family conditions; managed by Caritas Diocesana in Rome which has been used as model for other groups who have concentrated either on care, or on prevention (Italy)
- The newly co-funded by the NACP construction of the hospital-based day care centres with several advantages: to offer more personal services to patients seen by the same medical team, to feel safer and more responsible towards the hospital services, to decentralise and increase the accessibility to services, to avoid long costly stay and decrease the consequent negative psychological impact (Portugal)
- The recent agreement between the NACP and the Lisbon Santa Casa da Misericórdia for home support and residential shelters (Portugal)
- The HIV/AIDS home care programme of the Catalan NGO Actua (Spain)

Access to information

- 7 AIDS Reference Centres which provide answers to the physicians' or organisations' technical inquiries (Belgium)
- Home care and co-ordination of therapeutic housing (France)
- The offer of an overnight stay for 10 Fr. by the programme for drug users and the syringe exchange shops which give clients the chance to have a bath and consult a physician (France)
- All patients at the St James' Hospital Social Work Services are allocated a social worker or counsellor to discuss secondary prevention among the HIV positive persons on a one to one basis (Ireland)
- Day care services offered at the Open Heart House in Dublin for people living with HIV to provide support in taking control of their lives and overcoming isolation (Ireland)

Legal aspects

- Legalisation of resident status for any person suffering from HIV infection for full access to social security services facilitating in turn their access to treatment and care (France)

Support structures

- The National AIDS Strategy Committee is seen as a model for policy development and as a forum for developing consensus priorities allowing to nurture best practices (Ireland)

3.13.2 Northern, Central and Eastern Europe

Prevention: Information and communication

- The "Health in Schools" programme, launched in 1992-3, is part of a European network that aims to establish health education in schools. It is supported by the EU and WHO. A national network of schools that teach health promotion was established and later managed by an NGO. In 1999 40 schools and nursery schools were part of the network (Bulgaria).
- "Youth Health Centres" have an important task in the prevention of STDs and HIV/AIDS. This initiative started in 1998 and is to be expanded in future prevention programmes. Sexual health of adolescents and their knowledge of

STD and HIV-related contraception measures play a major role in the public health system (Lithuania).

- "Teenagers to Teenagers about AIDS" is a highly effective prevention measure where adolescents teach other adolescents about AIDS. For young people the "Europe against AIDS" summer camp is the most attractive and outstanding prevention campaign (Lithuania).
- Three "peer training programmes" were conducted by the National Committee on HIV/AIDS Prevention together with the National Reference Centre for HIV/AIDS Prevention, UNAIDS Focal Point, local health and social education institutions in various regions (Slovakia).
- The "I HAVE GOT AIDS" campaign was initiated and conducted by sociologists of the Dept. of Research on Social and Biological Communication, Slovak Academy of Sciences (Slovakia).
- Sex and human relations as part of the school curriculum, using improved teaching methods for this subject (Sweden).
- Distribution of so-called "Interrail bags" (filled with info material) to young people (Sweden).
- The Internet as a new prevention medium. RFSL's site has over 10,000 visitors a day (Sweden).
- Lessons and information events on HIV/STDs in schools and youth centres (Sweden).
- The "Stop AIDS Marathon" project, which aims to provide information and concentrates above all on individual government districts and not, like its predecessors, on the capital of Tallinn. Specialists work locally with target groups (Estonia).
- "Women in the age of AIDS": a project conducted in close co-operation with public broadcasting stations. The topic of HIV/AIDS was increasingly integrated in programmes specially targeted at women (Poland).
- "Safe Vacation" – information material to make school children and students aware of the topic; lots of copies were issued in tie-in lessons and during the holidays on the most heavily frequented train and bus routes (Poland)
- Publication of Sixteen magazine with a condom inserted in each issue (Finland).

Access to prevention offerings and counselling

- The "Spiral Project" instructs prostitutes on contraception methods (Sweden).
- Support measures for families affected by HIV (Sweden).

- The Stop AIDS Campaign in Denmark features a buddy service, with around 30 voluntary helpers visiting AIDS patients and lending them a helping hand (Denmark).
- The Finnish Slot Machine Association finances a project that offers home care as an alternative to in-patient hospital care for a term of three years (1993-19996) (Finland).
- Slovenia likewise has a network of around 700 district nurses who offer home care.
- In Denmark patient groups meet every month in larger hospitals nationwide and discuss the situation in the respective ward with medical staff and social workers.
- Latvia's State Infection Centre successfully offers so-called post-test counselling. In the case of a positive test result, it provides counselling and support, where needed, during a one-week stay (Latvia).
- The "Lighthouse" project – a self-help programme organised by the Czech AIDS support organisation (Czech Republic).
- In 1999 the Contact Centre for People with HIV in Norway added a hospice to its day-care centre, supported by funds of the city mission and the city of Oslo (Norway).
- The "Gaflon" project - anonymous telephone counselling for homosexuals (Slovenia).
- A nationwide 24-hour phone hotline, where doctors and psychologists offer advice (Poland).

Training and information for staff in the health sector

- The Phare LIEN Programme at Bucharest's Victor Babes Hospital is a training programme for employees, voluntary NGO staff and affected parents that is to give infected children a better quality of life and longer life expectancy. (Romania).
- In Sweden some clinics for infectious diseases have specially trained nurses, who can manage the organisation of home care offerings, where necessary. They liaise with local nursing staff, prepare them, where needed, for special requirements, and can be contacted at any time, thus creating a direct link with the clinic.

Risk minimisation

- The "Busing" project in Oslo. A bus calls at IDU hang-outs, distributes clean needles and condoms free of charge and offers counselling. The measure was evaluated in 1998 and rated as beneficial and cost-effective (Norway).

Access to information on treatment

- On the introduction of tri-therapy the ministry of health initiated a broad-based, popular information campaign, which was able to reach hitherto unco-operative patients. (Bulgaria).
- "Positive Outlook" is a self-help project organised by and for PLWAs and their relatives. (Estonia).

Legal regulations

- A positive AIDS test is expressly no reason to refuse an entry permit (Estonia, Czech Republic).
- Anti-discrimination laws are in force. The discrimination of homosexuals has been an offence since 1995 (Finland).
- Homosexual partnerships can be officially registered (Norway).
- The Communicable Diseases Act with its regulations and guidelines supports HIV-infected persons (Sweden).
- If in need, PLWAs are entitled to a pension (Sweden).
- Although there are no special regulations for immigrants, they are entitled to free treatment if they suffer from AIDS (Slovenia).

4. Conclusions and recommendations for actions and future research

The present inventory acknowledges the diversity and wealth of experiences of the European countries. The following conclusions to the research questions give evidence of the solidarity between European countries, eagerness to learn from each other as well as respecting their own characteristics.

The following recommendations for future research are based on the analysis of the Country Reports, and the second country collaborators meeting Berlin, 5-7 th. November 1999, and various inputs by individual country collaborators.

From the various analysis and country collaborators' feedback, a number of conclusions emerge which can be formulated as prospects and possibilities for action, and are complemented by recommendations for future research.

The countries have found the writing of their own Country Reports a very valuable and informative exercise, as well as a general feeling that it has raised the attention of governmental and non-governmental authorities to the HIV Prevention Policies in their country. As a side effect to the work, the country collaborators have found the exchange of information and experiences between countries and sub-regions quite useful, as illustrated in the animated debates of two the Country Collaborators' meetings. Finally, country collaborators have expressed interests to read other Country Reports to comprehend the lessons learnt from other countries, and understand better the situation in neighbouring or border countries.

4.1 History and chronology

An agenda for action

- Creating a favourable and permissive environment (e.g. legality of homosexuality and injecting drug use) among the public at large and the opinion leaders pave the way for HIV/AIDS prevention policies
- Large campaigns for the general population allow to inform the public at large of HIV transmission, and prevention measures, and must be combined with solidarity information
- Special direct communication channels (peer groups, special materials) can be effective to reach specific vulnerable groups
- The integration of HIV prevention and care activities, with other existing structures such as STDs, or Communicable Diseases, or sexual health, or

health promotion, as well as the geographical decentralisation, is a trend, and needs to be anticipated and nurtured carefully

Recommendations for future research

- By the example of the HIV/AIDS prevention policy the influence of different social systems on the development of health policies could be examined in the context of historical research work.

4.2   General policy on HIV/AIDS

An agenda for action

- Refining through the European Union the HIV prevention policies "golden" standards may stimulate and encourage countries in Europe to follow those with more exchange between policy-makers at an international level (for example through a Task Force)*
- Barriers faced presently in HIV Prevention Policies in Europe due to the normalisation of the disease, its professionalisation or medicalisation, the decreasing budgets, the medical advancements which are still unsatisfactory, and the loss of idealistic commitment, all need to be overcome*
- The States' commitment to HIV Prevention with sufficient funding is a condition sine qua non to a favourable environment for HIV Prevention policies*
- Prioritise HIV Prevention within the Health and Social Policy Sectors*
- To decentralise and stimulate the development of HIV Prevention Policies and dialogue to sub-regions (e.g. Western, Southern, Central and Eastern, Scandinavia, and the Baltic States)*
- The national plans under the form of strategic planning documents, or more flexible planning documents such as the "Evolving Strategy" in the UK, are essential guidance tools to translate HIV Prevention policies into reality
- Inter-sectoral and multi-disciplinary inputs are essential contributions to sound HIV prevention policies
- The involvement of local partnerships (local authorities and social organisations) through decentralised mechanisms are essential to facilitate the implementation of HIV prevention policies tailored to local needs

- Sound policy-making for HIV Prevention needs at all levels of the system the involvement of the voluntary sector, including representatives from the different vulnerable groups (People living with HIV, migrants...)
- Ensuring the support of the different churches to specific HIV/AIDS prevention policies can be instrumental in accelerating successful strategies
- Information campaigns need to address the key issues of modification of behaviours among populations most at risk, and to integrate HIV/AIDS health promotion in the broader sexual health messages to sustain the efforts
- A wider access to condoms, sterile injection materials can pave the way to successful HIV prevention policies, particularly for vulnerable groups (youth, IDUs, prison inmates...)
- More attention needed to the increasing drug scene with the early introduction of harm reduction and effective strategies and structured policies, and overcoming the main existing obstacles: converging legislation, training of professional in interaction with IDUs, acceptation of drug use by the general population, positive influence of the Churches*
- More attention needed to programmes addressing prostitution and sex tourism*
- Support projects which stimulate best practices to tackle the emerging vulnerable groups (women and youth, ethnic minorities or migrants)*
- Developing HIV prevention policies and responses for migrants spreading beyond borders, i.e. in the countries of origins as well*
- Applying WHO recommendations for testing policy from mandatory to voluntary, and get the right people to get tested and to profit from advances in treatment, identifying every new case as soon as possible (also by contact tracing)*
- Wide diffusion of the HIV Prevention Policies findings through national and international networks

Recommendations for future research

Future research in areas related to the making of HIV prevention policies may address the following questions:

- the mechanisms facilitating the local authorities' and voluntary sector's participation to the making of local and national HIV prevention policies
- the influences of the national and regional Parliaments and of the national laws to the making of HIV prevention policies
- the factors contributing or constraining the targeting HIV prevention policies to different vulnerable groups
- the role of epidemiology to inform policy at the national and local levels
- the churches influence in contributing actively or not to the development and implementation of HIV prevention policies
- the improved understanding of the mechanisms of integrating HIV/AIDS various dimensions, and using more horizontal approaches
- Analysis of the main individual factors/parameters (ref. Chap. 2 and Analytical Framework) influencing HIV prevention policies and of external factors (politics, social, economics factors)

4.3   Institutional structures of policy implementation

An agenda for action

- The involvement of essential partners from the more vulnerable groups in the various formal structures of the making of policies at different levels is key to the success of implementation of HIV prevention policies
- A well prepared and gradual decentralisation of HIV activities to the regions or local levels can provide more effective partnerships between the public and voluntary sectors
- A national Government commitment, with HIV/AIDS activities high in the agenda of public priorities, can encourage the various Ministries and the regions to implement HIV prevention policies more diligently
- Despite existing coordinating structures and mechanisms, and with the pressure of scarcer resources, more attention needs to be paid that the public and voluntary agencies do not duplicate tasks and activities

- The emerging vulnerable groups can be provided services if provision is made for a minimal earmarked fund, and if the share of roles between the public and the voluntary sectors is delineated

Recommendations for future research

- What is the most effective roles National AIDS Committees, and their equivalent in the local structures, in relation to the mix between policy development and implementation?
- How to institutionalise primary prevention in an environment of decentralisation and with less resources?
- What are the mechanisms of communication and policy implementation in newly decentralised structures?

4.4 Legal aspects

An agenda for action

- Updating and developing laws adapted to the new emerging vulnerable groups pave the way to sound HIV prevention policies
- Close examination of laws and regulations can reveal the loopholes and identify transparent solutions to implement HIV prevention policies even where existing laws are restrictive
- The introduction and adaptation of existing laws within a reasonable time period for HIV prevention policies is an indicator of Governmental commitment

Recommendations for future research

The legal aspects analysis point to the needs in the following areas of research:

- How to identify the most useful laws to facilitate the implementation of sound HIV prevention policies?
- What are the mechanisms which can accelerate the introduction or updating of laws facilitating HIV prevention policies in Europe, particularly among the new emerging vulnerable groups?
- What is the influence of larger EU treaties such as Maastricht or Schengen on setting a positive environment to the development of laws related to HIV

prevention policies in Europe, and is there room for more guidance of the EU in relation to legal developments?

- How are the WHO Guidelines, that are accepted by all EU members, put into practice in the different countries?
- How are laws introduced to combat the underlying factors increasing the vulnerability to HIV
- How is the transition from socialist to democratic social systems carried out referring to legal aspects which impact does this transition have on the prevention policies?

4.5 Epidemiology

An agenda for action

- Epidemiological data and documentation can often offer persuasive evidence for instituting measures aimed at the more vulnerable groups
- AIDS epidemiological data need to be complemented with HIV epidemiological data to facilitate the formulation of HIV prevention policies due to the recent development of new therapies
- The analysis of risk behaviours to complement the present epidemiological data is needed to tailor improved intervention strategies

Recommendations for future research

- How to improve the use of epidemiological data for decision-making at the local (regional, district...) level?
- How to link epidemiological HIV/AIDS data with information on risk behaviour?
- How to improve the reliability of the epidemiological data?

4.6 Surveillance systems

An agenda for action

- HIV-based surveillance systems, with decentralised regional sources of information, collecting data by transmission groups and/ or probable route of infection, including migrants, combined with compulsory and anonymous reporting are useful tools to monitor infection
- On the long run, the HIV/AIDS surveillance may be more sustainable and effective when improvements in reporting are striven for, and when integrated with other routine reporting systems, e.g. for infectious diseases
- Additional intelligent monitoring of needs and quality, including behavioural data, may add substantial operational benefits to develop an effective local response.

The following recommendations in chapter 4.6 are part of the EC funded report "HIV Testing in Europe: A Review of Policy and Practice" from the London School of Tropical Medicne and ORS PACA-INSERM, France.

- Surveillance should be part of a comprehensive strategy to prevent and control HIV/AIDS. HIV/AIDS surveillance should enable the assessment of epidemic trends and help to monitor the provision and effectiveness of prevention and care activities.
- HIV reporting should be continued and, where necessary, developed at national level and HIV reporting should be set up at European level to complement AIDS reporting (this recommendation has also been made by the WHO[142]). Reporting of cases of HIV infection has become a key element in HIV/AIDS surveillance in Europe, particularly since the introduction of highly active antiretroviral therapies which have markedly affected the course of HIV infection and, hence, the usefulness of AIDS surveillance for making inferences about HIV infection trends.
- AIDS reporting should be maintained; HIV infection and AIDS should be reported into an integrated HIV/AIDS surveillance system. AIDS increasingly becomes an indicator of failure of secondary (lack of access to HIV diagnosis or treatment) or tertiary (failure of HIV treatment) prevention.

---

[142] Hamers FF, for the group of experts and national coordinators of HIV/AIDS surveillance from the countries of the WHO European Region. Recommendations for HIV surveillance in Europe. Eurosurveillance 1998; 3:51

- Because of the chronic nature of HIV infection, the same individuals may be reported several times. HIV/AIDS surveillance systems should incorporate mechanisms to ensure effective elimination of duplicate reports and, also, to link reports of HIV, AIDS and death for a given individual. These mechanisms should ensure that confidentiality is strictly respected and should be devised taking into consideration the respective national environment including case load, degree of homogeneity among cases, risk for breaches in confidentiality, and existing public health surveillance structures.
- Monitoring of uptake of antiretroviral treatment is important to evaluate access to treatment, treatment effectiveness and survival; surveillance of recent infections is essential to estimate HIV transmission and to better target and evaluate prevention measures. Information on treatment and on disease stage including information allowing the characterisation of cases recently infected should be included in HIV/AIDS reporting systems.
- Numbers of reported HIV cases do not represent HIV incidence or HIV prevalence, and they are strongly influenced by HIV testing patterns (among populations at risk and over time). HIV reporting data should be carefully interpreted and disseminated through clear public health messages.
- The emergence and transmission of HIV strains that are resistant to antiretroviral drugs is a serious threat. Research on ways in which surveillance should be developed to address this is an EU-wide priority.

Recommendations for future research

- How to improve the use of the surveillance systems for decision-making at the local level?
- How to combine HIV/AIDS with behavioural surveillance data collection at minimum costs with maximum applications (i.e. the UNAIDS second generation surveillance system)?

4.7 System of primary HIV prevention

An agenda for action

- Find ways to adjust to the marginalisation of the epidemic: empowering instead of victimising vulnerable groups, acknowledging instead of narrowing solutions to health and materials needs*
- Beware of the possibility of a second wave and keep population vigilant and supportive without an unreasonable level of panic and fear*
- Action research and documentation of best practices can offer persuasive evidence for institutionalising HIV prevention policies and large-scale programmes for vulnerable groups
- The known gaps to address the vulnerable groups' needs must be urgently addressed in each country
- The power and dynamism of the voluntary sector and Non-Governmental Organisations' (NGOs) can have an impact on the formulation of HIV prevention policies at local and national levels through broad-based coalition, and the relationships and support of these partners must be therefore nurtured
- The integration of HIV prevention and AIDS activities with STDs, as well as Hepatitis activities are steps towards sustainable and more effective HIV prevention*
- Ensure equal access to services (people should know their rights and ways to enforce those)*
- Continue to address the prevention related to gay men, particularly in countries where there is no gay community*

Recommendations for future research

- What is the best mix of strategies to continue to inform the general population, and at the same time to reach the vulnerable groups, with scarcer resources?
- How to promote and use best practices experiences in each country to scale up efforts, and to disseminate those in other European countries?
- How to build-in action research in existing strategies, particularly for pioneer work with the emerging vulnerable groups?
- How can large scale efforts to train professionals in HIV prevention activities be more effective?
- What are the best prevention messages and strategies to reach the young female group in each country?

- What are the best mix of national and local structures to support the development and implementation of HIV prevention policies?

4.8 Social and economic measures of support for HIV positive persons

An agenda for action

- Ensuring the development of comprehensive policies at the national and local levels to support the social and economic measures for HIV positive persons, particularly the people in precarious situations, can pave the way for equitable and wider access of care and psycho-social services
- Promote and disseminate best practices experiences in the rapidly evolving field of social and economic measures for national large scale replication, and international diffusion

Recommendations for future research

- How to develop in each country a balanced and effective response from the public and voluntary sectors to support social and economic measures of support for HIV positive persons?
- What are the conditions which would facilitate the introduction of a system to levy national and local taxes to improve the sustainability of supporting social and economic measures?
- In which areas of support for HIV positives and people with AIDS are NGOs more effective than governmental institutions and vice versa?
- Does Normalization correspond to the needs of PLWAs in Europe also in the field of psycho-social support?

4.9 HIV/AIDS treatment and care

An agenda for action

- Guidelines, or continuing education through experts and discussion groups, provide a favourable environment to adapt and promote quality HIV testing and treatment among different professionals in a rapidly changing and complex field of intervention
- Closer examination of laws and regulations can reveal loopholes for some of the more vulnerable groups, e.g. destitute, IDUs, and particularly illegal migrants regarding their accessibility to treatment and care
- Best practices in each country can offer persuasive evidence for instituting legal policy and programme change both within and outside the country
- Adapt to continuous medical advances, especially in the field of care*

Recommendations for future research

- To measure the effectiveness of treatment and care in each country and identify the existing different bottlenecks and recommend solutions, in particular to the vulnerable groups
- How to facilitate compliance of treatments in the various different existing structures in each country?
- What are the factors necessary to scale up some of the Best Practices in each country?

4.10 Expenditures for HIV/AIDS

An agenda for action

- With the new HIV infections which have remained stable instead of decreasing, minimum HIV prevention budgets, particularly for communication activities of the general population or most vulnerable groups, must be safeguarded
- Alternatives financing sources can provide a relief for government budgetary constraints
- The monitoring of trends allocated to prevention activities vs. other activities (e.g. anti-retroviral treatment) may provide powerful argument to protect HIV prevention budgets

- Countries which are documenting a serious response to HIV prevention with their budget allocations (e.g. Greece, Spain, England) may be used as role models for others
- The challenge lies in using decreasing resources in the most effective manner: with the most effective prevention strategies, and curative strategies, and the correct mix and quantity of those*
- Support some of the countries in Europe suffering from financial resources limitations to mount HIV prevention policies efforts in their countries (particularly Eastern Europe) in a global world*

Recommendations for future research

- Urgent need for a comparative comprehensive costing study of the global costs (in ECU) of HIV/AIDS prevention activities in Europe
- Setting-up of monitoring of costing trends of HIV/AIDS prevention activities in each country
- Costing data as influential factor to model HIV prevention policies
- Research in prioritisation and cost-effectiveness to be able to use decreasing resources in the most effective manner*

4.11 Research on risk behaviour and behavioural changes

An agenda for action

- Countries which have encompassed as standard policies the development and regular use of consistent protocols for the measurement of risk behaviours and behavioural changes which encompass similar definition of terms, sample selection, have a comparative advantage in measuring changes and improving programme design and effectiveness over others which do not
- National campaigns still need to address adequately the stigmatisation surrounding HIV/AIDS, and stimulate solidarity with PLWAs
- Monitoring more carefully and regularly the risk behaviours and behavioural changes among the youth as early behavioural indicators can pave the way to future successful and sustainable HIV prevention programmes

- On-going monitoring of the various vulnerable groups' risk behaviours and behavioural changes, and of their proxy indicators, can be promoted as part of 'best practice' interventions
- Facilitating the exchange of "best practices" advancements between the countries in pioneer areas of interventions, e.g. IDUs in prisons, outreach to more vulnerable women groups, sexual health education in schools etc.*
- Promote the conversion of knowledge acquired through research into practice*
- Improve the quality of activities: reaching new groups where the information is insufficient (young gay men...)*
- Developing and promoting the exchange of new experiences through modern communication technologies through for example new on-line HIV/AIDS networks.

Recommendations for future research

- What are the trends in the sales of condoms reflecting in behavioural changes in Europe, and what are the major barriers to their use (costs, knowledge...)?
- How to keep up effective HIV prevention messages when the public is less interested to information campaigns?
- What are the figures and trends on HIV testing showing, and what are the main barriers to HIV testing, or motivations and behaviours for people who may need or wish to take the test, not to do so?
- How to develop more research on risk behaviour and behavioural changes which encompass an improved understanding of the contextual and social factors which influence the modes of behaviour using psycho-social and community constructs, and how these modes can be modified?
- How are the research results on risk behaviour and behavioural changes influencing national and international HIV prevention policies?
- Behavioural research on migrants' behaviours*
- Research related to the identification of the channels of communication with the various types of migrants between prevention services and their social environment (religious groups, sport teams etc.)*
- Research related to gay men (MSM) addressing particular problems (new perception of the disease, young MSM, the bi-sexual groups who do not relate to the gay men communities, reaching gay men in countries where there is no gay community)*

- Improved monitoring of HIV incidence in particular and risk behaviours, particularly in the more vulnerable groups*
- Develop indicators to measure and monitor the development of HIV prevention policies in Europe*

4.12 Perception of the system, current debates and likely policy changes

An agenda for action

- Concerted advocacy by the public and voluntary sectors to keep HIV/AIDS as a relevant and important theme is a condition sine qua non to the complete success of sustainable HIV prevention policies
- A sound HIV/AIDS situation analysis is instrumental to predict changes and apply timely measures, and needs to be complemented by well-defined HIV prevention policies, articulated around clear priorities which are in turn taking into consideration the limited existing resources available
- Countries can take stock of the proven existing successes for strategies used to reach vulnerable groups and rural populations in Europe, and policies need to promote an equal accessibility to the prevention and treatment for them
- Communication strategies that are evolving, innovative, mix, involving the clients in the design and implementation, tailored to the specific vulnerable groups' needs and understanding, age groups and time specific, promoting sustainable behavioural changes, addressing the pockets of stigmatisation, evaluated, all pave the way to positive results
- Incremental changes in structures supportive of HIV prevention policies and implementation (integration, decentralisation, health care reform, co-ordination, inter-sectoral co-operation, redefinition of roles in prevention and treatments at different levels, etc.), complemented with a well-informed public, create a supportive environment to positive results as well
- Improved methods and relevant and effective tools to implement HIV prevention policies need to be further developed with the beneficiaries' inputs tailored to each country specific needs and priorities
- Developing a vaccine for HIV Prevention for the benefits of the more vulnerable populations in Europe, as well as for the populations of developing countries*[143]

---

[143] we note here that, as of the end of 1999, it is known that most of the present AIDS vaccine candidates are against HIV-Subtype B found mostly in North America and Europe, whereas comparatively very little investment is going into vaccine candidates against HIV-Subtypes C, D and E found in developing countries

Recommendations for future research

- What is the impact made by prevention policies?
- What impact does the recent normalisation and medicalisation of HIV/AIDS, including the introduction of new treatments, have on changes in risk behaviours among the population, as a consequence, and what are the prevention policies and strategies implications?
- How to prioritise interventions among the multiple choices existing?
- How to develop effective risk reduction vulnerable group specific strategies, with the involvement of the interested parties, and sustain those efforts?
- Beyond the direct expected positive impact of large national campaigns on the target groups, what are the indirect long term side effects of those, in relation to the peoples' saturation of information, and consequent indifference, or negative attitude vis-à-vis HIV/AIDS related matters?
- What is the best mix of communication strategies, both cost-effective and sustainable, to keep the population at large on top of all HIV/AIDS issues (HIV/AIDS information, sexuality, sexual behaviours, awareness, attitude to PLWAs...)?
- What are the causes of failed positive behavioural changes among some individuals or vulnerable groups, despite the information, education, and communication brought to them?
- What is the best share of roles between the public and voluntary sectors to step up effective communication strategies at the national and local levels?
- How to bridge the gap of the lack of involvement and interests of the health care personnel in HIV prevention activities in some countries?
- How to accelerate and pave the way to a wide spectrum of positive structural changes (integration, health care system, co-ordination, co-operation, task forces) in the reform structures occurring in different countries which can facilitate HIV prevention policies and implementation?
- What minimal budget allocation is necessary to continue the HIV prevention in light of competing resources in the field of HIV/AIDS activities?
- How to develop a common set of valid indicators to measure HIV prevention?

References

Becker C, Guenther-Grey C, Raj A. Community empowerment paradigm drift and the primary prevention of HIV/AIDS. *Social Science and Medicine* 1998;**46**(7):831-842.

Broering G, van Duifhuizen R. AIDS prevention for mobile drug users in Europe: results of a pilot project. *International Conference on AIDS* 1996;**11**(2):187.

Burban Y. Legal aspects of AIDS prevention. *International Conference on AIDS* 1996;**11**(2):399.

Cattacin S, Panchaud C, Tattini V. Les Politiques de Lutte contre le VIH/SIDA en Europe de l'Ouest Du risque à la normalisation. Paris: L'Harmattan, 1997.

Chambers G. Inside the Labyrinth. *Eurohealth* 1996;**2**(3):7-11.

Cremer SE. HIV/AIDS Prevention Policies for Youth in Europe State of the Art. Woerden, The Netherlands: NIGZ Netherlands Institute for Health Promotion and Disease Prevention, 1998.

Danziger R. An overview of HIV prevention in central and eastrern Europe. *AIDS Care* 1996;**8**(6):701-707.

Dehne K, Khodakevich L, Hamers F, Schwarländer B. The HIV/AIDS epidemic in eastern Europe: recent patterns and trends and their implications for policy-making. *AIDS* 1999;**13**:741-749.

Dubois-Arber F. La prevention du sida dans une nouvelle phase de l'epidemie: questions et enjeux. 2eme conference europeene sur les methodes et les resultats des recherches en sciences sociales sur le sida 1998, Paris: 105-115.

European Centre for Epidemiological Monitoring of AIDS. HIV testing and HIV case reporting in Europe. Saint-Maurice, France: European Centre for Epidemiological Monitoring of AIDS, 1998.

European Centre for the Epidemiological Monitoring of AIDS. HIV/ AIDS Surveillance in Europe. Saint-Maurice, France: European Centre for the Epidemiological Monitoring of AIDS, 1998.

European Commission. The health situation of women in the European Community. Luxembourg: European Commission, 1997.

European Union. Eurobarometer 51. Brussels: E.U., 1999.

Franken I, Kaplan C. Risk contexts and risk behaviours in the euregion Maas-Rhein: the boule de neige intervention for Aids prevention among drug users. *AIDS Education and Prevention* 1997;**9**(2):161-180.

Gordenker L, al. e. International cooperation in response to AIDS. New York: Pinter Publishers, 1995.

Gostin L, Webber D. HIV infection and AIDS in the public health and health care systems: the role of law and litigation. *JAMA* 1998;**279**(14):1108-1113.

Hamers F, al. e. AIDS trends in Europe: decrease in the west, increase in the east. *Eurosynthèse* 1996.

Hamers F, al. e. Diversity of the HIV/AIDS epidemic in Europe. *AIDS* 1998;**12**((suppl A)):S63-S70.

Hamers F, Brunet J. Differences geographiques et tendances recentes de l'epidemie de VIH/ sida en Europe. 2eme conference europeene sur les methodes et les resultats des recherches en sciences sociales sur le sida 1998, Paris: 13-24.

Houweling H, al. e. An age-period-cohort analysis of 50 875 AIDS cases among injecting drug users in Europe. *International Journal of Epidemiology* 1999;**28**.

Hubert Mea. Sexual Behaviour and HIV/AIDS in Europe. London: UCL, 1998.

Jackson L, al. e. Frequency of Policy Recommendations in Epidemiologic Publications. *American Journal of Public Health* 1999;**89**(8):1206-1211.

Jowell T. Future public health agenda for Europe. *Eurohealth* 1997;**3**(Autumn 1997):11-12.

Kenis P, Marin B. Managing AIDS. Organizational Responses in six European Countries. Aldershot: Ashgate Publishing Company, 1997.

Kirp D, Bayer R, eds. AIDS in the Industrialized Democracies: Passions, Politics and Policies. New

Brunswick, 1992.

Kroneman M, Zee Jvd. Health policy as a fuzzy concept: methodological problems encountered when evaluating health policy reforms in an international perspective. *Health Policy* 1997(40):139-155.

Kübler D, Joye D, Hausser D. Implemention problems of harm-reduction policy in Switzerland: The politics of location. In: Friedrich D, Heckmann W, eds. Aids in Europe - The behavioural aspect. Sigma ed. Berlin, 1995: 109-116.

Lamptey P, Price J. Social marketing sexually transmitted disease and HIV prevention: a consumer-centered approach achieving behaviour change. *AIDS* 1998;**12**(2):1-9.

Laurisden M, Lund M. Public Health in the European Union -Status and Perspectives. *Eurohealth* 1996;**2**(1):25.

Luger L. HIV/AIDS prevention and 'class' and socio-economic related factors of risk of HIV infection. Berlin: WZB, 1998.

Müller W. Time-ordered Indicators: Useful and Efficient Tools for Steering the National HIV-Prevention Campaign in Germany. 12th World AIDS Conference 1998, Geneva.

NIH. Interventions to prevent HIV risk behaviors. *NIH Consens Statement* 1997;**15**(2):1-41.

Piot P. Mobilizing against the AIDS epidemic in the context of the International Conference on Population and Development. Statement in plenary. The Hague, 1999.

Prokop H. Politisch-administratives Handeln angesichts neuartiger Herausforderungen. In: Rosenbrock R, Salmen A, eds. Aids-Prävention. Sigma ed, 1990: 275-289.

Robert Koch Institute. Epidemiologisches Bulletin. Berlin: R.K.I., 1999.

Robert Koch Institute. Daten aus der HIV-Laborberichtsverordnung. Berlin: Robert Koch Institute (RKI), 1999.

Rosenbrock R. Ein Grundriß wirksamer Aids-Prävention. *Zeitschrift für Gesundheitswissenschaften* 1994;**2**(3):223-44.

Rosenbrock R. Gesundheitspolitik - Einführung und Überblick (daraus: Verhaltensprävention / Felder und Institutionen der Primärprävention / Gruppenbezogene Primärprävention S.32, 34, 38). Berlin, 1998.

Rosenbrock R, al. e. The Aids Policy Cycle in Western Europe. Berlin: WZB, 1999.

Saltman R, Figueras J, Sakellarides C, eds. Critical challenges for health care reform. Buckingham: Open University Press, 1998.

Sandfort T, Hubert M, Bajos N. Interet des etudes realisees en Europe occidentale sur le comportement sexuel, en termes de prevention du VIH. 2eme conference europeene sur les methodes et les resultats des recherches en sciences sociales sur le sida 1998, Paris: 99-104.

Schaeffer D, Moers M, Rosenbrock R, eds. Aids-Krankenversorgung. Sigma ed. Berlin, 1992.

Steffen M. The Fight Against Aids An international public policy comparison between four European countries France, Great Britain, Germany, Italy. Grenoble: Presses Universitaires de Grenoble, 1996.

Stimson G. AIDS and injecting drug use in the United Kingdom, 1987-1993: the policy response and the pevention of the epidemic. *Social Science and Medicine* 1995;**41**(5)**:**699-716.

UNAIDS. Taks Force on HIV Prevention among Injecting Drug Users in Eastern Europe and the Newly Independent States: Mission Statement. Geneva: UNAIDS, 1997.

UNAIDS. The UNAIDS Report. Geneva, 1999.

UNAIDS/WHO. AIDS epidemic update. Geneva: UNAIDS/WHO, 1998.

van de Water H, van Herten L. Health Policy on Target? Leiden, 1998.

Walt G. Health Policy: an Introduction to Process and Power. London: Zed Books Ltd., 1994.

Wellings K. General Population. *Sozial- und Präventivmedizin* 1994;**37**(Suppl 1)**:**S14-S46.

Wellings K, Field B. Stopping AIDS AIDS/HIV Public Education and the Mass Media in Europe. London and New York: Addison Wesley Longman Ltd., 1996.

WHO. Regionale Strategie zur Erreichung des Ziels "Gesundheit für alle bis zum Jahr 2000. Eur/RC 1981, 30/8Rev.

WHO Regional Office for Europe. Principles for preventing HIV infection among drug users. Copenhagen: WHO, n.d.

Publisher: Eliva Press Global Ltd

Email: info@elivapress.com

Eliva Press is an independent international publishing house established for the publication and dissemination of academic works worldwide. The company provides high quality and professional service to all our authors.

Our Services:
Free of charge, open-minded, eco-friendly, innovational.

-Free standard publishing services (manuscript review, step-by-step book preparation, publication, distribution, and marketing).
-No financial risk. The author does not have to pay any hidden fees for publication.
-Editors. Dedicated editors will assist step by step through the projects.
-Money paid to the author for every book sold. Up to 50% royalties guaranteed.
-ISBN (International Standard Book Number). We assign a unique ISBN to every Eliva Press book.
-Digital archive storage. Books will be available online for a long time. We don't need to have a stock of our titles. No unsold copies. Eliva Press uses environment friendly print on demand technology that limits the needs of publishing business. We care about environment and share these principles with our customers.
-Cover design. Cover art is designed by a professional designer.
-Worldwide distribution. We continue expanding our distribution channels to make sure that all readers have access to our books.
-Marketing tools. We provide marketing tools such as banners, paid advertising, social media promotion and more.

www.elivapress.com

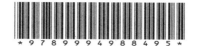

BV - #0011 - 110124 - C20 - 229/152/37 - PB - 9789994988495 - Gloss Lamination